BIOETHICS

CHILDLESSNESS AND ARTIFICIAL REPRODUCTION!?

BIOETHICS

CHILDLESSNESS AND ARTIFICIAL REPRODUCTION!?

An Enlarged Edition

Paschal Nwaezeapu

Leonine Publishers
Phoenix, Arizona

Nihil Obstat: Reverend Micheal Adebanjo
Diocese of Ijebu-Ode, Nigeria
29 April 2011

Imprimatur: ✠ Most Reverend Ayo-Maria Atoyebi
Bishop of Ilorin Diocese, Nigeria
29 April 2011

Published by Leonine Publishers LLC

ISBN-13: 978-0-9836740-4-7

Library of Congress Control Number: 2011934895

10 9 8 7 6 5 4 3 2 1

Printed in the United States of America

Visit us online at www.leoninepublishers.com
For more information: info@leoninepublishers.com

DEDICATION

To

His Holiness, Pope Benedict XVI and all the other members of the Sacred Congregation for the Doctrine of the Faith who prepared *Donum Vitae* (1987), a document that largely shaped my thought in Bioethics,

To

All my friends,

And to

All who value truth and true friendship.

ACKNOWLEDGEMENTS

My most profound gratitude goes to the Almighty God for His mercy and loving kindness, and for sustaining me, especially in the last three years (2007–2010) and during the period I struggled to write this book. I am extremely grateful to my bishop, Anthony Cardinal Okogie, for his support and for the opportunity to further my studies. I cannot find enough words to express my deep appreciation to my professors in Rome, especially Prof. Lucio Romano, M.D., Reverend Father (Prof.) Thomas Williams and my Dean at the Faculty of Bioethics, Reverend Father (Prof.) Gonzalo Miranda. Right Reverend Monsignor John Aniagwu and Mother Benedicta Prassino will always be a source of inspiration to me. I acknowledge the contributions of Sir Albert Oyenuga, Mrs. Bridget Itsueli, Dr. Mrs. Henrietta Williams and a prolific writer, Reverend Father (Prof.) Francis Oborji of Universita Urbaniana, Rome, who keeps encouraging me to write. I thank Prof. Giwa-Osagie and Dr. John Esangbedo for their contributions to the success of this work. I deeply appreciate the friendship and encouragement of my family and friends. Finally, I acknowledge my indebtedness to Dr. Mrs. Taiye Gefu and Dr. Anthony Okeregbe who were extremely gracious to read through the manuscript. Tony was equally generous to write the Introduction to this book. May God graciously bless and reward all of you!

Rev. Msgr. Paschal Chibuzo Nwaezeapu
11 January 2011

CONTENTS

CHAPTER 1
BIOLOGY OF HUMAN PROCREATION
PAGE 1

CHAPTER 2
THE PHENOMENON OF INFERTILITY
PAGE 29

CHAPTER 3
CHILDLESSNESS
PAGE 65

CHAPTER 4
THE ARTIFICIAL REPRODUCTIVE TECHNOLOGIES
PAGE 97

CHAPTER 5
ARTIFICIAL REPRODUCTIVE TECHNOLOGIES: THE NIGERIAN SITUATION
PAGE 131

CHAPTER 6
ART: RELATED TECHNIQUES
PAGE 151

CHAPTER 7
ETHICAL ISSUES IN ARTIFICIAL REPRODUCTIVE TECHNOLOGIES
PAGE 181

CHAPTER 8
ETHICAL ISSUES IN PGD, SEX SELECTION, AND HUMAN GENETIC ENHANCEMENT
PAGE 225

CHAPTER 9
THE RELIGIONS AND ARTIFICIAL REPRODUCTIVE TECHNOLOGIES
PAGE 247

CHAPTER 10
REFLECTING FURTHER ON THE ARTIFICIAL REPRODUCTIVE TECHNOLOGIES
PAGE 275

CHAPTER 11
WHAT CAN BE DONE? SOME RECOMMENDATIONS
PAGE 337

LIST OF ABBREVIATIONS

AAS	*Acta Apostolicae Sedis*
AI	Artificial Insemination
AID	Artificial Insemination by Donor
AIH	Artificial Insemination by Husband
ART	Artificial Reproduction Technologies
ATR	African Traditional Religion
Cf.	Confer
CT	JOHN PAUL II, *Catechesi Tradendae, On Catechesis in our Time,* Pauline Books and Media, Boston 1979
DV	CONGREGATION FOR THE DOCTRINE OF THE FAITH, *Donum Vitae,* Instruction on Respect for Human Life in its Origin and on the Dignity of Procreation: Replies to Certain Questions of the Day, Vatican City 1987
ed./eds.	Editor/Editors
et al.	and Others
EV	JOHN PAUL II, *Evangelium Vitae, The Gospel of Life,* Pauline Books and Media, Boston 1995
FC	JOHN PAUL II, *Familiaris Consortio, On the Role of the Christian Family in the Modern World,* Pauline Books and Media, Boston 1981
FSH	Follicle Stimulating Hormone
Gal.	Galatians

GIFT	Gamete Intra-fallopian Tube Transfer
GnRH	Gonadotropin Releasing Hormone
GS	*Gaudium et Spes* - On the Pastoral Constitution of the Church in the Modern World, published on 7 December, 1965, in FLANNERY, A. (ed.), *Vatican Council II, The Conciliar and Post Conciliar Documents,* Costello Publishing Company, Inc., Bandra Mumbai 1975
hCG	Human Chorionic Gonadotropin
Ibid.	The Preceding Work Cited
ICSI	Intra Cytoplasmatic Sperm Injection.
IUI	Intra Uterine Insemination
IVF	In Vitro Fertilization
IVF-ET/IVF and ET	In Vitro Fertilization and Egg Transfer
LH	Luteinizing hormone
N./No.	Number
Op. cit.	Work (already) Cited
PGD	Pre-Implantation Genetic Diagnosis
p. (pp.)	page(pages)
STD	Sexually Transmitted Diseases
Vol./Vols.	Volume/Volumes
ZIFT	Zygote Intra Fallopian Transfer

FOREWORD

MICHAEL J. RAYES, M.B.A.

Test-tube babies. Artificial insemination. In vitro fertilization. And it goes on and on. There is a confusing array of options bewildering modern married couples. These options present problems that should not be addressed without recourse to standards of faith and morals.

If you are faced with infertility, know that you are not alone. Thousands of couples today experience the same thing. Couples throughout history experienced infertility, and there are examples of "blameless" men and women in the Bible who were infertile (cf. Gen. 16:1-2; 17:16; also Luke 1:6-7). So the cause of infertility is not unworthiness or ungodliness.

Infertility is too big of a concern to handle by yourself. Do you wonder how you will ever know that your decision to handle infertility was a good one? Left to oneself, a person is like a piece of wood drifting at sea: lost, alone, going with the tide. A person who relies on the wisdom of faith and morality, however, is like a tree firmly planted on an island. The ocean waves come; storms pass, yet the tree remains tall and strong.

Some may argue that morality restricts freedom of choice. You are not choosing on your own, they say, if you must rely on the strictness of moral rules. But consider the weight of such a choice. Are you willing to go against moral standards to get what you want? Think about the long-term result of your decision. Wouldn't you rather feel at peace knowing you followed your conscience as it was informed by ethical standards of sexual morality?

Morality is actually freeing rather than restrictive. Moral guidelines can give you the comfort of knowing you have something on which to rely. When it comes to the larger issues in life, such as infertility, you can rest assured that your decisions to treat your syndrome are aligned with ethical standards.

You have every right to treat infertility and try to conceive a baby. Couples may seek help, both medical and psychological, to treat infertility. The desire to have a baby is legitimate and natural. Sometimes, however, children are viewed as mere commodities to make a potential parent feel complete as a human person. Married persons may wish to examine their own consciences to see if their desire for a child is born of the earnest impulse of love to share with a child, or a selfish craving to fill up one's own self-worth.

What should couples do if they are faced with infertility? First, pray. God loves you both and He understands the void you feel in your hearts. Remember, this is a biological phenomenon and you must not place blame on your partner.

Second, search for information. This book features a lot of information on reproductive technology and the various methods to treat infertility.

Next, talk with a spiritual leader you trust. Do not move forward alone. Share your problem with a spiritual guide who can help you sort out all the information and place it within the ethical framework you need. Finally, you will need to decide what to do, and to what extent you wish to treat your infertility.

In this book, a technical explanation of procreation is given first. The specific problem of infertility and medical solutions follow in several chapters. These chapters are presented in a "neutral" format so the solutions are given the most objective presentation possible. Later in the book, the solutions are weighed with Islamic, African Traditional Religion, and especially Catholic moral ethics. Some further reflections and recommendations are given in the final chapters.

What must be remembered when reading about these various procedures is that the only morally acceptable use of the human sexual act ("coitus" or sexual intercourse) is within marriage, and each act must end the natural way to allow for the potential of procreation. If a procedure to help the couple conceive a child can work within this context, it is moral. Most of what is objectively discussed in the following chapters do not meet these criteria, and are therefore immoral (for example: masturbatory acts; artificial insemination that results in the willful destruction of unwanted embryos, etc.). However, the procedures are presented in a narrative format so readers have as much information as possible.

They will gain a fuller understanding of the problematic nature of these methods as they continue reading the book.

For the person interested in human biology and the particular problem of reproductive infertility, this book is presented to shed light on a sensitive and important topic.

INTRODUCTION

PROLEGOMENA TO BIOETHICAL INQUIRY ON ARTIFICIAL REPRODUCTIVE TECHNIQUES (ART)

Inclinatio naturalis quod homo in societate vivat.[1]

– St. Thomas Aquinas

BY ANTHONY OTOME OKEREGBE, PH.D.

Department of Philosophy, University of Lagos

All over the world, across all cultures and races, the birth of a child is celebrated with feast and festivity. And one reason for this stems from a cultic insinuation that the newborn is the community's link between yesterday and tomorrow in the manifold world of human existence. But in a more arcane sense, the arrival of children is the natural response to the biological imperative of propagation of the human species and the furtherance of social continuum. Therefore, however pretentious a society may be about its values, one aspect of human life this pretention can barely be sustained is on the issue of children. Given the premium accorded the birth and nurturing of children, childlessness, and especially involuntary childlessness, is usually regarded as a frustration of this biosocial process, and thereby injurious to the lifeworld of the community. To the one who is childless, the attendant feeling of inadequacy and incompleteness, sadness and self-denigration could be a harrowing experience with very dire emotional and psychological consequences.

Cognizant of the effects of childlessness on the overall well-being of the individual, as well as the biological dimension associated with its challenges, scientists, in the last few decades, have come together to positively address this problem by designing assisted reproductive

---

[1] Aquinas, *Summa Theologica*, I. II, 94, 2.

programmes otherwise called Artificial Reproductive Techniques (ART). These techniques are a bio-technological design that simulates the process of procreation to a greater extent outside the natural environment of, and procedures for procreation. When any of these techniques is successfully carried out on an infertile or childless couple, or on a woman for that matter, it is argued that a great good would have been done. At the end, the shackles of infertility are broken and the encumbrance of childlessness is banished; the erstwhile victims of childlessness and infertility are happy, and humankind is blessed.

If this happy narrative suggests the ability of the empirical sciences to solve human problems, why then is this book, *Bioethics: Childlessness and Artificial Reproduction!?* necessary? By the author's use of an exclamation and a question mark in the book title, there seems to be a registration of both an alarm and a probe. Childlessness! Ah! Artificial Reproduction? What does this mean? Can a natural process known as procreation be artificial? And this putative headliner presents the problem statement of the book, which is that Artificial Reproductive Techniques (ART) raise certain fundamental questions that cannot be wished away without subjecting them to the purifying fire of rational scrutiny. So, to properly interrogate ART and ART-related techniques, Paschal Nwaezeapu approaches the debate within the context of childlessness and infertility.

This contextualization is very apt because it falls within the ambit of the author's research in Bioethics, a discipline with varied conceptions. From a narrow perspective, Bioethics tends to be viewed as an applied professional ethics akin to medical ethics, and as such domiciled in the faculties of the life sciences (biology, medicine, genetics). This misleading conception of Bioethics is responsible for the fragmented ethical and philosophical evaluation of the life sciences; and given this situation the profundity of bioethical reflections are greatly hampered and devoid of the richness contributable by other disciplines which have life as their object of inquiry. To properly interrogate ART and ART-related techniques, Bioethics has to reflect its intellectual ancestry as an axiological inquiry that is not delimited by the restrictive methodologies of the empirical sciences, and thereby earn its rightful place as "the philosophical study of the ethical controversies brought about by advances in biology and medicine."[2] In this wise, the focus of Bioethics becomes "the broad terrain of the moral problems of the life sciences, ordinarily taken to encompass medicine, biology, and some important aspects of the environmental, population and social sciences. The traditional domain of medical ethics would be included within this array, accompanied now by many other topics and problems."[3]

Putting our object of inquiry in proper perspective, the fundamental research questions that come to the fore in this regard include the following: What are the ethical implications of the so-called artificial reproductive technologies? Are they morally justifiable? Do they promote or compromise the dignity of the human person? Again, can a natural process be 'artificialized' as the term Artificial Reproductive Technologies suggests? In response to these questions, this work argues the thesis that, within the purview of bioethical reflections, Artificial Reproductive Techniques (ART) are a questionable technological facility for assisting procreation because they undermine the dignity of the human person, her right to life, integrity and respect, while their moral assumptions are based on consequentialist reasoning.

In furtherance of this thesis, the approach of this book subsists on a medley of narrative methodologies with tinges of inductive research. It is expository, analytical, synthetic and critical, while it also employs reported real-life scenarios in the media, and simulations from home videos as case studies. Its expository nature is observed in the author's task of bringing to light perceived flaws and fallacies in the ethical principles of ART proponents. To do this, the author embarks on a quarrying exercise that subjects the grandiose ART complex to some atomization process for easy understanding, in a bid to build up an alternative ethical structure for a fuller understanding and holistic appreciation of the life sciences.

The first step towards this fuller understanding comes in the form of a reflection: Can chance create the complexity that is human procreation? To respond to this question, we recall the above quoted header attributed to St. Thomas Aquinas. When the Angelic Doctor in his influential

---

2 "Bioethics," Available at: http://en.wikipedia.org/wiki/Bioethics.

3 *Encyclopedia of Bioethics*. Rev. ed. Toronto: Simon & Schuster Macmillan; Prentice Hall International, 1995, p. 250.

Summa Theologica, penned this immortal truth about human society, he was not just reiterating a mere sociological truism that expresses man as a social animal, but he was also more importantly affirming a teleology of human existence that transcends man's concrete actualization in society. At face value, teleology may appear as a simple principle that establishes a conscious, deliberate or goal-directed progression of an action or event; in short, purposefulness. However, within this simple principle of teleology is the explanation of the facts about the complexity of nature, society, and thought.

This principle is better appreciated in the first chapter of the book titled, Biology of Human Procreation, where the complex human reproductive system is described as a natural process, thereby downplaying the misleading concept of reproduction which conveys the idea of artificiality in human conception. To underscore the naturalness of human conception, the author delves into modern biology to explain the character of the human reproductive system and how the intricacies involved in sex cells formation and fusion provide the blueprint for the propagation of species.

Despite the fact that the author is not a biological scientist, much less an expert in reproductive biology or obstetrics, he traces the process of human conception from the germinal stage of sex cell formation and fusion, through the catalystic function of hormonal action, to fertilization. In all this, the complex phenomena and processes that beget each tissue of each organ, and each organ of the structures that form the human reproductive system, are painstakingly described.

Notwithstanding the teleology and intelligence evinced by the ingenuous complexity of the biology of human procreation, the human reproductive system is far from being a totally efficient one. Like every concrete phenomenon, it is dogged by the imperfection, defect, and inefficiency reflective of cosmological contingencies and human finitude. One area where this is greatly felt is in the failure of fertilization, or pregnancy to occur, even after the two gametes, namely, the sperm and the ovum have intermingled following coitus. This incident, conventionally known as infertility, has posed a major challenge to the realization of the desire of people to procreate and form a family, and thereby embark on the teleological quest to propagate the human species. With frightening statistical data that cut through every human taxonomy, the book goes to explain that infertility has been known to emotionally and physiologically emasculate childless couples, and pose serious mental health problems. It is also a subject of serious consideration in many communitarian societies and traditional cultures, where life is celebrated as a community property.

Yet, as Paschal Nwaezeapu would want us to bear in mind and take to heart, infertility is not inconsistent with mortality; it is not a curse. Neither is it a phenomenon that is below the dignity of the human person. Amidst the categorization of the numerous causes of infertility into male factors, female factors and unexplained factors, he urges us to understand that infertility may arise from factors that may be related to endocrinology, physiology, neurological disturbances, inability of the female to carry a pregnancy to term, sickness or even the consequence of a particular lifestyle. However, in general statistical terms, the major causes of infertility in couples are outlined as: ovulatory dysfunction – 15%, tubal and pelvic pathology – 35%, male factor – 35%, unusual problems including uterine factors – 5%, and unexplained infertility – 10%.

Whatever the major causes of infertility, the predictable consequence is childlessness; childlessness that is made all the more obvious when the affected couple desire to bear their own biological children. As in many societies, notwithstanding the challenges of modern socio-economic living, cultural preferences and religious sentiments tend to have favoured, more than not, the desire of married couples to have children. However, this quest is very pronounced in African societies, including Nigeria, which forms the case study in this chapter. According to this book, the Nigerian society, just as it loathes any deliberate or voluntary form of childlessness in marriage, is contemptuous of married couples who are victims of involuntary childlessness. Oftentimes, this uncharitable gesture towards childless married couples is characterized by stigmatization of the couples and their families, ostracization from social circles, threat to marital and interfamily relations, psychological suffering, identity crisis, and exposure to dehumanizing, intrusive fertility overloads, amongst others. And in the minds of those who view procreation as an advance in the teleology of social existence, childlessness would seem antithetical to man's natural inclination of living in society, and of propagating his species. However, apart from being problems in themselves, this representation of childless married couples constitute a moral tension that raises fundamental questions concerning the moral worth of the human person as well as interrogate the rationale behind what is socially acceptable or permissible by public morality.

Consequently, to address the problem of infertility and prevent the stigma associated with childlessness, many are trying to understand and embrace the succour provided by science and technology in the name of Artificial Reproductive Techniques (ART). Technically, this group of techniques refer to "any treatment or procedure for assisting reproduction, which includes the handling of human eggs, sperm or embryos." Driven by the goal of achieving conception and establishing an uncomplicated pregnancy that will lead to the birth of a healthy baby, providers of ART embark on treatments or procedures that range from a seemingly simple procedure of assisted insemination to the more complex and strenuous procedure of *in vitro* fertilization. Notwithstanding their varied complexity and ethical problems, these techniques can be grouped under two broad headings: assisted insemination and assisted fertilization. In the first, fertilization occurs *in vivo* (inside the womb) while in the latter it takes place outside the womb. As the book observes, the latter techniques have made the human embryo amenable to a variety of laboratory manipulations. Prominent among the standard IVF protocols examined in this book are Cryopreservation of embryo, its advantages, risk and success rates; Gamete Intra-Fallopian Tube Transfer (GIFT); Zygote Intra-Fallopian Transfer (ZIFT); surrogacy practice; Intra-Cytoplasmic Sperm Injection (ICSI) represents one of the most significant breakthroughs in the history of ART; Microsurgical Epididymal Sperm Aspiration (MESA) and Testicular Sperm Aspiration (TESA); and egg donation.

Given the success of the IVF technology, there have been increased possibilities for infertile couples to have children. Yet, the IVF procedure carries several potential risks, some of which could be mild or severe; and this book groups them under three main headings: maternal/donor's risks, maternal/foetus risks, and risk to embryo/foetus or offspring. However, beyond these risks is an ethically problematic situation arising from cryopreservation of fertilized eggs for future use. This scenario is rendered by Nwaezeapu thus: "Some couples who undergo IVF and other ART procedures requiring egg retrieval often produce a good number of eggs, which are usually fertilized and cryopreserved for future use should the current cycle fail or should they desire to have more children in the future. Sometimes, some successful IVF couples may no longer require the cryopreserved embryos, leaving them with the option to either destroy them or to donate them to research. But since some find these options morally unacceptable, subsequent attempts to remedy the situation gave rise to embryo donation, which involves the donation of one's spare embryo anonymously to other IVF couples, with no right over the potential child that will result." This kind of situation generates some probing questions for the reflective mind: How do I feel as a parent whenever the thought that the child I call mine is a donated embryo? How would the child feel if he or she comes to know that she is really not an offspring of 'love' but a product of an artificial procedure from a freezer?

Beyond these there are other ART-related techniques which combine biotechnology and genetic engineering to aid procreation. Two of those treated in this book are Pre-implantation Genetic Diagnosis (PGD) and sex selection techniques. As the author asserts, PGD, an aspect of human genetic engineering, is a technique used to determine genetic defects in embryos created in the laboratory with IVF or ICSI techniques before implanting them into a woman for gestation. While the therapeutic use of these techniques may seem laudable, it does not foreclose the possibility of their non-therapeutic employment, since they have the prospect of being available to facilitate the creation of superhuman beings or designer babies; offsprings whose corporeal qualities owe their emergence to the cosmetic specifications dictated by the mundane caprices of their parents.

All the aforementioned scenarios together raise fundamental questions of philosophical common sense, by interrogating the metaphysical underpinning upon which the practitioners of ART and ART-related techniques and the consumers of their services situate their conception of being *vis-à-vis* the notion of person. They raise epistemological questions by probing into the justification and validity of the methods and methodologies advanced by the scientific philosophy of ART and ART-related technologies, and by examining whether or not biological sciences are epistemically neutral in their truth judgement. They also bring to the fore some ethical implications and human rights issues.

However, glossing over the first two philosophical inquiries, this book, in Chapter 7, throws its intellectual weight on the ethical implications and perceived human rights issues which these techniques and their clinical indications raise. In order to put this chapter in perspective, Paschal Nwaezeapu brings to light the arguments in favour of, and against ART. The basic argument of those who subscribe to ART lies in the utilitarian consideration that ART maximizes the pleasure of the greatest number of peoples, and also provides a pragmatic response to the problem of childlessness. The argument here is that, infertility is a painful state of living and ART may be the only medical option open to many infertile couples desirous of having children to realize that desire, thereby alleviating their sufferings and making them happy. Supporters of ART also justify their use as a right, more or less akin to reproductive right. In this sense, the use of these techniques is posited as a promotion of the autonomy of the individual, or an exercise in the expression of the freedom of choice.

In the next 40 pages of this chapter the author romances the arguments put forward by opponents of ART, which are as follows: that ART are a deliberate manipulation and destruction of human embryos; that they reduce human beings, women especially, to commodities, that they reify and undermine the psycho-social integrity of the future child. On the other hand, surrogacy is conversely argued as a degradation of the phenomenon of pregnancy and childbirth, just as it weakens the virtues of family lineage as well as undermining the taboos of adultery and incest.

This same structure of argument is verily sustained in chapter 8, where the ethical issues of PGD, sex selection and human genetic enhancement are exhaustively analyzed. In this analysis, three main positions are put forward. The first position argues that PGD, sex selection and human genetic enhancement are morally unacceptable and should not be permitted for certain reasons. Advocates of the second position claim that these techniques are morally acceptable if their application is limited to medical conditions, while the third position finds PGD for both medical and non-medical reasons ethically permissible. Just as in ART and ART-related techniques, the moral justification for PGD, sex selection and human genetic enhancement rests on pragmatic and utilitarian considerations; conversely, they are criticized for reification of the human person and undermining her spiritual essence. Thus, while PGD may be therapeutically valuable in preventing genetic diseases, its reliance on the IVF technology leaves it open to the ethical problems associated with IVF and related techniques.

Now, why this fuss about the human person? What is so special about personhood that requires such expeditious dissipation of logic to establish its defence against the onslaught of consequentialism, pragmatism and ancillary theories? To respond to these queries, this book borrows strength from religion. Beside the academic defence of the person, some of the greatest implications of ART have a bearing with religious beliefs. Is life entirely somatic and emotional? Is there no spiritual, mystical dimension to it that delimits the biomedical scientist's authoritarian pronouncement on life? For the religious mind, there are many dimensions about life that transcend the inquiring capability and competence of the biomedical sciences, and these, it is claimed, ART have glossed over.

Mindful of this fact, the book tells us that, while situating her interrogation of ART within the context of both a Christian anthropology that views man as an incarnate spirit and marriage, the Catholic Church "insists on respect for three fundamental goods: the intrinsic value and dignity of a human being and the right of every human being to life and physical integrity from conception to natural death and man's corresponding duty to preserve it; the unity of marriage, which implies respect for the exclusive right of a couple within marriage to become a father or mother only with one another; and the specifically human values of sexuality which require a responsible means of procreation." Though the church endorses medical assistance to infertile couples who cannot procreate normally due to medical conditions, she rejects any form of artificial insemination or fertilization that either substitutes the marital act or resorts to donated gametes because the introduction of a third party into procreation violates both the reciprocal fidelity of couples, the dignity of procreation, and is harmful to the child who has a right to be conceived and brought into the world in and from marriage.

Unlike the seeming difficult pronouncement of the Church on the extent of medical assistance permissible to infertile couples, the Islamic religion endorses ART in certain conditions where pregnancy cannot be established through sexual intercourse. However, it is vehemently against techniques that require third party involvement to establish pregnancy. This position differs slightly from the African traditional standpoint, which culturally harbours a home-grown surrogacy as a way of assisting not only infertile couples but also fertile couples whose prospect of bearing and rearing their own children have been truncated by some mishaps.

Having done justice to both God and Caesar in exposing an enlightened common sense assessment, and a religious evaluation of the ethical implications of ART, Paschal Nwaezeapu, in Chapter 10, pursues a further reflection that embodies his personal views. Under his critical searchlight, the first moral assumption to develop cracks is the consequentialist reasoning that characterizes utilitarian ethics, upon which proponents of ART erect their moral edifice. Consequentialist theories of morality, such as utilitarianism state that the rightness or wrongness of an action is judged by the goodness or badness of the actual consequences, but the author argues that "an action is not justified solely by its consequence." In the same vein, he denounces as a misnomer the use of the term "Artificial Reproduction" or "Assisted Reproduction" in the human procreation process, because it pre-establishes a biological reductionism that denies the spiritual nature of the human person. The same efficiency is sustained as he delves deeper into the issue pertaining to the respect for the dignity of human procreation. Here he shines his ethical searchlight on the issue of masturbation in ART, the involvement of a third party in the conception of a child, the interest and right of the child, the question of commercialization, and the moral status of the embryo, amongst other resultant moral issues.

In conclusion of his exposition, analyses and evaluation of the ethical implications of ART, Paschal Nwaezeapu takes a bow by making some recommendations. Firstly, he canvasses the need for a curative technique for infertility as a way of solving the real problem of infertility. The confidence behind this recommendation is borne out of the conviction that a curative rather than circumventive technique is more readily attuned to tackle the problem of infertility from the perspective of the total man. To this end, he calls for the population of the Natural Procreative Technologies (NaPro Technology), a holistic curative therapy that neither replaces the conjugal act, nor makes the agent perpetually dependent on the physician or the surgeon and his scalpel. While he recommends an all-involving health education campaign to prevent infertility, he canvasses the need for laws to guide assisted procreation in Nigeria in order to control and regulate infertility.

In terms of cultural orientation, he urges a rediscovery of the positive attribute of solidarity, the creation of support groups, and the need for sexuality education, the use of the communication media, workshops and seminars for balanced information about ART. To fight the evils in ART, he recommends the strong arm of the law to effect provisions that outlaw third party conception and commercialization, restrict the use of ART, and limit the amount of embryos created, amongst others. He also recommends the protection and strengthening of the family, the promotion of pre-marriage preparatory course, the introduction of a post-confirmation class to bridge the inactivity between confirmation and marriage. Other recommendations include the creation of a conducive atmosphere for children's wholesome development, rethinking the issues of abortion and child abuse, and adoption of children.

The significance of this work lies on the fact that this is a novel and highly commendable effort at producing a very comprehensive work on the complex issue of infertility and Artificial Reproduction Techniques (ART), as they relate to our people. An added value is the case study, which is Nigeria; and here the book treads a familiar terrain by excavating from our cultural history traditional African practices that become raw material for bioethical investigations. Although the bias of the empirical sciences has been noted to becloud a complete understanding of bioethics, since positivistic axiology and philosophy of science seemed to be the drivers of popular bioethical studies, little or no work has come from this part of the world despite promising case studies. In view of the bias and promises, this work is a welcome literature that complements our understanding of bioethics and its objects of inquiry.

The work is also significant because of its futuristic appeal. Statistics state that infertility rates are on the increase. Owing to the effects of technology and mass media, access to ART, which used to be restricted to the affluent, is creeping down the social ladder. It is envisaged that concurrent with widespread infertility would be the availability of, and unrestricted access to, ART and related technologies. This work, as an innovatory piece in the intricate field of bioethics, is a book in the waiting for the professional whose counsel would be morally authoritative in the intentions of aspiring ART users. In a country like ours, where all sorts of professionals double as moral counselors and soul-menders, and therefore may want to pontificate on bioethical issues such as ART and infertility, this book is an expository material to the questions, scope of study and delimitation of bioethics as it concerns infertility and ART.

Throughout the pages of this work, the author has insisted that the ethical implication of many of the Artificial Reproductive Techniques is centred mainly on one theme—the moral status of the human embryo. Is the human embryo an *'Imago Dei'* (image of God) and as such a person? Or is it just a nondescript being? His last words in the concluding chapter telegraphs his position: "Whatever conclusion we seek to hold, following an ethical appraisal of ART, depends largely on the values we hold dear in ethical judgment, and especially on our stand concerning the moral status of the human embryo. If we deny the personhood of the early embryo or evaluate the moral rightness of an action solely from the standpoint of the utility it offers the agent or on the basis of respect for procreative autonomy understood in an absolute sense, then all the artificial 'reproductive' technologies will be morally acceptable. But, if we say that the early human embryo has a right to life or enjoys a personal status and insist on the criteria for moral rightness that evaluate an action from the perspective of the goodness of the end of the agent, the moral object and the circumstances (of which the consequences for the child, family and society are important), then we are bound to reject most of the ART procedures currently in use."

In fidelity to his calling as a pastor, and within the limits of his epistemic capacity, the author has chosen a personalist standpoint in his evaluation of the moral status of the embryo. Personalism, the philosophy that upholds this standpoint, is a thinking that attempts to place persons and personal relationships at the centre of theory and practice.[4] According to Erazim Kolak, a proponent of this school, "Personalism is a philosophy predicated upon the irreducibility and primacy of personal categories, that is, the kind of categories that govern the meaningful interaction among personal beings – categories of meaning rather than cause, of respect rather than force, of moral value rather than efficacy, of

---

4 Shaun Gallagher, "Personalism: A Brief Account," On-line Bibliographies, Available at: http://www.philosophy.ucf.edu/pers.html, 1996, p. 1.

understanding rather than explanation."[5] Since it considers persons as larger than the universe, theistic personalism, in its investigations, gives primacy to ethical or moral dimensions of human endeavours, such that in matters like ART, morality takes precedence over utility; in politics, persons and their lifeworlds take precedence over systems and structures.

However, the personalist standpoint of this work is theistic in vision, and invokes the Church's magisterium to accentuate, and minister to grey areas bordering on faith. At the core of this standpoint is the recognition of human embryos as persons, rather than as things, biological materials or beings that just exist. In line with this tradition, a proper understanding of human teleology as a project of divine intelligence is attained when we recognize human embryos are persons who have an inviolable dignity of transcendent quality; intrinsic value and dignity that finds credence in the theistic vision that man is created rational and in the image and likeness of God. Against this standpoint is the reductionist thinking that views persons as agents and vehicles of systems and structures, or as dispensable means for a goal. Recognizing human embryos as persons rejects this depersonalization process which technology and biomedical mercantilism promote.

By embarking on this work, the author has dared the champions of today's neo-capitalist, consumerist and postmodern ideologies, whose criticisms are often uncharitable to works of this nature. Whatever the kind of criticism that will trail this work, one factual assessment is that critics will hardly be able sustain their argument publicly, because this work is unbeatable in its objectivity, rich in facts and figures and sound logic, even as it minimizes appeal to apologetics. This work displays courage without being sophistically controversial; it aims at truth without scholarly arrogance: the truth about infertility, ART and their ethical implications, which we seek to know; and the courage to act aright based on enlightened decision.

---

[5] Ibid., p. 2.

CHAPTER 1

BIOLOGY OF HUMAN PROCREATION

Man is the most complex of organisms, for in addition to his being biological, he is also a thinking being who is always seeking to understand himself and his habitat as a step towards mastering the earth. From antiquity, he has shown keen interest in the nature and mechanisms of human generation. At different epochs in history, Aristotle, Vesalius, and a host of others made significant strides in understanding and explaining the biology of human generation. Significant discoveries were made in the latter part of the nineteenth century; in recent times, the rapid advances in science and technology have equipped man with tremendous potential to redefine and control reproduction in animals and, to a limited extent, in humans.

Here, our primary objective is to describe the natural process of human conception as a prelude to our discussion of the causes of infertility, the problems of childlessness, and Artificial Reproductive Techniques (ART). While we will embark on this discourse strictly from the standpoint of modern biology, we must also note from the outset that man is not merely simple matter and cannot be reduced thereto. Any sound discourse on human procreation must take into account both its biological and anthropological aspects. Hence, the use of the phrase "human reproductive biology" in this book does not suggest that human beings are merely reproduced as are the animals.

THE TWO MODES OF REPRODUCTION: ASEXUAL AND SEXUAL

From a layman's perspective, we cannot think of reproduction without sex, because, in the mind of many people, reproduction and sex are two inseparable realities. However, this is not in consonance with our knowledge of reproductive biology. Although the two are inextricably interwoven in many multi-cellular organisms, they are two distinct processes. In biology, there are two primary approaches to reproduction: sexual and asexual. The main difference between them is that sexual reproduction involves meiosis and fertilisation, while asexual reproduction does not.[1]

ASEXUAL REPRODUCTION

In the early years of life on the earth, living organisms reproduced either through binary fission or budding. In the first case, which was common with many bacteria, a cell grows, divides in half, and shares its genetic contents equally among the parts.[2] The latter involves the "budding off" of one or more cells from the parent organism to give rise to another genetically identical organism.[3] Thus, a characteristic feature of asexual reproduction is that each new cell that results is genetically identical to the parent cell and is therefore its clone. We can observe asexual reproduction in plants and animals as well. Even though it is uncommon in vertebrates, especially mammals, it does occur; a good example is the case of identical twins. According to George Seidel Jr., "The duplication that occurs when one embryo produces two individuals is asexual reproduction, albeit superimposed on sexual reproduction."[4]

SEXUAL REPRODUCTION

The connection between sex and reproduction can be traced to the emergence of sexually reproducing organisms about 1.5 billion years ago.

---

[1] G. SEIDEL JR., "Cloning" in S. POST (ed.), *Encyclopaedia of Bioethics, 3rd Edition, Vol. 1,* Macmillan Reference USA, New York 2004, p. 447.

[2] R. PINON JR., *Biology of Human Reproduction,* University Science Books, Sausalito, California 2002, p. 27.

[3] Ibid., pp. 27-28.

[4] G. SEIDEL JR., "Cloning..., *op. cit.,* p. 448.

In this more complex mode of reproduction, two cells from two different organisms of the same species fuse to produce a new organism that is genetically distinct from the parents. The offspring are not clones of the parent organisms as in asexual reproduction.[5] The unicellular eukaryotes were the first organisms to reproduce sexually. In this case, there was no distinction between germ cells and somatic (body) cells, since each cell in the organism was responsible for the reproduction of the whole organism. However, the distinction between germ cells and somatic cells developed with the emergence of multi-cellular organisms.[6] This led to a situation in which the germ-line cells gave rise to the whole organism, while the somatic cells reproduced the organism's tissues and organs.[7] This way, the propagation of the species came to depend on the fusion of the germ cells from two distinct organisms of the same species. The genetic code of each organism carried the information that specified how its cells, tissues, and organs would develop. Moreover, this genetic code, or genome, distinguished it from other species and served as the generational link between parent and child.[8] Among humans, male and female parents contribute 50% of their genetic resources (that is, 23 chromosomes) to each of their children, whereas in some species the male does not contribute genetic resources to its progeny.[9]

ROLE OF STEROID SEX HORMONES IN REPRODUCTION

The body of an animal is composed of cells, tissues, and organs, which need to interact constantly to coordinate and regulate each other. This interaction, which allows the organism to function effectively, is

---

[5] R. PINON JR., *Biology of Human Reproduction, op. cit.*, p. 28.

[6] Ibid. See also L. SPEROFF – M. FRITZ, *Clinical Gynecologic Endocrinology and Infertility, Seventh Edition,* Lippincott Williams and Wilkin, Philadelphia 2005, p. 4. Eukaryotic cells (e.g. human cells) contain a nucleus as distinct from prokaryotic cells (e.g. bacteria), which do not have a nucleus and reproduce by cell division.

[7] See R. PINON JR., *Biology of Human Reproduction, op. cit.*, pp. 28, 41.

[8] Ibid., p. 28.

[9] Ibid., p. 40. In such cases, some evolutionary biologists claim that sex introduces a disadvantage of 50% because a female that reproduces asexually would normally contribute 100% of her genes to her offspring.

realized through the nervous system and the endocrine system. The primary function of the endocrine system is to produce hormones, which are chemical messengers with a specialized function.[10] The endocrine system comprises glands—such as the pituitary, hypothalamus, and thyroid—that secrete hormones directly into the bloodstream. The hormones are carried to all other parts of the body, where they activate specific organs and tissues to grow, to change their physiological activity, or to control an important bodily function. This global mode of hormonal action is known as *endocrine*. But hormones can also act locally in two ways, *paracrine* and *autocrine*. In the former, as Pinon explains, since the secretor and the cells that are targeted are neighbours, the hormone is secreted into the intercellular spaces instead of the circulatory system. By contrast, in the latter, the secretor and the target cells are homologous, and the hormone is secreted into the exterior of the cell to exert the required action on it.[11] In general, only specific cells in the body respond to each hormone. This is because the cells of the target tissues have hormone receptors in their cytoplasm or nucleus that respond only to a given hormone.[12] Although hormones carry out many important functions in the organism,[13] we are only interested in those of the steroid sex hormones, which are associated with reproduction.

Steroids are molecules[14] derived from cholesterol. In multicellular organisms, they regulate the activities of the different tissues. In mammals, the steroid sex hormones refer to the female sex hormones,

---

[10] A. EHRLICH – C. SCHROEDER, Medical *Terminology for Health Professions, Fifth Edition,* Thomson Delmar Learning, New York 2005, p. 368.

[11] R. PINON JR., *Biology of Human Reproduction, op. cit.,* p. 54-55.

[12] R. JONES, *Human Reproductive Biology, Second Edition,* Academic Press, San Diego, California 1997, p. 5.

[13] C. AMMER, *The New A to Z of Women's Health, Fifth Edition,* Checkmark Books, New York 2003, p. 197. Ammer asserts that although all the functions of hormones are not completely understood at present, some of the vital ones include regulating growth, sexual development, reproduction, blood composition, maintaining life (e.g. insulin), transmitting messages in the CNS (brain and spinal cord) and so on.

[14] See 'Molecule' in *BBC English Dictionary,* Harper Collins Publishers 1992. A molecule is the smallest amount of a chemical substance which can exist.

progestins and *oestrogens*, and the male sex hormones, *androgens*.[15] They are socalled because they are produced primarily by the gonads. Progestins and oestrogens are derived primarily from the ovary and placenta, while androgen has the testis as its primary source.[16] While the steroid sex hormones carry out many important functions, those connected with reproduction are the most significant. For instance, androgen and oestrogen hormones play a vital role in *spermatogenesis* in the male and *oogenesis* in the female and are essential for the development of secondary sex characteristics. Progesterone prepares the woman's uterus for implantation after fertilisation and maintains it during pregnancy.[17]

THE ROLE OF THE BRAIN IN REPRODUCTION: THE H-P-G AXIS

Despite the important role of the gonads in human reproduction, scientists in the twentieth century have concluded that the brain is "the final arbiter and determinant of the reproductive activity in animals."[18] More specifically, the hormones secreted in a pulsatile manner by the hypothalamus and pituitary glands sequentially control the activities of the gonads.

THE HYPOTHALAMUS

The hypothalamus is a small but important area in the base of the brain, next to and above the pituitary gland.[19] It forms part of the endocrine system and the central nervous system (CNS)[20] and secretes

---

[15] R. PINON JR., *Biology of Human Reproduction, op. cit.,* p. 60. Steroids are molecules derived from cholesterol. In multi-cellular organisms they regulate the activities of the different tissues. *Progestins, androgens* and *oestrogens* are subfamilies within the larger steroid hormone family.

[16] Ibid., p. 60.

[17] Ibid., p. 62.

[18] Cf. Ibid., p. 163.

[19] See C. TURKINGTON – M. ALPER, *Understanding Fertility and Infertility*, Checkmark Books, New York 2003, p. 146.

[20] See C. AMMER, *The New A to Z of Women's Health, op. cit.,* p. 206.

neurohormones.[21] In addition to its role in reproduction, it fulfils vital physiological functions, such as the regulation of blood pressure, body temperature, and sugar metabolism; complex behavioural activities like eating, drinking, sleeping, and sexual behaviour; and even emotions like anger, fear, joy, love, and hate. However, all of its activities belong to the unconscious level, meaning that we cannot control them consciously.[22]

THE PITUITARY GLAND OR HYPOPHYSIS

The pituitary gland, also known as the *hypophysis*, is a small, round ball of tissues located at the base of the brain. It is below the hypothalamus and connected to it by a structure called the pituitary stalk.[23] It produces important hormones, such as follicle stimulating hormone (FSH), luteinizing hormone (LH), and prolactin. The pituitary controls the activities of the gonads, but it does so only in conjunction with the hypothalamus. Therefore, it is not an autonomous organ, because its ability to fulfil its proper function depends on its connection with the hypothalamus. It secretes a particular hormone according to the signals it receives from a hypothalamic-releasing hormone. The pituitary comprises anterior and posterior lobes.[24] In the past, scientists saw the anterior pituitary, or the *adenohypophysis,* as the "master gland" of the endocrine system. Recent discoveries, however, indicate that most of its functions are controlled by the hypothalamus.[25] Nevertheless, it

---

[21] See A. EHRLICH – C. SCHROEDER, *Medical Terminology for…, op. cit.,* pp. 370-371. According to Ann Ehrlich and Carol Schroeder, neurohormones differ from hormones in the sense that they are secreted by, or act on, a part of the nervous system.

[22] See R. PINON JR., *Biology of Human Reproduction, op. cit.,* p. 164. Pinon maintains that the hypothalamus, which is present in all vertebrates, is connected to other parts of the brain and its numerous functions are accomplished by groups of neurons (called hypothalamic nuclei) located in its different parts.

[23] C. TURKINGTON – M. ALPER, *Understanding Fertility and Infertility, op. cit.,* p. 146.

[24] Ibid., p. 165. The primary role of the pituitary is to secrete hormones that control the activities of the other endocrine glands.

[25] See R. JONES,*Human Reproductive Biology, op. cit.,* p. 3. The *neuro-hypophysis* or posterior pituitary also has its own functions. Two hypothalamic hormones, *oxytocin*, which stimulates uterine contractions during childbirth,

is an important gland of the endocrine system; we can summarize its main functions as the following: "to encourage and maintain the body's secondary sexual characteristics and to promote fertility."[26]

THE GONADS: OVARY AND TESTIS

The testis and the ovary are specialized tissues that determine the difference between the male and the female and produce the germ cells necessary for the propagation of the species.[27] Sex determination and foetal sexual differentiation are distinct phenomena that are dependent on two different processes. While the former is determined by the genes and takes place at fertilisation, the latter depends on the brain. In humans—and mammals in general—the formation of the gonads and the internal and external genitalia begins very early in the development of the embryo and is completed before birth.[28] The ovary produces the eggs for reproduction and secretes the steroid sex hormones oestrogen and progesterone, which together orchestrate the menstrual cycle. The testis produces sperm and secretes hormones that determine the male body type.

HYPOTHALAMUS-PITUITARY-GONADAL (H-P-G) AXIS

The H-P-G axis refers to the Hypothalamus-Pituitary-Gonadal axis. It primarily comprises the hypothalamus, the pituitary gland, the gonad, and certain elements of the CNS.[29] To carry out their reproductive function, the hypothalamus, the pituitary, and the gonads interact through hormones. In both the male and the female, the hypothalamus secretes a hormone called gonadotropin-releasing hormone (GnRH). The pituitary gland responds to the hypothalamic stimuli by secreting the gonadotropic hormones, LH and FSH, which target the gonads. In response to the action of gonadotropins, the gonads produce the steroid

---

and *vasopressin*, which has effect on the blood vessel, uterus and kidney, are stored here.

[26] C. TURKINGTON – M. ALPER, *Understanding Fertility and Infertility, op. cit.,* p. 146.

[27] R. PINON JR., *Biology of Human Reproduction, op. cit.,* p. 6.

[28] Ibid., p. 6.

[29] Ibid., p. 7.

sex hormones needed for the production of the egg or the sperm.[30] These, in turn, regulate the activities of the hypothalamus and pituitary through feedback mechanisms. The feedback is negative when it inhibits the secretion of a pituitary hormone, and it is positive when it produces an increase in its secretion. This regulatory mechanism ensures that the hormones required for reproduction are always available.[31] Describing this complex regulatory network, Pinon maintains that the H-P-G axis

> Describes a complex regulatory network that includes control of gonadal function by the hypothalamus and pituitary, feedback regulation of the hypothalamus and pituitary by the gonadal hormones, and modulation by internal and external (environmental) stimuli.... In both cases, the central nervous system (CNS) plays a critical role in modulating the H-P-G axis.[32]

In the woman, the finality of this complex interaction between the hypothalamus, pituitary, and ovary is ovulation, which usually occurs in the middle of the woman's menstrual cycle.

THE GNRH PULSE GENERATOR

The secretion of GnRH by the hypothalamus, as well as of the LH and FSH by the pituitary, occur in a pulsatile fashion. Experiments with animals suggest that the LH pulsatility follows immediately from that of the hypothalamus, which secretes GnRH every 60 to 90minutes. Thus, LH pulsatility depends on the ability of the GnRH neurons to secrete GnRH in a synchronized fashion.[33] Pulsatile secretion of LH occurs in many mammals, but the pulse frequency differs from one species to another and does not depend on input from other regions of the CNS. Rather, it is a property of the GnRH pulse generator, which is a set of

---

[30] Ibid. Pinon explains that these hormones account for the somatic differences between the male and the female, such as body, shape, distribution of body hair, and perhaps even differences in behaviour.

[31] C. TURKINGTON – M. ALPER, *Understanding Fertility and Infertility, op. cit.*, p. 146.

[32] R. PINON JR., *Biology of Human Reproduction, op. cit.*, p. 164.

[33] Ibid., p. 168.

neurons in the hypothalamus that can be called the central regulator of reproductive activity in the organism.[34]

[34] Ibid., pp. 170-171.

GAMETOGENESIS: FORMATION OF THE GAMETES

Following sexual intercourse, the male and female gametes need to fuse to create the zygote, which is the product of fertilisation. Before this occurs, the gametes need to be formed in their respective male and female environments. In the next section we will discuss how this is accomplished.

THE GAMETES: SPERM AND OVUM

In Greek, the word *gamos* means "marriage."[35] In both humans and animals, the two types of gametes are the sperm and the ovum (also known as the egg or oocyte). The gonads are responsible for the formation of the gametes. The production of eggs for reproduction takes place in the ovary, while the production of sperm takes place in the *seminiferous tubules* (ST) in each of the testes.[36] Naturally, the two different gonads come from the male and the female. In some animal species, however, it is possible to have both gonads in the same individual; this individual would be described as monosexual or hermaphroditic.[37]

The body of the human adult is made up of cells, which can be divided into two broad categories: somatic cells and germ cells. The term "somatic," a derivative of the Greek *soma*, means body. Thus, somatic cells refer to our body cells. They make up the different tissues of the body and can be differentiated cells or stem cells.[38] On the other hand, the highly specialized germ cells give rise to the gametes for the propagation of the species. While the somatic cells are diploid cells containing 46

[35] Ibid., p. 28.

[36] Cf. A. EHRLICH – C. SCHROEDER, *Medical Terminology for Health..., op. cit.*, p. 395.

[37] R. PINON JR., *Biology of Human Reproduction, op. cit.*, pp. 29-31.

[38] See R. LUCAS LUCAS, *Bioetica per Tutti,* Edizione San Paolo s.r.l., Milano 2002, pp. 81-82. The major parts of the cells of the body are differentiated cells—nervous, muscles, bones, blood and so on. The stem cells are not fully differentiated cells that can produce other differentiated cells of the organism. They can be of two broad classes: embryonic stem cells (from early embryos, miscarriages or aborted foetuses) and adult stem cells from adult tissues, placenta, umbilical cords and so on.

chromosomes (23 maternal and 23 paternal), the germ cells are haploid cells with only 23 homologous chromosomes.

In both male and female mammals, gametes are formed from the primordial germ cells. These latter differentiate into gamete precursor cells called *spermatogonia* in the male and *oogonia* in the female,[39] both of which are diploid cells with 23 pairs of chromosomes.[40] To prepare for fertilisation and reproduction, they must first undergo a process of maturation known as *gametogenesis*.

GAMETOGENESIS: FORMATION AND MATURATION OF THE GAMETES

Gametogenesis is the process of the formation and maturation of the gametes for fertilisation and propagation of the species. This process, known as *spermatogenesis* in the male and *oogenesis* in the female, is achieved through a type of cell division known as meiosis.[41] The timing of this process differs in the male and the female.[42]

SPERMATOGENESIS: FORMATION OF THE MALE GAMETE

During foetal life, a pool of spermatogonial cells is present in the seminiferous tubules of the testes. After birth, these remain dormant in the prepubertal testis and only become active at the onset of puberty, during which time they begin to increase in number in response to signals from the hypothalamus.[43] Spermatogenesis is the process whereby these spermatogonia transform into mature sperm for reproduction. The purpose is to form reproductive cells (sperm) containing half of the individual's 46 chromosomes. These reproductive cells can fuse with a

---

[39] W. LARSEN, *Human Embryology, Third Edition,* Churchill Livingstone, Philadelphia 2001, pp. 1-4.

[40] To ensure that the normal chromosomes of the cells of the human body remain 46, the chromosome complement of the germ cells will have to be halved to 23 to form haploid cells, which will later unite at fertilisation to restore the diploid character in the zygote.

[41] See K. MOORE – T. PERSAUD, *The Developing Human: Clinically Oriented Embryology, 7th Edition,* Saunders, Philadelphia, Pennsylvania 2003, p. 16.

[42] W. LARSEN, *Human Embryology…,op. cit.,* p. 4.

[43] See K. MOORE – T. PERSAUD, *The Developing Human…., op. cit.,* pp. 16-19; See also R. PINON JR., *Biology of Human Reproduction…, op. cit.,* p. 143.

functionally mature ovum to generate a new life.[44] In cellular terms, this purpose is accomplished through meiosis.

Spermatogenesis occurs in the three following stages and continues until death: proliferation and regeneration of the stem cell population, meiosis, and spermiogenesis.[45] Following several mitotic divisions, the germ cells differentiate into spermatogonia. These are later transformed into primary spermatocytes, secondary spermatocytes, spermatids, and finally mature spermatozoa.

OOGENESIS: FORMATION OF THE FEMALE GAMETE

The term oogenesis refers to the development and formation of the female gamete. It is the process by which oogonia are transformed into mature oocytes. This process begins during foetal life and continues throughout the reproductive life. *Oogonia* are present during foetal life and proliferate by mitotic divisions to form primary oocytes before birth. During the fifth month of pregnancy, the total number of oogonia reaches its maximum. The number then begins to decrease irreplaceably until menopause because of "follicular atresia," which consists in the degeneration of both the follicle and the oocyte. Usually, the oogonia commence their first meiotic division to form primary oocytes then immediately enter a state of meiotic arrest until puberty.[46] Thus, the female acquires during foetal life all the primary oocytes she will possess throughout her

---

[44] See C. NIEDERBERGER – D. LAMB "Spermatogenesis in the Adult" in L. LIPSHULTZ – S. HOWARD, *Infertility in the Male, Third Edition,* Mosby Publication, St. Louis 1997, p. 106.

[45] See R. PINON JR., *Biology of Human Reproduction, op. cit.,* pp. 144-148; See also K. MOORE – T. PERSAUD, *The Developing Human…, op. cit.,* p. 20; See also W. LARSEN, *Human Embryology…, op. cit.,* p. 3. In the first stage, the spermatogonial cells which are the precursors of the gamete begin to differentiate and proliferate. In the second stage, the B spermatogonia differentiate into primary spermatocytes. These undergo meiotic division to form secondary spermatocytes. Following a second meiotic division, these produce four spermatids. In the third stage, the spermatids are gradually transformed into mature spermatozoa without any further division, even though they undergo certain changes. In the end, the spermatozoa move to the lumina of the ST, from where they are later transported to the *epididymis* where they are eventually stored and become functionally mature.

[46] Ibid., p. 1.

reproductive life. The maturation of primary oocytes into secondary oocytes begins at puberty and continues until menopause, when the ovarian reserve of the woman is emptied, usually between 48 and 55 years of age.

MEIOSIS: MITOTIC AND MEIOTIC DIVISIONS

Every normal cell of the human being contains the same number of chromosomes. The somatic cells as well as the primordial germ cells, from which the male or female gametes are formed, contain 23 pairs of chromosomes, making 46 chromosomes total. To keep the human chromosome complement constant at 46, the germ cells need to be halved, that is, reduced from diploid to haploid cell in preparation for reproduction. This is achieved through a process known as meiosis. At the beginning of meiosis, the spermatocytes and primary oocytes replicate their DNA such that each of the chromosomes is duplicated into sister *chromatids.*[47]

Mitosis or Mitotic Division: Mitosis is a type of cell division that pertains to all the somatic cells of the body. One diploid cell undergoes a single division, producing two diploid daughter cells that are genetically identical to the parent cell.[48] Each will have the full complement of 23 maternal chromosomes and 23 paternal chromosomes. This first division involves DNA replication and recombination in the interphase.[49]

Meiosis or Meiotic Division: According to William Larsen, "meiosis is a specialized process of cell division that occurs only in the germ cells"[50] to give rise to functional male and female gametes for fertilisation. It involves two qualitatively different cell divisions. The first is a reduction division; the second is a separation, in which the chromosomes separate just as in mitosis. At the end of the second meiotic division in the male, four mature, identical haploid *spermatids* are produced from one spermatocyte. When they are transformed into spermatozoa, each one can fuse with a functionally mature egg to produce a new life. In the female,

---

[47] T. SADLER, *Langman's Medical Embryology…, op. cit.,* p. 6.

[48] L. SPERROF – M. FRITZ, *Clinical Gynecologic…,op. cit.,* p. 4.

[49] See T. SADLER, *Langman's Medical Embryology…, op. cit.,* pp. 5-6.

[50] Ibid., p. 5. DNA replication takes place in mitosis as well as in the first meiotic division to yield double stranded chromosome.

the meiotic divisions are unequal because they produce a single, massive, mature haploid oocyte for fertilisation and one small non-functional cell (called a polar body),[51] which will eventually degenerate as it has no role in reproduction.

Importance of Meiosis: By halving the chromosome number of the germ cells to 23, meiosis ensures that the normal human chromosome number remains 46 from generation to generation. Without this, the chromosome number of every child would be different from that of its parents.

In addition, meiosis allows for the random redistribution of the maternal and paternal chromosomes. It reorganizes the segments of the maternal and paternal chromosomes through the process of "crossing over" (of the segments), which "shuffles" the genes and produces a recombination of the genetic material. This process ensures that every individual is genetically unique (except in the case of identical twins).[52] This creates genetic variability within the general population.

---

[51] Ibid; See also K. MOORE – T. PERSAUD, *The Developing Human....*, *op. cit.*, p. 16. The first meiotic division is a reduction division because it involves the reduction of the chromosome complement of the cell from diploid to haploid. What takes place here is similar to what happens at the mitotic division, the only difference being that the chromosome number of the cells that undergo the second meiotic division is haploid and not diploid as in the case of mitotic division.

[52] See T. SADLER, *Langman's Medical Embryology...*, *op. cit.*, p. 6. The process of "crossing over" and the random exchange of segments of maternal and paternal chromosomes assure the uniqueness of the individual that results from each cell because each spermatozoon or ovum that is formed is genetically different from any other, a phenomenon that guarantees genetic viability.

THE HUMAN REPRODUCTIVE SYSTEM

Despite the differences in the reproductive systems of male and female humans, both systems are intended for the same goal. We will examine them briefly.

THE MALE REPRODUCTIVE SYSTEM

The function of the male reproductive system is to produce millions of sperm every day and to deposit them in the female reproductive tract during sexual intercourse. Here, one of the sperm must fuse with a functionally mature secondary oocyte to give rise to a new life.

THE FEMALE REPRODUCTIVE SYSTEM

The fertility of a woman consists of a cycle covering her fertile and infertile periods. The average length of the menstrual cycle is 28 days, but it can vary from 24 to 35 days.[53] The production of gametes takes place within this cycle, and what happens here is significantly different in comparison to the male. While sperm production is a continuous exercise with millions produced every day, only one ovum is produced roughly every month.[54] The woman's cycle is divided into two phases. The first phase, known as the follicular phase, involves the production of eggs, which are released at the time of ovulation. The other phase is the luteal phase, during which the uterus is prepared for implantation of the fertilized egg.[55]

THE FOLLICULAR STAGE: EMERGENCE OF THE DOMINANT FOLLICLE

The follicular stage is characterized by the development and selection of the dominant follicle. Beginning from puberty, a cohort of follicles contains primary oocytes that resume their maturation process within a woman's menstrual cycle. This occurs in response to gonadotropic

---

[53] R. PINON JR., *Biology of Human Reproduction, op. cit.,* p. 110.

[54] See Ibid., p. 110.

[55] Although there is no clear separation of the two phases, the two important events that indicate the transition from one phase to the next in the operational sense are the LH surge and the ovulation that occurs about thirty-six hours after.

hormones the pituitary secretes in response to the stimulation by the hypothalamus. Among these follicles, usually only one becomes dominant and ovulates, that is, expels the mature egg, now called a secondary oocyte.[56] The development of the dominant follicle that will eventually ovulate passes through three phases: initiation, recruitment, and selection.[57]

The dominant follicle is the follicle that is ovulated, and hormonally it is considered the most important structure in the ovary. It emerges in one of the two ovaries; once this happens, it quickly registers in the other ovary with the help of the oestrogen it produces,[58] leading to the suppression of further follicular development. Normally, only a single egg is ovulated per cycle. Occasionally, however, two or more eggs are ovulated, implying that two or more dominant follicles must have been selected. This may result in the birth of fraternal twins if the two are fertilised.[59] During the follicular phase of the woman's cycle, the dominant follicle is responsible for the production of most of the steroid sex hormone output in the female.

THE LUTEAL PHASE

The luteal phase is characterized by the formation, maturation, and demise of the *corpus luteum*. Ovulation occurs when the wall of the follicle breaks down and expels the secondary oocyte from the follicle. Following this, *granulosa* cells, which remain after the rupture of the follicle wall, along with cells of the *theca interna,* form a new structure called the endocrine corpus luteum. This new structure secretes large quantities of oestrogen and progesterone to prepare the endometrium for

---

[56] Once this process is initiated, two things are possible: a follicle—but sometimes more than one egg—may either be ovulated at the appropriate time in the cycle (usually the 14th day) or go into altresia.

[57] R. PINON JR., *Biology of Human Reproduction, op. cit.,* pp. 124-126. As Pinon observes, it is estimated that the development of the primordial follicle to the late Graafian stage takes about nine months. Usually, in the end, only one of the tertiary follicles selected from the recruited follicles will become dominant and ovulate.

[58] This is made possible by the vascular connections of the dominant follicles.

[59] R. PINON JR., *Biology of Human Reproduction, op. cit.,* p. 126.

implantation. If either fertilisation or implantation does not occur, the *corpus luteum* will degenerate after about 14 days.[60]

[60] W. LARSEN, *Human Embryology…,op. cit.,* p. 17.

THE HUMAN REPRODUCTIVE STRUCTURE

Human beings have various reproductive structures, which differ according to the sexes. Because of their importance to our subsequent discussion on infertility, we shall examine them briefly.

MALE REPRODUCTIVE STRUCTURE

The primary structures of the male reproductive system include the testes, the internal genitalia (the epididymis, vas deferens, prostate, seminal vesicles, and bulb urethral glands), the penis, and the scrotum.

THE MALE GONADS OR TESTES

The male gonads refer to the testes or testicles, which are two glandular organs in the scrotal sac below the penis.[61] They develop inside the body and then migrate to the scrotum outside the body either before birth or shortly thereafter. The postpubertal testes carry out two important functions: the production of the spermatozoa, which takes place at a lower temperature than that of the body, and the synthesis and secretion of androgens, especially the male hormone testosterone, which determines and maintains male characteristics.[62]

THE PENIS AND THE TUBES

The penis is the external sex organ of the male and contains the urethra canal traversing its length.[63] The tubes refer to the vas deferens, epididymis, and ejaculatory ducts. Sperm that is produced in the seminiferous tubules of the testes are stored in the epididymis, although it is also stored in the first portion of the vas deferens. In addition, sperm matura-

---

[61] Among other things, they comprise the *seminiferous tubules* where sperm are formed and the interstitial tissue containing the *Leydig* cells, which are the principal source of testosterone hormone.

[62] See R. PINON JR., *Biology of Human Reproduction, op. cit.,* pp. 139, 143. As Pinon explains, it is important to note that *androgen* that is produced by the testes is responsible for the formation of all the anatomical elements of the male reproductive system (i.e., the internal and external genitalia) and functionally maintains them.

[63] L. KAPLAN – C. KAPLAN, "Natural Reproduction and Reproduction-Aiding Technologies," in K. ALPERN, (ed.), *Ethics of Reproductive Technology,* Oxford University Press, New York 1992, p. 16.

tion is completed in the epididymis. The vas deferentia are long paired ducts that conduct or transport sperm from the testes to the penis during ejaculation. The urethra is the tube that removes urine from the bladder and the channel through which sperm is expelled during ejaculation.

THE ACCESSORY SEX GLANDS

There are different glands along the ejaculatory duct, such as the prostate gland, seminal glands, and bulb urethral glands. These contribute secretions to form the seminal plasma that mixes with the spermatozoa; this mixture constitutes the semen at the time of ejaculation. The energy supplied by these substances supports the spermatozoa's locomotion. Additionally, the milky fluid produced by the prostate protects the sperm from the high acidity of the vagina.

SPERM FOR FERTILISATION

About 200 million sperm are produced by the testes[64] every day. The concentration of sperm required for reproduction is at least 20 million per milliliter, and at least 40% must show vigorous swimming. Each mature sperm cell contains 23 chromosomes—22 autosomes and one sex chromosome, denoted XY.

FEMALE REPRODUCTIVE STRUCTURE

The primary structures of the female reproductive system include the ovary, fallopian tubes, uterus, and vagina. We will discuss them briefly.

THE FEMALE GONAD: THE OVARY

The ovaries[65] are two reproductive organs located on the right and left sides of the lower abdomen of a female. The eggs (secondary oocytes) for fertilisation develop here and are expelled during ovulation.[66] We can distinguish four stages in the development of the ovary: the prenatal

---

[64] R. JONES, *Human Reproductive Biology, op. cit.,* p. 165.

[65] See R. PINON JR., *Biology of Human Reproduction, op. cit.,* p. 102. As Pinon explains, in the past, the uterus was regarded as the most important organ in female anatomy and physiology, but this opinion changed around the middle of the nineteenth century. With a better understanding of its vital role, the ovary came to be recognised as the most prominent organ that distinguishes a woman. A woman has two ovaries located on either side of the uterus.

[66] Cf. K. MOORE – T. PERSAUD, *The Developing Human…, op. cit.,* p. 22.

ovary, the postnatal and prepubertal ovary, the postpubertal ovary, and the postmenopausal ovary.[67] The postpubertal ovary fulfils two important functions: first, the periodic maturation of primordial follicle into the female gamete and its release in ovulation; second, the synthesis and secretion of oestrogens and progesterone to prepare the endometrium for implantation.[68]

THE FALLOPIAN TUBES OR OVIDUCTS

The fallopian tubes (also called oviducts or uterine tubes) connect each of the ovaries to the uterus. Fertilisation occurs here, after which the zygote travels through these tubes to the uterus.

THE UTERUS

The uterus or womb is the site where the embryo implants and develops. After fertilisation, the embryo implants on the endometrium, which is the inside lining of the uterus wall. The superficial part of the endometrium sheds during each menstrual cycle due to a decrease in progesterone level, but if pregnancy occurs, it will not shed. In this case, the endometrium undergoes important modifications related to thickness and gland morphology and secretion.

THE CERVIX AND THE VAGINA

The cervix is a canal connecting the uterus to the vagina. During coitus, millions of sperm are deposited in the vagina; they are then transported to the site of fertilisation through the cervix and its mucus.

---

[67] R. PINON JR., *Biology of Human Reproduction*, *op. cit.*, p. 102.

[68] The activity of the ovary during post-pubertal period is not limited to the female reproductive function alone. It is connected to other non-reproductive functions as well.

PROCESS OF FERTILISATION IN HUMANS

The sperm and the ovum are living cells, but each on its own cannot give rise to a human being. First, they need to fuse to form a new diploid cell. Fertilisation is the fusion of these two highly specialized germ cells to form a single diploid cell known as a zygote.[69] In this section we will describe the process of fertilisation, but first, let us briefly review the process that leads to it.

Prior to fertilisation, the gametes need to meet and fuse. Naturally, ovulation and coitus are the first steps in this process. At the time of ovulation, the fimbriae of the fallopian tube cover the surface of the ovary, probably to ensure that the extruded ovum lands in the tube. The ovum is transported to the ampullary-isthmic junction, which is the widest region of the tube and the site of fertilisation. The transportation to this region results from the movements of the tubes.[70] The sperm, aided by the beating of their tails, have to move from the vagina towards the secondary oocyte at a swimming rate of about 3mm per minute. Usually, they travel a distance of 15cm in the 30 minutes after ejaculation. Out of the estimated 100 to 300 million sperm deposited in the vagina, only about 200 to 500 eventually reach the ovum at the site of fertilisation.[71]

The beating of the sperm tail is not actually of great importance in the journey through the uterus and the fallopian tube. This is demonstrated by the fact that both live and dead sperm reach the tube at the same time. This, perhaps, is due to the contraction of the muscles in the female reproductive tract, which facilitate sperm movement.[72] During their transport to the site of fertilisation, sperm are subjected to a rigorous selection process. This process is meant to ensure that only those sperm with the highest motility have the opportunity to fertilise the egg. Both

---

[69] T. SADLER, *Langman's Medical Embryology…, op. cit.,* p. 3.

[70] R. PINON JR., *Biology of Human Reproduction, op. cit.,* p. 274. The blocking of the oocyte at the ampullary-isthmic serves a functional purpose and the sperm for fertilisation may be ejaculated either shortly before or after ovulation.

[71] See Ibid. p. 282; See also T. SADLER, *Longman's Medical Embryology…, op. cit.,* p. 38.

[72] Cf. K. MOORE – T. PERSAUD, *The Developing Human…, op. cit.,* p. 39.

the coagulum and the cervical crypts appear to play a vital role in this process.[73]

THE PROCESS OF FERTILISATION

Fertilisation is a complex biochemical process whereby a sperm gradually penetrates various layers of the egg.[74] The process takes about 22 to 24 hours, beginning with the first contact of the sperm with the plasma membrane of the secondary oocyte and culminating in the formation of the zygote.[75] The process leading to fertilisation is characterized by a complex interaction between the sperm and the secondary oocyte, which has been primed to receive it. This complex interaction can be divided into the following phases: capacitation; acromosome reaction; fusion of the sperm and oocyte membranes and zona reaction; formation and fusion of the male and female pronuclei; and syngamy.

CAPACITATION OF SPERM

Although spermatozoa undergo certain changes in the epididymis that increase their fertilizing ability, humans (and many other mammals) require further capacitation. This means that the sperm ejaculated during coitus need to undergo a further process of maturation to be able to fertilize the egg. This additional period of maturation is called capacitation.[76] This process involves some modifications of the surface characteristics of the sperm and lasts for approximately seven hours.[77] Although the sperm do not undergo morphological changes during this period, the components of their membrane are extensively altered, making them more active.[78] Usually, the sperm are capacitated in the uterus and

---

[73] See R. PINON JR., *Biology of Human Reproduction, op. cit.,* p. 282.

[74] Cf. T. SHANNON – A. WOLTER, "Reflections on the moral status on the Preembryo," in T. SHANNON – J. WALTER, *The New Genetic Medicine,* Rowman and Littlefield Publisher Inc., Maryland 2003, p. 44.

[75] N. FORD, *When Did I Begin?* Cambridge University Press, New York 1998, p. 103.

[76] See R. PINON JR., *Biology of Human Reproduction, op. cit.,* p. 275.

[77] T. SADLER, *Langman's Medical Embryology..., op. cit.,* p. 38.

[78] Cf. K. MOORE – T. PERSAUD, *The Developing Human..., op. cit.,* p. 31.

fallopian tubes by substances secreted by these organs,[79] but some authors suggest that the process is initiated as the sperm pass through the cervical mucus.[80] Sperm acquire the following during capacitation: the ability to undergo acromosome reaction, the ability to bind to the zona pellucida (ZP), and the necessary hyper-motility to penetrate the cumulus cells and ZP.[81] Thus, capacitation matures the sperm and increases their motility and attraction to the oocyte. After undergoing capacitation, sperm display a new pattern of movement called hyper-activated motility. They acquire greater speed and better direction.[82]

ACROMOSOME REACTION

Following capacitation, the sperm make contact with the *corona radiata* surrounding the secondary oocyte; here they undergo acromosome reaction, which makes them capable of fusing with the oocyte.[83] The acromosome reaction is the means by which "the *lytic* enzymes in the sperm are released so that they can facilitate the passage of the sperm through the egg coverings."[84] In spite of the maturation of sperm in the epididymus and the capacitation that takes place in the female reproductive tract, not all the sperm that reach the egg are able to fertilize it.[85]

---

[79] Ibid.

[80] See L. SPEROFF – M. FRITZ, *Clinical Gynecologic..., op. cit.,* p. 238.

[81] See Ibid., pp. 237-238.

[82] Ibid., p. 236.

[83] K. MOORE – T. PERSAUD, *The Developing Human..., op. cit.,* p. 31. During their contact with the *corona radiata* surrounding the secondary oocyte, the sperm undergo complex molecular changes that result in the development of perforations in the acromosome.

[84] B. CARLSON, *Patten's Foundation of Embryology, 5th Edition,* McGraw-Hill New York, 1988, p. 134; See also J. BEDFORD, "Capacitation and the Acromosome Reaction in Human Spermatozoa" in L. LIPSHULTZ – S. HOWARDS, *Infertility in the Male..., op. cit.,* p. 133; The acromosome reaction provides the enzymes that will facilitate sperm penetration of the zonapellucida.

[85] See L. SPEROFF – M. FRITZ, *Clinical Gynecologic..., op. cit.,* p. 238.

FUSION OF THE SPERM/OOCYTE MEMBRANES AND ZONA REACTION

After reaching the oocyte, the sperm eat through the cumulus cells and bind their heads to the ZP[86] surrounding the oocyte. This occurs in a way that is highly specific to each species, which is meant to make it impossible for the sperm of one species to fertilise the oocyte of another species.[87] Next, the sperm try to digest a pathway through the ZP and penetrate the egg by the action of enzymes released from the acromosome. According to Sadler, "Both the binding and the penetration of the sperm are mediated by the ZP3, a zona protein."[88]

Usually, many sperm reach the oocyte, but only one fertilises it. As the sperm enters the cytoplasm of the secondary oocyte with its head and tail, it leaves its plasma membrane behind, which then fuses with that of the oocyte. Following this contact, the cortical granule reaction occurs. Thousands of small cortical granules lining the plasma membrane of the oocyte release *lysosomal enzymes* into the space between the oocyte and the ZP. These interact with the ZP in a way that alters the structural properties of the sperm receptor molecules, causing the zona to harden and to become impenetrable to any other sperm. This mechanism prevents the fertilisation of the oocyte by more than one sperm, a rare occurrence known as *polyspermy*. This condition is detrimental to the health and survival of the embryo.[89]

The entrance of the sperm head into the ooplasm of the oocyte activates the second meiotic division begun at ovulation, resulting in the formation and extrusion of the second polar body.[90] It is only at this

---

[86] W. LARSEN, *Human Embryology…, op. cit.,* p. 18. The zonapellucida facilitates the penetration of the sperm by producing molecules ZP1, ZP2 and especially, ZP3.

[87] See R. PINON JR., *Biology of Human Reproduction,op. cit.,* p. 286. As Pinon explains, the mechanism involved in this process is not completely known.

[88] T. SADLER, *Langman's Medical Embryology…, op. cit.,* p. 38.

[89] Cf. Ibid., p. 18, 39; See also R. JONES, *Human Reproductive Biology, op. cit.,* p. 165, 175; See also R. PINON JR., *Biology of Human Reproduction, op. cit.,* p. 286. Zona reaction is the alteration of the structural appearance and chemical properties of the ZP to make the membrane of the oocyte impenetrable to any other spermatozoon that may also have penetrated the ZP.

[90] Cf. R. PINON JR., *Biology of Human Reproduction, op. cit.,* p. 286.

point that the oocyte is reduced to a haploid cell and is called an *ootid.*[91] One of the resulting daughter cells becomes the definitive oocyte with 22 autosomes and an X sex chromosome. The other daughter cell, which receives only a little cytoplasm, becomes the second polar body.[92] As this has no biological role in the development of the embryo, it eventually degenerates.

FORMATION/FUSION OF THE MALE/FEMALE PRONUCLEI AND SYNGAMY

Over the next few hours, the sperm head (or male nucleus) decondenses and enlarges within the oocyte to form the male pronucleus within its own nuclear envelope; the tail detaches and degenerates. Next, a membrane develops around the female chromosomes to form the female pronucleus. Usually, the male and female pronuclei are morphologically indistinguishable.[93] As they grow and move toward each other in the next 6 to 10 hours, they replicate their DNA. Subsequently, as they move into close proximity in the centre of the ovum, their nuclear membranes break down. Thereafter, the mixing of the maternal and paternal chromosomes takes place, a process known as syngamy. This produces a single highly specialized diploid cell called a zygote. As Speroff and Fritz explain, the chromosomes are then arranged on a spindle, setting the stage for cell division.[94]

IMPORTANCE OF FERTILISATION

The exact time of fertilisation *in vivo* is not known, but in general, it is seen as a process that occurs within 22 to 24 hours. We shall describe what happens after fertilisation in a later chapter, when we discuss the status of the human embryo. For now, it suffices to state that the zygote is a genetically unique human organism; it contains a new combination of chromosomes that is different from that of the mother or father.[95] At this juncture, it is clear that fertilisation is the first major step in

---

[91] R. JONES, *Human Reproductive Biology, op. cit.,* p. 172.

[92] T. SADLER, *Langman's Medical Embryology…, op. cit.,* p. 39.

[93] K. MOORE – T. PERSAUD, *The Developing Human…, op. cit.,* p. 33.

[94] L. SPEROFF – A. FRITZ, *Clinical Gynecologic…, op. cit.,* p. 235.

[95] K. MOORE – T. PERSAUD, *The Developing Human…, op. cit.,* p. 33.

the development of the human organism.[96] It accomplishes four major things, which are described below.

1. During fertilisation, the haploid cells (sperm and ovum) unite to form a new diploid cell—the zygote—thereby restoring the normal 46-chromosome complement of the human person.

2. The sex of a child is determined at fertilisation, depending on whether the ovum is fertilised by the X chromosome female-producing sperm or the Y chromosome male-producing sperm. Specifically, it is determined by the presence or absence of a "particular gene on the Y chromosome."[97]

3. Fertilisation establishes the genetic uniqueness of every new human. This results from the process of meiosis, which occurs prior to fertilisation.

4. Fertilisation initiates the cell divisions of the new zygote. To be able to implant, the zygote must undergo several cell divisions to reach the blastocyst stage. If fertilisation does not occur, the secondary oocyte degenerates 24 hours after ovulation.[98]

THE SEX OF OFFSPRING

The sex of a child is determined at fertilisation. As we have already noted, this depends on whether it is the Y-carrying sperm or the X-carrying sperm that fertilises the oocyte. Regarding chromosome constitution, there are two types of normal sperm (23, X and 23, Y), whereas there is only one type of normal secondary oocyte (23, X). Usually, each gamete contains 23 chromosomes: 22 autosomes and a sex chromosome, which is XX for female offspring and XY for male offspring.[99] The sex chromosome of a sperm could be X (female) or Y (male), but that of the ovum is

[96] The product of fertilisation is called zygote. From the first cleavage of the zygote to end of the eighth week it is called embryo. From the ninth week to the time of birth it is called foetus.

[97] C. AMMER, *The New A to Z of Women's Health...*, *op. cit.*, p. 173.

[98] T. SADLER, *Longman's Medical Embryology...*, *op. cit.*, p. 40.

[99] Cf. THE REPORT OF THE PRESIDENT'S COUNCIL ON BIOETHICS, *Human Cloning and Human Dignity*, Public Affairs, New York 2002, p. 66.

always X. Thus it is the man, not the woman, who determines the sex of the couple's offspring.[100]

[100] At the end of spermatogenesis the male produces four *spematids:* two Y-male bearing sperm and two X-female bearing sperm. During intercourse, the female supplies the X sex chromosome always, while the male supplies X or Y. Any of these has a 50 percent chance to fertilise the ovum after coitus and determine the sex of the child. The sex of offspring is determined by the presence or absence of the Y chromosome bearing sperm. In its absence, the embryo will be female.

CHAPTER 2

THE PHENOMENON OF INFERTILITY

The human genes have been frequently described as "selfish genes" by virtue of the strong natural desire in human beings to procreate and form a family. Infertility poses the ultimate challenge to the fulfilment of this desire and to the survival of the family and the human race; it is thus a traumatizing experience for most couples and is therefore a serious human problem worth investigating.

INFERTILITY IN GENERAL

As we noted in the previous chapter on biology, human beings reproduce sexually[1] through the union of the sperm and the ovum. Following coitus, these two gametes unite to form a new diploid cell called a zygote, thus setting the stage for the development of a new human being. The problem is that fertilisation, and consequently pregnancy, does not occur with every exposure of the egg to sperm. Though our aim in this chapter is to discuss the numerous causes of infertility, we will first clarify the meaning of the term itself.

CLARIFICATION OF TERMS

To aid our understanding of this chapter, we must clarify the following terms: fertility, fecundity, fecundability, infertility, and sterility. Fertility refers to the reproductive ability of living beings. Fecundity is the probability to achieve a live birth with one menstrual cycle. Fecundability, estimated to be 20% to 25% in non-sterile couples, is the probability of achieving a pregnancy within one menstrual cycle.[2]

Infertility is conventionally defined as one year of unprotected coitus without conception.[3] Here, we can distinguish between primary and secondary infertility. The former refers to the infertility of those who have never conceived, while the latter refers to the infertility of those who have previously conceived.[4]

---

1 In the real sense, the phrase 'reproduce sexually' is only applicable to the biological aspect of human procreation. It does not encompass everything that takes place in the generation of a human being who also has a spiritual, non-biological dimension.

2 See L. SPEROFF–M. FRITZ, *Clinical Gynecologic…*, *op. cit.*, p. 1013.

3 See Ibid., p. 1013. Some authors find this definition a little inadequate and prefer to lay some emphasis on frequency of intercourse and live birth. Hence, they define infertility as one year of "regular unprotected coitus without conception." Considering that the inability to have a child is what is at stake in every case of childlessness, it may be better to see it as the inability of a couple to achieve a pregnancy the woman can carry to term after one year of regular unprotected coitus.

4 Cf. L. KAPLAN – C. KAPLAN, "Natural Reproduction..., *op. cit.*, p. 19.

Sterility refers to a permanent inability to reproduce that cannot be overcome by therapeutic intervention. This would apply to a couple that cannot have children[5] because the woman has no ovaries or the man has no testes.[6] The difference between infertility and sterility is that the former can possibly be rectified, whereas the latter is a permanent condition.

INCIDENCE OF INFERTILITY: A WORLDWIDE PHENOMENON

Today, infertility is commonplace all over the globe. Although its incidence worldwide cannot be determined with certainty, many studies reveal that more and more people are becoming infertile. What appears to be the medical consensus is that infertility affects 15% of couples in the industrialized world[7] and 30% of couples in Africa and the developing nations.[8] Some authors report that infertility is as high as 40% for couples in Africa.[9]

In the United States, some estimate that 20% of couples in child-bearing age experience infertility,[10] while others estimate 15%.[11] In 1987,

---

[5] Cf. P. MAHLSTEDT, "Psychological Issues of Infertility and Assisted Reproductive Technology" in L. LIPSSHULTZ – S. HOWARDS, *Infertility in the Male…, op. cit.,* p. 46.

[6] See L. KAPLAN – C. KAPLAN, "Natural Reproduction…, *op. cit.,* p. 30.

[7] Cf. L. SPEROFF – M. FRITZ, *Clinical Gynecologic…, op. cit.,* p. 1013.

[8] See P. BUTLER, "ART in Developing Countries – A Response to Individual Need or a Social Priority?" in J. KHANNA, Progress in Reproductive Health Research, by WHO, No. 63, 2003, p. 2.

[9] See I. POLLARD, *Life, Love and Children: A Practical Introduction to Bioscience Ethics and Bioethics*, Kluwer Academic Publishers, Boston 2002, p. 108. Beyond this general figure cited above, the incidence of infertility does not only vary from continent to continent, country to country, but it may also vary in different areas in the same country.

[10] See M. McCLURE, "Infertility," in F. SHENFIELD – C. SUREAU (eds.), *Encyclopedia of Applied Ethics,* Vol. 2, Academy Press, San Diego 1998, p. 673.

[11] See P. CATALDO, "Beginning of Life Issues: Catholic Teaching on Reproductive Technologies," in P. CATALDO – A. MORACZEWSKI (eds.), *Catholic Health Care Ethics: A Manual for Ethics Committees,* Part III, The National Catholic Bioethics Center, Boston Massachusetts 2001, 9\6.

a total of one billion US dollars was spent on fertility treatment by couples seeking professional assistance to resolve their infertility.[12] In the United Kingdom, the story is similar. An extensive study by Fiona McAllister and Lynda Clarke at the Family Policy Studies Centre reveals that "growing childlessness" is widespread in Europe with the United Kingdom having one of the highest fertility rates.[13] The situation in Africa is not much different. Friday Okonofua, an obstetrician and gynaecologist in Nigeria, estimates that 20% to 30% of the population of Africa has fertility problems.[14] In Nigeria, infertility is a major health problem: various studies indicate that the incidence of infertility is high and is increasing.[15]

INEFFICIENCY OF HUMAN REPRODUCTION

The human reproductive system is somewhat inefficient, especially when compared to the reproductive systems of other species. While some species ovulate with every intercourse and have multiple pregnancies with minimal miscarriages, human beings have low fertility coupled with higher rates of spontaneous abortion.[16] Fertilisation does not occur with every exposure of the egg to sperm; when it does occur, there is no certainty that the fertilised egg will implant and lead to a successful birth. For instance, the probability of achieving a live birth in one cycle of unprotected coitus is generally estimated to be below 30%. Of non-sterile couples engaged in unprotected sex, 25% conceive within one month, 63% conceive within six months, 75% conceive within nine months, 80% to 90% conceive within one year, and only

[12] See L. KAPLAN – C. KAPLAN, "Natural Reproduction..., *op. cit.,* p. 19.

[13] See F. McALLISTER– L. CLARKE, "Choosing Childlessness," in *Findings by the Family Policy Studies Centre,* July 1998, Ref. 738.

[14] F. OKONOFUA, Quoted in "Health, IVF: An African Dream," in *BBC News World Edition,* July 2003. See http://news.bbc.co.uk/2/hi/health/3086273.stm. (downloaded April 24, 2005).

[15] Cf. "The Difficulties Encountered in the Management of Male Infertility in Nnewi, Nigeria," *The Nigerian Medical Journal,* 45, 2003: 1.

[16] Cf. O. RODRIGUEZ-ARMAS "Infertility: The Problem and its Prevention" in O. RODRIGUEZ-ARMAS – B. HEDON – S. DAYA, *Infertility and Contraception,* The Pantheon Publishing Group, New York 1998, p. 1.

an additional 5% conceive after six more months.[17] As L. Kaplan and C. Kaplan observe, when the sperm reaches the egg in the fallopian tube, about 84% are fertilised out of which 69% implant in the uterus. Of this number, 42% survive the first week of pregnancy and only about 31% survive until birth.[18]

[17] See G. BENTLEY – C. MASCIE – TAYLOR (eds.), *Infertility in the Modern World: Present and Future Prospects,* Cambridge University Press, Cambridge 2000, p. 47. Here, these authors cited R. WILLIAMSON – S. ELIA, "Infertility and Pregnancy Loss?" in R. KING – J. ROTTER – A. MOTULSKY (eds.), *The Genetic Basis of Common Diseases,* Oxford University Press, New York 1992, pp. 577-595.

[18] See L. KAPLAN – C. KAPLAN, "Natural Reproduction..., *op. cit.,* 19.

CAUSES OF INFERTILITY

In the last twenty years, there has been remarkable progress in understanding the causes of infertility, although many factors still remain unknown. Infertility affects both males and females, and the factors responsible for it are many and varied. While a comprehensive discussion of the possible causes is beyond the scope of this book, we will attempt to categorize the numerous causes into male factors, female factors, combined male/female factors, and unexplained factors. In general, infertility may arise from factors related to endocrinology, physiology, neurological disturbances, sickness, or even the consequences of a particular lifestyle.[19] The major causes of infertility and their frequency of occurrence are summarized as follows: ovulatory dysfunction, 15%; tubal and pelvic pathology, 35%; male factor, 35%; unusual problems including uterine factors, 5%; and unexplained infertility, 10%.[20]

FEMALE FACTOR INFERTILITY

One of the primary functions of the female reproductive system is the periodic production and release of a mature oocyte. Other functions include the transportation of eggs from the ovary to the fallopian tube, the transportation of the embryo to the uterus, the production of steroid sex hormones to prepare the uterus for implantation and embryo development, parturition, and the production of milk to feed the child after birth.[21] However, problems can arise at any stage of the female reproductive system and impair a woman's fertility. The causes of infertility in the female are discussed below.

OVARIAN FACTOR INFERTILITY

The ovary is indispensable to female reproductive function, but to some extent it is also, as Pinon states, that on which the day-to-day well-being of the female depends.[22] Accordingly, serious disturbances in the

---

[19] See R. PINON JR., *Biology of Human Reproduction, op. cit.,* p. 400.

[20] See L. SPEROFF – M. FRITZ, *Clinical Gynecologic…, op. cit.,* p. 1028.

[21] Cf. A. EHRLICH – C. SCHROEDER, *Medical Terminology for…, op. cit.,* p. 401.

[22] See R. PINON JR., *Biology of Human Reproduction, op. cit.,* p. 120.

ovaries can lead to the loss of a woman's fertility and impact her general health and comfort.

Ovarian dysfunction is one of the leading causes of infertility in women. Approximately 20% or more of female factor infertility is related to the ovulatory factor.[23] The five key hormones that control the functions of the ovary are the sex steroids (oestrogen and progesterone) and the gonadotropins (LH, FSH, and prolactin).[24] Ovulation is governed by complex, well-synchronized hormonal interactions between the CNS, hypothalamus, pituitary, and ovary. If anything goes wrong in these complex hormonal interactions, ovulation will not occur, meaning that no egg will be available for fertilisation.[25] Other factors can also affect ovulation, such as a radical change of diet, excessive exercise, and severe stress. But the most serious cause of absence of ovulation is premature ovarian failure, or premature menopause, in which the woman's body absorbs all the eggs in her ovaries until they are depleted. This usually occurs before age 40, whereas the typical age for menopause is 48 to 55 years. This condition (about 1% to 3% incidence according to some studies)[26] is clearly linked to infertility because no egg will ever be ovulated during the woman's cycle. Ovulatory factor infertility may also result from several other conditions, including congenital absence of the ovaries from birth and chromosomal abnormalities such as Turner Syndrome, in which the ovary contains only a few follicles. It can be caused by ovarian antibodies in the woman that attack and deplete the follicles, by removal

---

[23] Cf. Z. BEN-RAFAEL – R. ORVIETO, "Infertility due to Defective Ovulation," in O. RODRIGUEZ-ARMAS – B. HEDON – S. DAYA, *Infertility and Contraception,* The Pantheon Publishing Group, New York 1998, p. 22. Sometimes, some authors cite about 30% for ovulatory factors. However, it is the second highest cause after the tubal factor.

[24] See R. PINON JR., *Biology of Human Reproduction, op. cit.,* p. 120.

[25] See Z. BEN-RAFAEL - R. ORVIETO "Infertility due to Defective..., *op. cit.,* p. 22. Ovulation refers to the extrusion of a secondary oocyte from a dominant follicle and it is triggered by an increase in the number of the hormone often known as the LH surge. Ovulatory dysfunction may be caused by reduced weight, chronic anovulation, endometriosis, impending ovarian failure and so on.

[26] See Ibid., p. 34.

of the ovaries due to ovarian cancer, or by physical damage to the ovaries during treatments such as chemotherapy and radiotherapy.

AGE AND FEMALE INFERTILITY

The age of a woman has a strong yet complex influence on her reproductive function. Maximum fertility in the female occurs around age 24 and then begins to decline gradually. This decline is clearly observed in the late 30s and becomes more rapid from age 40 to 50, at which point the number of women that can achieve a pregnancy is almost zero.[27] A large-scale study in France indicated that women under 31 years had a pregnancy rate of 74%; those from age 31 to 35 had a rate of 62%; and those over 35 years had a rate of 54%.[28] During perimenopause,[29] women can experience decreased fertility, higher risk of diseases, higher risk of spontaneous abortion, higher risk of having a child with chromosomal abnormalities, higher risk of stillbirth, and a gradual dismantling of the H-P-O axis.[30] Age adversely affects fertility in women in several ways, such as those listed below.

Endocrinology and Age: By endocrine we mean a system of glands—such as the hypothalamus, pituitary, and thyroid—that secrete hormones directly into the bloodstream. The endocrine system plays an important role in reproduction and changes with age. A woman's ovary develops during foetal life. During the first 16 to 20 weeks of pregnancy, the number of germ cells produced reaches six to seven million. From this time onward, the germ cell content starts to diminish irretrievably through atresia. There are approximately one million germ cells at birth and only 300,000 at puberty. During the woman's reproductive life, only 400 to 500 oocytes will ovulate. In the last 10 to 15 years before

[27] Cf. G. BENTLEY – C. MASCIE – TAYLOR (eds.), *Infertility in the Modern World…, op. cit.,* p. 47.

[28] See R. PINON JR., *Biology of Human Reproduction, op. cit.,* p. 402.

[29] The perimenopause in females, also known as climacteric, refers to the period of physiological decline of the H-P-O axis. This usually occurs from the late 30s to age 50. Menopause refers to the last menstrual cycle of a woman usually determined in retrospect. Some attribute it to the depletion of primordial follicles.

[30] See R. PINON JR., *Biology of Human Reproduction, op. cit.,* p. 242.

menopause, these are depleted by atresia until only a few hundred are left.[31] At menopause, all the follicles are depleted. The rate of loss from birth to age 38 remains relatively constant, but after this time, it doubles. Reduced ovarian reserve is associated with a lower probability of conception and a higher probability of miscarriage.[32]

Age and the Woman's Reproductive System: The quality of the eggs for reproduction is crucial. As a woman ages, her reproductive system degenerates. Although her ovary continues to expel an egg in every cycle, its reproductive quality or potential diminishes. There is a decline in the egg's capacity to be fertilised, to implant, and to survive during pregnancy.[33] Experiments involving the artificial reproductive technologies have repeatedly demonstrated that pregnancy delivery rates in women over 40 years of age are one-third to one-half of the rates in younger women.[34] Aging can affect fecundability and fecundity and increase the probability of spontaneous abortion and chromosomal anomalies. Aging also leads to hormonal fluctuations, which impair fertility by causing irregular menstruation and infrequent ovulation.[35]

Age and Diseases: An older woman is more likely to experience diseases and medical conditions that impair fertility, such as endometriosis, fibroids, and tubal damage.

Age and Complications during Pregnancy: Older women have an increased risk of experiencing complications during pregnancy. For instance, recent studies suggest that women over 35 years of age develop high blood pressure twice as often as women in their 20s.[36] This can affect the outcome of pregnancy and thereby reduce fertility.

---

[31] See L. SPEROFF– M. FRITZ, *Clinical Gynecologic…, op. cit.*, p. 1017.

[32] See S. BAYER – M. ALPER– A. PENZIAS, *The Boston IVF Handbook of Infertility,* The Pantheon Publishing Group, New York 2002, p. 11.

[33] Cf. L. SPEROFF– M. FRITZ, *Clinical Gynecologic…, op. cit.*, pp. 1016-1017.

[34] Ibid., pp. 1015-1017.

[35] C. TURKINGTON – M. ALPER, *Understanding Fertility and Infertility, op. cit.*, p. 10.

[36] See J. BARTON – N. BERGAUER *et al.*, "Does advanced maternal age affect pregnancy outcome in women with mild hypertension remote from

GENETIC FACTOR INFERTILITY: SPONTANEOUS ABORTION

A remarkable feature of human reproduction is the prevalence of spontaneous abortion, which affects both younger women in their optimal reproductive age and older women.[37] Even when conception and implantation are successful, the body may still reject the embryo. Spontaneous abortion is a problem both in natural[38] and artificial reproduction. This problem may be associated with smoking, excessive consumption of alcohol, or exposure to certain chemicals. But studies indicate that most early spontaneous abortions that occur after age 35 are due to chromosomal anomalies in the embryo; the rate of such anomalies increases with maternal age. From a genetic standpoint, as a woman advances in age, so do her eggs. This increases the chances of having embryos with chromosomal abnormalities; most of these embryos will result in spontaneous abortion and thereby decrease fertility. For instance, the risk of clinically recognized spontaneous abortion increases from 10% in most women under age 30 to 18% in the late 30s and 34% in the early 40s.[39] Additionally, spontaneous abortion can occur before or after implantation. Recent human chorionic gonadotropin (hCG) studies indicate a post-implantation pregnancy loss rate of 45%

---

term?" *American Journal of Obstetrics and Gynecology,* Vol. 176, Issue 6, June 1997, 1234-1240.

[37] See G. SHER – V. DAVIS – J. STOESS, *In Vitro Fertilisation: The A. R. T. of Making Babies, Updated Edition,* Facts on File Inc., New York 1998, p. 95. These authors maintain that about 20% to 25% of embryos conceived by younger women naturally or through IVF are chromosomally defective whereas this increases to 50% to 80% when they are over 40 years.

[38] See R. JONES, *Human Reproductive Biology, op. cit.,* p. 321. A high rate of spontaneous abortions is associated with the normal reproductive process in humans. One possible explanation for this is offered by Richard Jones. He maintains that, under normal circumstances, a mother does not immunologically reject her developing embryo as a foreign tissue. Although her immune system recognises the foetus as foreign, rather than expel it, it produces antibodies which, paradoxically protects it against rejection. However, in some cases of miscarriage, the foetus is not different enough from its mother genetically, so she does not produce enough protective antibodies, leading to its expulsion.

[39] See. L. SPEROFF – R. GLASS – N. KASE, *Clinical Gynecologic…, op. cit.,* p. 1015.

in women in the optimal reproductive ages and of over 90% in women approaching menopause.[40] This shows that chromosomal abnormalities increase with advancing maternal age. At age 20, the risk is one for every 526 live born infants; at age 35, it is one for every 192; and at age 40, it is one for every 66.[41]

Spontaneous abortion is considered the greatest obstacle to a live birth for older pregnant women.[42] Studies of trisomy 16 indicate that the association between maternal age and trisomy is caused by diminished recombination.[43] As Moore and Persuad maintain, the majority of these early abortions appear to be a kind of mechanism to prevent the development of abnormal embryos. This natural screening of embryos greatly reduces the incidence of infants born with congenital abnormalities.[44] L. Kaplan and C. Kaplan corroborate this view by asserting that "the most serious factor relating to spontaneous abortion is the body's rejection of embryos with chromosomal defects as a natural safeguard against the development of defective embryos."[45] *Mosaicism* can also impede fertility, and the risk of this condition is higher with advancing maternal age.[46]

---

[40] See D. HOLMAN – K. O'CONNOR – J. WOOL, "Age and Female Reproductive Function: Identifying the Most Important Determinants" in C. SAUVAIN-DUGERDIL *et al.* (eds.), *Aging – From culture of Nature,* Clarendon Press, Oxford 2000, Cited in G. BENTLEY – C. MASCIE-TAYLOR, (eds.), *Infertility in the Modern World..., op. cit.,* 47.

[41] S. BAYER – M. ALPER – A. PENZIAS, *The Boston IVF Handbook of..., op cit.,* p. 46.

[42] See L. SPEROFF – R. GLASS – N. KASE, *Clinical Gynecologic..., op. cit.,* p. 1015.

[43] See T. HASSOLD *et al.*, "Recombination and Maternal Age-Dependent Non-disjunction: molecular Studies of Trisomy 16," *American Journal of Human Genetics* 57:867-74.

[44] See K. MOORE – T. PERSUAD, *The Developing Human..., op. cit.,* p. 40.

[45] L. KAPLAN–C. KAPLAN, "Natural Reproduction..., *op. cit.,* p. 22.

[46] See S. MUNNE – M. SANDALINAS *et al,* "Chromosome mosacism in cleavage-stage human embryos: evidence of a maternal age effect" *Reprod-BioMed Online,* 4:223, 2002. Sometimes, during the early cleaving stage of the embryo, one or more of the cells or blastomeres may have chromosome numbers that are different from the others. This condition is described as mosaicism. It implies that the result from a genetic analysis of one cell may

TUBAL FACTOR INFERTILITY

Tubal factors are the most common cause of infertility in women, accounting for approximately 35% to 40% of female infertility. Fertilisation takes place in the fallopian tubes. If one or both of these tubes are damaged, blocked, or absent, the extruded egg may not be fertilized because the sperm may not be able to reach it. In like manner, if the walls of the tubes are damaged or blocked, they may fail to effectively move the embryo to the uterus, thus impeding implantation. Tubal factor infertility can be caused by scarring from a sexually transmitted disease (STD), rupture of the appendix, an asymptomatic pelvic infection, previous use of Intra-Uterine Devises (IUDs), previous ectopic pregnancy, irritation, and other accidents.[47]

CERVICAL FACTOR INFERTILITY

Cervical factor is responsible for infertility in less than 5% of couples. To reach the egg in the fallopian tube where fertilisation takes place, the sperm need to pass through the cervix and its mucus, which can either facilitate or prevent such access. Earlier in the follicular phase of a woman's cycle, the mucus is thick, viscid, and opaque due to low oestrogen levels;[48] this is meant to protect the uterus against infections. Any sperm deposited in the vagina at this time will be unable to penetrate this poor-quality mucus and will die in the vagina within a few hours because of its high acidity.[49] But shortly before ovulation and in the days after ovulation, rising oestrogen levels cause the mucus to become thin

---

not be truly representative of the condition of the others from the genetic point of view.

47 See S. BAYER – M. ALPER – A. PENZIAS, *The Boston IVF Handbook...*, *op. cit., p.16.*

48 L. SPEROFF – M. FRITZ, *Clinical Gynecologic...*, *op. cit.*, p. 1037. The mucus is thick, viscid and opaque earlier in the follicular phase of the cycle due to low oestrogen output and later in the luteal phase when progesterone counteracts the effect of oestrogen. Cervical mucus is said to be hostile when it impedes the natural passage of sperm through the cervical canal.

49 See S. BAYER – M. ALPER – A. PENZIAS, *The Boston IVF Handbook...*, *op. cit.*, p. 13. We should note that the acidic environment of the female reproductive tract can inhibit sperm motility. A hostile cervical mucus can act as an effective barrier to sperm movement from the vaginal/cervix into the uterus.

and stretchy, thereby facilitating sperm penetration and viability. If the mucus fails to become thin and stretchy, the impaired sperm penetration can contribute to infertility.[50]

A weak or incompetent cervix can also impair fertility because the pressure of a developing foetus can lead to miscarriage or premature birth.[51] Cervical problems may arise from a malformed cervix at birth, cervical malformation after a medical treatment, the production of inadequate or poor-quality mucus, and infections.[52]

UTERINE FACTOR INFERTILITY

Dysfunction of the uterus can impair female fertility. Motility of the sperm is an important factor of fertility, but sperm transport through the uterine and fallopian tubes is not dependent on sperm motility. Rather, the contraction of the uterus produces waves that move the sperm to the site of fertilisation. If such waves are weak, infrequent, or improperly directed, a woman's fertility will be impaired.[53] Congenital absence of the uterus or its removal due to disease and the condition of uterine fibroid, which occurs in about 15% to 20% of women over age 35, can affect fertility.[54]

LUTEAL PHASE INFERTILITY

Once ovulation occurs, the rupturing ovarian follicle is transformed into a new structure called the *corpus luteum*. This structure secretes large quantities of progesterone and significant quantities of oestrogen. These hormones, especially the former, act on the endometrium (the wall of the uterus) to prepare it for both the implantation of the embryo and the

---

[50] See L. KAPLAN–C. KAPLAN, "Natural Reproduction..., *op. cit.,* p. 21. The inability of the sperm to penetrate the mucus does not arise exclusively from poor quality mucus because it can also result from poor quality sperm.

[51] See C. TURKINGTON – M. ALPER, *Understanding Fertility and Infertility, op. cit.,* p. 97.

[52] Ibid., pp. 100-101. The cervix, the opening into the uterus and the vagina, prevents foreign bodies from entering into the female reproductive tract.

[53] Ibid., p. 10.

[54] See S. BAYER – M. ALPER – A. PENZIAS, *The Boston IVF Handbook…, op. cit.,* p. 21. Fibroids can grow outside the uterus, in the uterine wall and in the cavity, with the last one having the greatest impact on fertility.

support of its subsequent development.[55] If the production of progesterone is delayed or inadequate, the uterine wall may not be prepared when the implanting embryo reaches the uterus, thus preventing implantation. Furthermore, implantation problems may result from damage to the endometrium due to Pelvic Inflammatory Disease (PID) or damage to the uterine lining from a previous abortion with dilation and curettage (D&C). Chromosomal anomalies also impede embryo implantation.

USE OF CONTRACEPTIVES

Although contraceptives are used to control fertility, some of them can increase the chances of tubal damage and decrease fertility. Some authors suggest that previous use of an intra-uterine device (IUD) and of oral contraceptives could cause a woman to become infertile earlier.[56] Moreover, IUDs increase the risk of PID and can result in the perforation of the uterus. These conditions can decrease the chances of establishing and maintaining a pregnancy.[57] Steven Bayer *et al.* maintain that women who have previously used an IUD are two times more likely to experience infertility than women who have used other types of contraception. Ashley and O'Rourke claim that IUDs can make women permanently sterile or cause other bodily harm.[58] J. Daling *et al.* suggest that the Dalcon shield IUD increases the risk of infertility six-fold.[59]

[55] Cf. K. MOORE – T. PERSUAD, *The Developing Human...*, *op. cit.*, p. 28. Progesterone causes the *endometrium* to thicken so that it can support the implantation and the growth of the embryo. The progesterone produced by *corpus luteum* maintains the pregnancy for about eight weeks after which the placenta takes over this role. If fertilisation does not occur, *corpus luteum* degenerates and the secretion of *oestrogen* and *progesterone* decreases gradually and then ceases.

[56] See E. BILLINGS – A. WESTMORE, *The Billings Method, Revised Edition,* Gracewing Publishing, Herefordshire, UK 2000, p. 115.

[57] See R. JONES, *Human Reproductive Biology, op. cit.*, p. 277. Severe pelvic infection in the form of PID can cause scarring of the uterus and fallopian tubes. Also, it can increase the risk of entopic pregnancy, which further impairs fertility.

[58] See B. ASHLEY – K. O'ROURKE, *Ethics of Health Care, Third Edition,* Georgetown University Press, Washington, D.C. 2002, p. 132.

[59] See J. DALING – N. WEISS – B. METCH, *et al.*, "Primary Tubal Infertility in Relation to the use of an Intrauterine Device," *N. Engl J. Med* 1985; 312: 937-41.

Cohabitation before marriage may indirectly augment the incidence of infertility by encouraging the increased use of contraceptives. Such prolonged use of contraceptives, including IUDs, may increase the risk of tubal factor infertility.

BODY MASS INDEX (BMI) – A WOMAN'S WEIGHT

Body Mass Index (BMI) is an estimate of the amount of fat an individual has. BMI is calculated by dividing the weight in kilogrammes by the square of the height in metres.[60] The range of body weight required for reproductive function in women is 86% to 119% of normal. Extremes of weight (being less than 86% or over 119% of the normal body weight) can increase the risk of infertility. Women that are overweight or grossly underweight are more likely to experience a delay in conceiving. On this topic, Onuekwuesi writes the following:

> Being grossly underweight can prevent ovulation altogether. But also, being overweight can distort menstrual cycles. In severe cases, there may be excessive oestrogen from fat tissue causing delayed ovulation and irregular cycles.[61]

As Pinon explains, reproduction requires energy provided by food, and fat is a useful way to store energy.[62]

NUTRITION AND INFERTILITY

Nutrition is critical to both general and reproductive health. With regard to the latter, it can affect both the achievement and maintenance of pregnancy. Malnutrition on the part of the woman can cause miscarriage or premature delivery.[63] Pinon explains that while malnutrition may

---

[60] See C. TURKINGTON – M. ALPER, *Understanding Fertility and Infertility, op. cit.*, p. 93.

[61] N. ONUEKWUESI, "Special Issues on Infertility," A paper presented at the Training of Trainers Workshop on Natural Family Planning for Catholic Health Services Workers and Family Life Promoters, Lagos, Nigeria, October 25, 2002, p. 5.

[62] R. PINON JR., *Biology of Human Reproduction, op. cit.*, p. 227.

[63] See R. JONES, *Human Reproductive Biology, op. cit.*, pp. 210-234. During pregnancy, a woman needs to maintain, not just her own health, but also that of the foetus. Hence, being malnourished harms her and the foetus.

only adversely affect men when it is severe, relatively minor malnutrition or reduced food intake can cause ovulation dysfunction and luteal phase defects in women. Severe dieting (or even moderate dieting and weight loss) can suppress ovulation in women with normal cycles. Even if a malnourished woman succeeds in ovulating and conceiving, she may be unable to carry the pregnancy to term or to survive herself.[64]

ABORTION AND FERTILITY

Abortion refers to the expulsion of the foetus before it is viable. Induced abortion is the voluntary termination of pregnancy by artificial measures, whereas spontaneous abortion occurs naturally. An induced abortion does not have any direct effect on a woman's future fertility. However, its side-effects, such as infections and cervical damage, can negatively affect fertility.[65] In addition, it has been suggested that bone fragments left embedded in the uterus after an induced or spontaneous abortion can lead to irritation, making it impossible for future embryos to implant and grow.[66] This problem can arise when the abortion occurs after about 12 weeks of gestation. Kimberly Elford and Paul Claman recommend that this problem can be treated by performing endovaginal ultrasound on all women who present with secondary infertility and have a history of at least one abortion.

DELAYING MARRIAGE AND CHILDBIRTH

We can identify two trends under this factor. The first tends towards delaying marriage until later in life, and the other tends towards postponing childbearing until later in marriage. The former trend is more prevalent in Nigeria, while the latter is more common in the United States and Europe. Both trends have underlying economic motives, even though other contributing factors may be cited. People who are

---

[64] See R. PINON JR., *Biology of Human Reproduction, op. cit.,* pp. 227-228.

[65] See R. JONES, *Human Reproductive Biology, op. cit.,* p. 315. We should note that frequent abortions may increase the risk of infertility.

[66] See NATIONAL RIGHT TO LIFE COMMITTEE, "Bone Fragments Left from Aborted Babies Can Cause Infertility," *National Right to Life News (Magazine/Journal), Vol. 30, Issue: 50*, May 1, 2003, p. 27. This finding was published in the April 2003 issue of *Fertility and Sterility* by Kimberly Elford and Paul Claman, who are researchers with the division of Reproductive Medicine at Ottawa Hospital.

conscious of the challenges of raising a family try to earn enough money to guarantee the family a decent living. This practice impacts indirectly on female fertility, which decreases with age.

MALE FACTOR INFERTILITY

Male factor infertility refers to any condition in the man that adversely affects the chances of a couple to achieve a pregnancy. The primary function of the male reproductive system is to produce millions of sperm and deliver them into the female reproductive tract during coitus. When this action takes place, conception may still fail due to certain anomalies in the male's reproductive system, endocrine, and lifestyle. The male factor accounts for about 40% of infertility.[67] Some of the factors responsible for male infertility are described below.

HORMONAL FACTOR

The hormones that govern reproduction in a man are under the control of the H-P-G axis. When this axis is not functioning normally, the production of these hormones may be impeded, which can compromise his fertility. Also, the malfunction of the testes may adversely affect his fertility. Since the testes are responsible for the production of sperm, testes dysfunction may lead to the complete absence of sperm or inadequacy in its production. This condition may arise from a number of factors, such as the effect of disease on the testis, physical injury, genetic defect, or excessive heat.[68]

SPERM QUALITY

Good sperm quality is critical to male fertility. The factors that determine the quality of the sperm include sperm count, volume, motility, and morphology. These vary greatly between individuals. We will discuss these factors in detail.

Sperm Count, Sperm Volume, and Seminal Fluid: Sperm count, or sperm concentration, is the total number of sperm in the semen specimen. *Oligoospermia* refers to low sperm concentration in a semen

---

[67] See L. CHARLESWORTH, *The Couple's Guide to In Vitro Fertilisation,* Da Capo Lifelong Books, Massachusetts 2004, p. 14. The figure is usually given as about 35% to 40%.

[68] Cf. L. KAPLAN – C. KAPLAN, "Natural Reproduction..., *op. cit.,* p. 22.

specimen. The majority of the cases of male sub-fertility arise from low sperm count.[69] The normal sperm count for reproduction is 20 million to 120 million per milliliter.[70] If a man consistently produces a sperm count that is below 20 million per milliliter, fertility may be impaired. In addition, if the sperm volume or the seminal fluid is low, fertility may be impaired, because this condition can decrease the ability of the sperm to reach the cervix and fail to adequately protect them from the high acidity of the vagina.

Another factor that can have an adverse effect on male fertility is a condition known as *azoospermia*, in which the semen contains the seminal fluid without any sperm. It is present in approximately 1% of all men and 10% to 15% of infertile men.[71] Azoospermia can be either obstructive or non-obstructive. In the former condition, normal production of sperm takes place, but it cannot be ejaculated during intercourse. In the latter case, spermatogenesis is reduced or completely absent.[72] These conditions may arise because a man's hypothalamus, pituitary gland, or H-P-G axis is functioning below normal levels.[73] But it may also arise from intrinsic testicular disease (primary testicular failure), congenital anomalies, severe injury, or other conditions.[74]

Sperm Motility (Asthenospermia): Sperm motility refers to the sperm's ability to move or swim. *Asthenospermia*, one of the main causes of male infertility, is a condition of impaired sperm motility that prevents

[69] Ibid., p. 20.

[70] Sperm concentration refers to the number of sperm cells per milliliter of semen. When the number of sperm in the ejaculate is given as the number of sperm per milliliter it is more accurately known as sperm concentration or sperm density.

[71] See G. WILLOT, "Frequency of *Azoospermia,*" *Forensic Sci. Int.* 20:9, 1982; See also J. JAROW – M. ESPELAND – L. LIPSHULTZ, "Evaluation of the *Azoospermia* Patient," *J. Urol* 142:62, 1989. *Azoospermia* is a condition of absence of sperm in the ejaculate.

[72] See L. SPEROFF – M. FRITZ, *Clinical Gynecologic.., op. cit.,* p. 1145.

[73] See R. JONES, *Human Reproductive Biology, op. cit.,* p. 322.

[74] Ibid.

their transport through the cervical mucus.[75] The movement of the sperm from the vagina to the uterus depends on sperm motility. To avoid being trapped in the coagulum as they swim towards the egg, the ejaculated sperm should be able to propel themselves in a straight direction within 60 minutes of ejaculation,[76] especially as they have a limited time of survival in the acidic cervical mucus. Normal sperm motility is given as more than 50%. If more than half of the sperm are slow or have difficulty moving straight forward, fertility is likely to be impaired.[77] Abnormal sperm movement in the mucus can be caused by the presence of sperm antibodies on the sperm head, impaired flagellar function, genital tract infections, *varicocele*, and prolonged abstinence.[78]

Sperm Morphology (Teratospermia): Sperm morphology refers to the shape, size, and structure of the sperm. *Teratospermia* refers to abnormal sperm morphology and is one of the main determinants of the reproductive capacity of a man. All men produce abnormal sperm, but the degree varies from person to person and may increase with age. Some sperm are dead, have abnormal heads or tails, or have joined heads or middle pieces; all of these conditions can impair their motility, their ability to penetrate the mucus, and their ability to fertilise an ovum. As Moore and Persuad maintain, most morphologically abnormal sperm are unable to pass through the cervical mucus.[79] For fertilisation to occur, at least 30% of the sperm should have a morphologically normal form. If the percentage of normal sperm is consistently lower than 30%, fertility may be impaired. However, Kruger gives the "strict criteria" as 14% or higher,[80] which is similar to the recent World Health Organization

[75] Cf. P. MORALES *et al.*, "The Relationship between the motility and morphology of spermatozoa in human semen," *Fertile Sterile* 54: 513, 1990.

[76] See R. PINON JR., *Biology of Human Reproduction, op. cit.,* p. 281.

[77] See L. SPEROFF – M. FRITZ, *Clinical Gynecologic...,op. cit.,* p. 1146.

[78] See Ibid., p. 1146.

[79] See K. MOORE – T. PERSUAD, *The Developing Human..., op. cit.,* p.22.

[80] See T. KRUGER *et al.*, "Predictive value of abnormal sperm morphology in vitro fertilisation," *Fertil Steril*, 49:112, 1988.

(WHO) criteria for the evaluation of sperm morphology.[81] Moore and Persuad claim that X-rays and anti-spermatogenic agents may increase the number of abnormally formed sperm.[82]

PATERNAL AGE AND INFERTILITY

Although men retain fertility until their 70s, their reproductive capacity can decrease with advancing age. A recent study suggests that male fertility begins to decline after age 24. Even in fertile couples, the probability that it will take more than 12 months to conceive nearly doubles from around 8% when the man is under age 25 to around 15% when he is over 35.[83] Furthermore, the quality of a man's sperm tends to diminish after age 40. At this age, men have an increased risk of germ cell mutation during spermatogenesis, which leads to a greater risk of transmitting genetic mutations to their offspring. Bayer, Alper and Penzias allude to this when they assert that

> In contrast to oogenesis, spermatogenesis is an ongoing process that continues throughout a man's life and it has been estimated that sperm stem cells divide 23 times each year.... This increased frequency of divisions increases the chance of errors that can result in new mutations. This has been referred to as 'copy error' which can result in the stem cells accumulating a mutation with each division.[84]

---

[81] See WORLD HEALTH ORGANIZATION, *Laboratory Manual for Examination of Human Semen and Sperm-cervical Mucus Interaction, 2nd Edition,* University Press, Cambridge 1992; Cited in L. SPEROFF – M. FRITZ, *Clinical Gynecologic..., op. cit.,* pp. 1144, 1147.

[82] K. MOORE – T. PERSUAD, *The Developing Human...,op. cit.,* p. 22.

[83] See http://www.statlander.com\reuters\repro\1407170017.html (Downloaded 2/7/2006); See also *Hum Reprod,* August 2000; 15:1703-1708. From a study of 8,500 couples in Bristol, Dr. Chas Ford of the University Division of Obstetrics and Gynaecology at St. Michael's Hospital, Bristol and his colleagues claim that as a man advances in age, it would take a longer time for the couple to conceive.

[84] S. BAYER – M. ALPER – A. PENZIAS, *The Boston IVF Handbook..., op. cit.,* pp. 45-46.

Corroborating this view, Speroff and Fritz state that "semen volume, sperm motility, and the proportion of morphologically normal sperm (but not sperm concentration), decrease gradually as a man's age increases."[85]

GENETIC FACTOR INFERTILITY

Recent studies indicate that certain cases of primary infertility have a correlation with genetic disorders or structural abnormalities in the male.[86] These include micro-deletions of the Y chromosome, congenital absence of the vas deferens, *cryptorchidism,* retrograde ejaculation, and other congenital malformations of the male reproductive system. All these conditions can cause infertility in males.[87] Depending on its severity, the disorder can result in mild to extreme reduction in sperm count or complete absence of sperm. For instance, serious impairment of fertility may result from the deletion of certain genes on the Y chromosome, which directs the spermatogonial stages of spermatogenesis.[88] In addition, infection of the prostate and congenital absence or blockage of the vas deferens can contribute to infertility in some males.[89] This

---

[85] L. SPEROFF – M. FRITZ, *Clinical Gynecologic…, op. cit.,* p. 1139. Here, Cited S. KIDD – B. ESKENAZI – A. WYROBEK, "Effects of Male Age On Semen Quality and Fertility: A Review of the Literature," *Fertile Steril,* 75:237, 2001.

[86] Cf. R. PINON JR., *Biology of Human Reproduction, op. cit.,* p. 407. Pinon maintains that studies involving *azoospermic* males have revealed that severe disturbances of the *seminiferous tubules* function may result in the inability of the male to produce sperm. Partial or complete deletion of the Y-chromosome may be associated with low sperm count or the absence of sperm in an ejaculate respectively. Men with Cystic Fibrosis (CF) have congenital absence of the *vas deferens* and are usually sterile. Also, absence of sperm may arise from retrograde ejaculation in which case sperm are forced backwards into the bladder during coitus (and mix with urine) instead of flowing out through the urethra. This condition may be caused by a dysfunction of the muscles of the urethra during ejaculation.

[87] Cf. A. BITTLES – L. MATSON, "Genetic Influences on Human Infertility" in G. BENTLEY – C. MASCIE-TAYLOR (eds.), *Infertility in the Modern World…, op. cit.,* p. 46.

[88] See R. PINON JR., *Biology of Human Reproduction, op. cit.,* p. 407.

[89] See R. JONES, *Human Reproductive Biology, op. cit.,* p. 324.

blockage does not allow sperm to pass through the penis during sexual intercourse; however, this condition can be corrected with surgery.

Male infertility can also arise from testes dysfunction. Since sperm are produced by the testes, any dysfunction here will affect their production and contribute to infertility. This problem may result from old age or exposure to radiation.[90] Moreover, abnormalities in the testes can arise from physical injury to the testes or as a result of cryptorchidism (that is, undescended testes), which can be either unilateral or bilateral. It is unilateral if only one of the testes fails to descend and bilateral if both fail to descend. Bilateral cryptorchidism is associated with infertility. Because the production of sperm usually occurs at a temperature lower than the normal body temperature,[91] varicocele, a genetic defect involving enlarged and twisted veins in the scrotum can raise the temperature of the testes. This can cause infertility by compromising sperm production, morphology, and motility.

MALE/FEMALE FACTOR INFERTILITY

The reproductive activity of humans is influenced by a variety of factors. In some cases, a combination of male and female factors may be responsible for a couple's infertility; these cases will be our focus here.

OCCUPATIONAL AND ENVIRONMENTAL HAZARDS

Spermatogenesis is sensitive to heat. The temperature of the scrotum is 2°F to 3°F lower than that of the core body. Thus, occupations that expose men to excessive heat can increase the temperature of the testes and reduce fertility. High scrotal temperatures reduce both the sperm quantity and quality in fertile men.[92] Situations involving ovens, tight clothing, or hot tubs can affect sperm production by exposing the genitals to excessive heat. As such, plant and machine operators, as well as men who frequently expose themselves to radiant heat from welding equipment, have an increased risk of oligoospermia.

---

[90] Ibid.

[91] See A. EHRLICH – C. SCHROEDER, *Medical Terminology for…, op. cit.*, p. 395.

[92] See P. THONNEAU *et al.*, "Occupational Heat Exposure and Male Fertility: A Review," *Human Reproduction,* 13(8) (1998) 2122-2125.

Environmental pollutants pose a potential threat, not only to general human health, but also to human fertility. Some pesticides and other environmental toxins can decrease fertility in male workers. In like manner, frequent exposure to such chemicals can cause delay in achieving pregnancy among the female partners; these women may also experience an increased incidence of spontaneous abortion.[93] Cumulative exposure to occupational and environmental hazards[94] could also reduce fertility in women as they advance in age.[95] Documented evidence shows that a higher rate of spontaneous abortion occurs in operating room personnel that are exposed to the inhalation of anesthetic gases; this higher rate of spontaneous abortion is present even when only the male partners are exposed to the gases. Likewise, exposure to mercury, dry cleaning chemicals, bleaches, and chemicals employed in beauty salons can decrease fertility in women.[96] Harmful chemicals can also cause low sperm count in males and miscarriages and birth defects in pregnant females. However,

---

[93] See G. PETRELLI – A. MANTOVANI, "Environmental Risk and Male Fertility and Reproduction," *Contraception,* 65 (2002) 297-300.

[94] Cf. R. PINON JR., *Biology of Human Reproduction, op. cit.,* p. 46. Pinon adds that besides decreasing fertility, environmental toxins, such as pesticides, household products, industrial chemicals, cosmetics and the sort are also chemical mutagens that can penetrate the gonads and cause mutations in the germ cells of those who are exposed to them at a high dosage. That is to say, such mutations, which can be transmitted to their offspring, can only occur if the exposure is so high that these agents succeed in penetrating the germ cells to the point of damaging their DNA. In general, exposures to such compounds in the general population are known to be low, except in the case of workers in chemical industries.

[95] Cf. L. SPEROFF – R. GLASS – N. KASE, *Clinical Gynecologic..., op. cit.,* p. 1015.

[96] See S. BAYER – M. ALPER – A. PENZIAS, *The Boston IVF Handbook of..., op cit.,* pp. 5, 40-41. As Bayer and others suggest, from a fertility perspective, the male is more suspectible to the effects of frequent exposure to chemicals or toxins considering that sperm production occurs on a daily basis. The high exposure to anaesthetic gases in operating rooms can affect both male and female fertility and can cause spontaneous abortions in women and congenital anomalies in their offspring even where only the male partners are exposed to them.

the danger of each case will depend on the extent and frequency of such exposure and the particular chemical or toxin in question.[97]

A study by Danish scholars suggests that a group of chemicals known as *xenoestrogens* can cause infertility in men by reducing their sperm count. They claim that these chemicals have caused a continuous decline in human sperm counts over the last 50 years, a decline which will eventually lead to widespread infertility. However, their impact on fertility has been a subject of controversy; opponents claim that the results from experiments with animals cannot be extrapolated to humans because some animal species are more sensitive to toxic effects from certain chemicals. Hence, they recommend extreme caution in applying the results of animal experiments to human beings.[98]

LIFESTYLE FACTORS

A person's lifestyle is important to both general and reproductive health. Lifestyle factors refer to the use of drugs, tobacco, alcohol, caffeine, and intensive physical exercise, all of which can have a significant impact on male and female fertility.

Smoking and Infertility: Besides the well-known effect of smoking on pregnancy and general health, studies suggest that both male and female tobacco use pose a great risk to fertility; smoking is therefore considered a reproductive toxin.[99] Since smoking can alter ovarian function and contribute to early menopause, it follows that the chemicals in smoke may be directly toxic to the ovaries.[100] Apart from this, fecundity is reduced in men and women who smoke, and the risk is greater when smoking begins at an early age.[101] One finding posits that smokers have

[97] See C. TURKINGTON – M. ALPER, *Understanding Fertility…, op. cit.,* pp. 102-103.

[98] See G. BENTLEY, "Environmental Pollutants and Fertility…, *op. cit.,* p. 85.

[99] Cf. AMERICAN COLEGE OF OBSTETRICIANS AND GYNECOLOGISTS, "Smoking and Women's Health," *Education Bulletin,* No. 240, 1997.

[100] See S. BAYER – M. ALPER – A. PENZIAS, *The Boston IVF Handbook…, op. cit.,* p. 6.

[101] See R. STILLMAN – M. ROSENBERG – B. SACHS, "Smoking and Reproduction," in *Fertility and Sterility,* 46 (1986) 545; See also S. LAURENT – S. THOMPSON *et al.*, "An Epidemiologic Study of Smoking and Primary Infertility in Women," *Fertility and Sterility,* 57 (1992) 565.

a conception rate of 6.3% compared to a rate of 16.8% for non-smokers.[102] Couples who smoke have a lower rate of conception, and women who smoke have a higher risk of miscarriage.

Furthermore, there is a dose-response relationship between the number of cigarettes smoked and the length of time it takes to conceive. The risk increases if either the woman or the man has been smoking for more than five years at any point in his or her lifetime. Female smokers are 60% more likely to be infertile than non-smokers.[103] Men who smoke one or more cigarettes per day have lower total sperm count, reduced motility, and an increased number of morphologically abnormal sperm.[104] Also, smoking has a correlation with greater risk of tubal pregnancy, high rates of spontaneous abortion, premature birth, and defects in the physical, intellectual, and emotional development of the child. There is also new evidence that smoking, particularly paternal smoking, can contribute significantly to genetic disorders and childhood cancer, perhaps because the gonads tend to absorb tobacco smoke.[105]

Effect of Alcohol Consumption on Fertility: The likelihood of conception is slightly lower for women who drink more than two glasses of wine per week and for men who drink more than ten glasses of beer or six glasses of liquor per week. Moderate to heavy alcohol consumption by women may increase the risks of two categories of infertility: the ovulatory factor and endometriosis.[106] In general, the more alcohol a woman consumes, the greater the impact on her ability to conceive. Increased levels of alcohol can alter oestrogen and progesterone levels, cause irregularities in the menstrual cycle, and lead to early onset of menopause.[107]

---

[102] See R. HAKIM, *et al.*, "Alcohol and Caffeine Consumption and Decreased Fertility," *Fertility and Sterility*, 70(4) (1998) 632-637.

[103] See C. AUGOOD, *et al.*, "Smoking and Female Infertility: A Systematic Review and Meta-analysis," in *Human Reproduction*, 3(6) (1998) 1532-1539.

[104] See R. KUNZLE, *et al.*, "Semen Quality of Male Smokers and Nonsmokers in Infertility Couples," *Fertility and Sterility*, 79(2) (2003) 287-291.

[105] See R. PINON JR., *Biology of Human Reproduction, op. cit.*, pp. 46-47.

[106] See F. GRODSTEIN, *et al.*, "Infertility in Women and Moderate Alcohol Use," *American Journal of Public Health*, 84(9) (1994) 1429-1432.

[107] See A. WISOT – D MELDRUM, *Conceptions and Misconception, Second Edition*, Hartley & Marks Publishers, Point Roberts, W.A. 2004, p. 256. The

However, it is important to note that these conclusions may not apply to everybody. For instance, Parazzini claims that alcohol consumption is not related to infertility among Italian women.[108] Pinon supports this view, asserting that there is documented evidence of alcoholic women achieving pregnancy and giving birth. He explains that in some women, the H-P-O axis can develop tolerance to the effects of chronic alcohol consumption. However, he contends that chronic alcohol abuse by women can result in irreversible impotency, and children born to them may present with a higher risk of some physical and developmental problems.[109] Bayer and others add that high levels of alcohol intake during pregnancy can cause foetal alcohol syndrome, which is associated with altered foetal growth and mental retardation.[110]

Effect of Caffeine Consumption: Although there is no scientific evidence that caffeine seriously reduces fertility, it has been suggested that excessive caffeine consumption may delay conception.[111] Women who drink the equivalent of a half cup of coffee daily would likely have a delayed conception compared to others who do not. Also, the partners of men who consume more than one cup of coffee daily have two times

authors state that some researches suggest that women who consume one to five alcoholic drinks a week will have about 40% reduction in the odds of conceiving, while this rises to about 66% reduction for those who consume more than ten drinks per week.

[108] F. PARAZZINI, *et al.*, "Alcohol Consumption is not related to fertility in Italian women," *British Medical Journal* (1999) 318-397.

[109] See R. PINON JR., *Biology of Human Reproduction, op. cit.,* pp. 400-412. Pinon contends that chronic alcohol consumption is associated with such reproductive problems like anovulation, amenorrhea, luteal phase dysfunction, ovarian pathology, and *hyperprolactinemia* in women. In males, alcohol consumption may affect testicular function, cause erectile dysfunction and infertility depending on whether the dose is acute or chronic. Alcohol suppresses testosterone synthesis in the testis indirectly.

[110] See S. BAYER – M. ALPER – A. PENZIAS, *The Boston IVF Handbook…, op. cit.,* p. 26.

[111] R. HAKIM, *et al.*, "Alcohol and Caffeine Consumption…, *op. cit.,* 70(4) (1998) 632-637.

greater likelihood of a multiple birth.[112] Bayer and others assert that a dose-dependent relationship exists between caffeine consumption and reduced fertility.[113] However, some investigators suggest that the effect on fertility may not be due to caffeine itself, but rather to tannins, which are compounds contained in caffeine and caffeinated soft drinks.[114]

Effect of Drugs on Fertility: As we noted previously, human reproductive activity is under the control of the GnRH pulse generator. Frequent use of drugs can interfere with the function of the GnRH pulse generator or its stimulation of the pituitary; it can also disrupt the H-P-G axis or the function of the gonads.[115] The frequent use of drugs such as marijuana, opium, anabolic steroids, and cocaine negatively affects every aspect of human reproduction and gives rise to male and female infertility. For instance, drug abuse can cause ovarian dysfunction and amenorrhea in female addicts and loss of libido and erectile dysfunction in male addicts.[116] In particular, frequent use of marijuana leads to lower serum testosterone levels and decreased sperm counts,[117] and cocaine abuse reduces spermatogenesis.[118] However, the degree of the effect depends on the amount taken, the frequency of use, and the duration of use.

---

[112]See A. WISOT – D. MELDRUM, *Conceptions and Misconceptions..., op. cit.,* p. 257. On the other hand, Wisot and Meldrum contend that daily consumption of more than one-half cup of caffeinated tea may increase women's odds of conceiving whereas the polyphenolic compounds in the tea probably promote fertility by reducing chromosomal abnormalities in embryos and the attendant incidence of spontaneous abortion. But the major reason may be that tea consumption promotes healthier lifestyle that enhances fertility.

[113]See S. BAYER – M. ALPER – A. PENZIAS, *The Boston IVF Handbook..., op. cit.,* p. 30.

[114]See R. PINON JR., *Biology of Human Reproduction, op. cit.,* p. 413.

[115]See Ibid., p. 410.

[116]See Ibid., pp. 177-178.

[117]See S. BAYER – M. ALPER – A. PENZIAS, *The Boston IVF Handbook..., op. cit.,* p. 27.

[118]See L. SPEROFF – M. FRITZ, *Clinical Gynecologic..., op. cit.,* p. 1023.

SICKNESS AND MEDICATION

Decline in fertility is common among men and women who suffer from certain illnesses, such as insulin-dependent diabetes, which tends to damage blood vessels and nerves. Diabetes may cause erectile dysfunction or impotence.[119] Spinal cord injuries are associated with decline in sperm quality, ejaculatory problems, and even impotence. Injury to the vas deferens due to surgery can impair normal spermatogenesis.[120]

Certain medications and medical treatments can decrease sperm production, decrease sperm quality, or even cause impotence. For instance, chemotherapy and radiotherapy used in cancer treatment affect ovarian function and often render the female permanently infertile.[121] In males, they can cause irreversible damage to spermatogenesis. Medications for treating hypertension can lead to inability to ejaculate and male impotence.[122] According to Bayer and others, the use of anabolic steroids can result in significant oligoospermia and sometimes azoospermia, while other medications used to treat mood disorders can interfere with erectile function and ejaculation.[123]

THE PRESENCE OF ANTIBODIES TO SPERM

Infertility can arise from the presence of antibodies to sperm in either the female or the male himself. Antibodies are proteins in the body. In a woman, antibodies to her husband's sperm may attach to the sperm and inhibit their motility, their ability to penetrate cervical mucus, and their ability to fertilise an oocyte.[124] They may even destroy the sperm

[119]Cf. C. TURKINGTON – M. ALPER, *Understanding Fertility…, op. cit.*, pp. 102-113. Such therapeutic drugs or medications that can affect the female fertility cycle include tranquilizers, antibiotics, antidepressants and the like.

[120]See S. BAYER – M. ALPER – A. PENZIAS, *The Boston IVF Handbook…, op. cit.*, p. 14.

[121]See R. PINON JR., *Biology of Human Reproduction, op. cit.*, p. 415.

[122]See O. RODRIGUEZ-ARMAS "Infertility: The Problem and its Prevention…, *op. cit.*

[123]See S. BAYER – M. ALPER – A. PENZIAS, *The Boston IVF Handbook…, op. cit.*, p. 14.

[124]See C. TURKINGTON – M. ALPER, *Understanding Fertility…, op. cit.*, pp. 7-9. The point of attachment to the sperm matters. If the antibodies

deposited in the vagina during coitus. Furthermore, a condition known as auto-immunity may arise in some women and cause premature ovarian failure; in this case a woman's immune system attacks and destroys her own germ cells before the normal onset of menopause.[125] A man may also produce antibodies to his own sperm,[126] which can result in infertility.

INFECTIONS AND SEXUALLY TRANSMITTED DISEASES (STDS)

Infections play a role in both male and female infertility. Among the viral or bacterial diseases that can significantly impede female fertility, pelvic inflammatory diseases (PIDs) are prominent. For instance, a PID can cause scars inside the fallopian tubes, which may subsequently damage or block the tubes or cause ectopic pregnancy. A study of 25 developed and developing countries suggested that PID was the primary cause of tubal factor infertility, causing 38% of cases in some European countries and 64% of cases in some African countries.[127] PIDs are mainly caused by STDs, primarily gonorrhea and chlamydia;[128] these diseases can adversely affect fertility—irrespective of the age or sex of the indi-

---

attach to the heads or tails of the sperm, they may cause them to stick together and can impede their motility, and consequently, their ability to penetrate and fertilize the egg.

[125]Ibid., p. 9.

[126]Ibid., pp. 7-9, 76. Antibodies to sperm are substances in their immune systems that identify any sperm deposited in the vagina as foreign proteins and then attack them. This happens when the natural barrier or protective mechanism that prevents any contact between sperm and blood break down, accidentally allowing them to be exposed to each other (for instance, during a surgery or an injury to the testicles, *cryptorchidism* or hernia repair, vasectomy, and so on). In this case, the body may misinterpret the sperm as foreign, causing the immune system to develop antibodies against them. Although this can also occur in women, the chances are much lower, occurring less than 5% in infertile women.

[127]See O. RODRIGUEZ-ARMAS "Infertility: The Problem and its Prevention..., *op. cit.,* p. 1.

[128]See R. PINON JR., *Biology of Human Reproduction, op. cit.,* pp. 293-294, 434. Chlamydia and gonorrhea are common bacterial STDs, which can be transmitted through unprotected sex and from mother to child at birth. For women, the more serious infections occur in the cervix, uterus and the fallopian tubes and can decrease fertility. They make conception increasingly difficult and raise the risk of ectopic pregnancy and premature birth.

vidual—at the time of occurrence, after occurrence, or even after treatment. They can easily damage a woman's fallopian tube and thus impair fertility. Other diseases that are associated with infertility include endometriosis and fibroid.[129]

Furthermore, in the male, bacteria can infect the epididymus and cause scarring and blockage, thus preventing sperm from leaving the duct or being ejaculated during intercourse. Also, a man's semen specimen may contain bacteria, which can compromise its fertilisation capacity.[130] The presence of harmful bacteria may damage the testicles, thereby compromising sperm production and quality.[131]

FREQUENCY AND TIMING OF INTERCOURSE

Other essential factors in both male and female fertility relate to the frequency and timing of intercourse. Infrequent coitus reduces the chances of conceiving. Some authors suggest that having coitus four times per week is optimal, whereas others see thrice a week as a better compromise because more frequent ejaculation could decrease sperm concentration and the volume of the ejaculate.[132] The lifetime of the ovulated secondary oocyte is only about 24 hours. Similarly, the survival period of the ejaculated sperm in the fallopian tube is only about 48

---

[129]See R. PINON JR., *Biology of Human Reproduction, op. cit.,* pp. 405-407. Pinon explains that endometriosis refers to a condition whereby the endometrial tissue grows in the fallopian tube, abdominal cavity and so on instead of the uterine, which is the normal site. It occurs 30% to 45% in women with infertility and about 10% in fertile women. Although pregnancy is possible in this condition, if a woman has a severe form of it in the fallopian tube, ovaries or the pelvic regions, it can impact her fertility due to severe scarring of the ovaries and/or tubes. On the other hand, uterine fibroid may interfere with the implantation of an embryo.

[130]See L. CHARLESWORTH, *The Couple's Guide To In Vitro Fertilisation, op. cit.,* p. 177.

[131]See A. TOTH, *The Fertility Solution,* The Atlantic Monthly Press, New York 1991, p. 27.

[132]See S. DAYA "Definitions and Factors Affecting Infertility," in O. RODRIGUEZ-ARMAS – B HEDON – S. DAYA, *Infertility and Contraception, op. cit.,* p. 5. Here he cites R. LEVIN – J. LATIMORE – A. WEIN *et al.* "Correlation of Sperm Count with Frequency of Ejaculation" *FertilSteril* 1986; 45: 732-734.

hours.[133] Consequently, couples who wish to achieve pregnancy need to time their intercourse for a period in which the egg and the sperm are available for fertilisation.

THE IMPACT OF STRESS ON FERTILITY

Chronic stress can cause sexual dysfunction and indirectly impact fertility in both men and women, but there are no conclusive scientific studies that establish it as a cause of infertility.[134] Nonetheless, it is clear that chronic or severe stress can lead to the suppression of sexual activity, irregular ovulation, and reduced sperm production, all of which can impair fertility. This happens by boosting the levels of stress hormone, which then inhibit GnRH, a reproductive hormone.[135] Additionally, stress can increase the level of another reproductive hormone known as gonadotropin-inhibitory hormone (GnIH), which interferes with reproduction by inhibiting GnRH secretion.[136] Hence, according to Pinon, "an important consequence of stress is the suppression of the GnRH secretion."[137] In other words, stress can affect the functional unity of the H-P-O axis.[138]

Stress can also contribute to infertility by reducing the frequency of intercourse. Some researchers claim that the stress that couples undergo during fertility protocols can render such treatments ineffective.[139]

---

[133]See Ibid., p. 5.

[134]See C. TURKINGTON – M. ALPER, *Understanding Fertility and Infertility, op. cit.,* p. 203. Scientists are divided on this. While some claim that negative emotions can contribute to the inability to conceive, others disagree that they cause infertility.

[135]See E. KIRBY – U. BERKELEY, "How Stress Causes Sexual Dysfunction, Infertility," in THE GUARDIAN, *Vol. 26, No. 11, 145,* July 2, 2009, p. 29.

[136]Ibid., p. 29.

[137]R. PINON JR., *Biology of Human Reproduction, op. cit.,* pp. 179, 216, 223. Both physical stress (strenuous physical exercise) and emotional stress can impact the H-P-G axis in the female and suppress the menstrual activity.

[138]Cf. Z. BEN-RAFAEL – R. ORVIETO "Infertility due to Defective Ovulation…, *op. cit.,* p. 23.

[139]See E. KIRBY – U. BERKELEY, "How stress causes sexual..., *op. cit.,* p. 29.

UNEXPLAINED INFERTILITY

Cases of unexplained infertility may also arise. This refers to a situation in which the cause of a couple's infertility cannot be established after clinical investigations. Such a condition may imply the presence of some undetected reproductive defects.[140] However, it is important to note that a person who is infertile with one partner may be fertile with another; the reason for this may be difficult to explain.[141]

[140] Ibid., p. 2.

[141] See A. TOTH, *The Fertility Solution, op. cit.,* p. 24.

INFERTILITY IN NIGERIA: A BRIEF REVIEW

Nigeria is the most populous country in Africa with a population of about 140 million people and about 250 ethnic groups. Here we will provide an overview of the infertility situation in Nigeria.

INCIDENCE OF INFERTILITY IN NIGERIA

Infertility is considered a common and widespread health problem in Nigeria, although there are no definitive studies or official statistics to confirm this view.[142] The Nigeria Fertility Society (NFS) suggests that about 12 million Nigerians—12% of couples—are affected by infertility.[143] The number could be higher, however, because infertile couples tend to hide their infertility to avoid being stigmatized.

PREVALENCE OF PRIMARY INFERTILITY

Primary infertility is more prevalent than secondary infertility,[144] and the incidence of male factor infertility is high.[145] This view is supported by a review of the records of all cases of male infertility at the Urology Clinic of Nnamdi Azikwe University Teaching Hospital (NAUTH) between 1996 and 2000. Of the 46 cases that were studied, 65.2% had primary infertility and 34.8% had secondary infertility.[146] In

[142]Cf. R. AJAYI "Nigeria" in Fertility World.org: Country – Reports, http://www.fertilityworld.org/content/doc_8/o/en/version_i/doc.asp. (23/12/2005). Ajayi is the managing director of the Bridge Clinic, which practises in ART in Nigeria.

[143]See NIGERIAN FERTILITY SOCIETY, "Communiqué from the First International Workshop on Assisted Conception," Held on 7th to 9th of November, 2005, at The Eko Hotel, Lagos, Nigeria, p. 1.

[144]Cf. "The Difficulties Encountered in the Management of Male Infertility in Nnewi, Nigeria," *The Nigerian Medical Journal,* 45, 2003: 1. The name of the author was omitted.

[145]Cf. J. IKECHUKWU – J. ADINMA *et al.*, "High Prevalence of Male Infertility in Southeastern Nigeria," *Journal of Obstetrics and Gynecology*, 2003; 23 (6): 657-659.

[146]See A. NWOFOR – A. UGEZU (eds.), "The Difficulties Encountered in ..., *op. cit.,* 1.

another study involving 114 couples, 70 presented with primary infertility and 44 with secondary infertility.[147]

CAUSES OF INFERTILITY IN NIGERIA

In Nigeria, male infertility is as high as female infertility,[148] contrary to the popular belief in society. The study of 133 couples by J. Ikechukwu and others shows that male factor was 42.4%, female factor was 25.8%, combined male/female factor was 20.7%, and unexplained infertility accounted for 11.1%.[149] Ndi Onuekwusi, a gynaecologist in the western part of Nigeria, also asserts that the male factor contributes as much to infertility as the female factor.[150]

Tubal problem is the single most common cause of infertility in couples, followed by oligoospermia and then the combination of tubal and male factors.[151]A foremost gynaecologist in Nigeria, Giwa-Osagie, asserts that tubal factor infertility accounted for over 60% of cases in most IVF treatment protocols, followed by oligoospermia and azoospermia.[152] One study to determine the causes of male factor infertility in 46 patients showed that 45% of the cases were due to varicocele, 21.7% were due to testicular problem, 19.6% were linked to erectile dysfunction, 6.5% were

[147]See W. CHUKWUDEBELU – N. ESEGE – U. MEGAFU, "Aetiological factors in infertility in Enugu, Nigeria." *Pub Med: Infertility* 2, 1979, (2): 193-200.

[148]Cf. Ibid.

[149]See J. IKECHUKWU – J. ADINMA *et al.*, "High Prevalence of Male Infertility ..., *op. cit.,* 657-659.

[150]See N. ONUEKWUSI, "Special Issues on Infertility..., *op. cit.,* p. 4.

[151]See O. GIWA-OSAGIE *et al.* "Aetiologic Classification and Sociomedical Characteristics of Infertility in 250 Couples," *International Journal of Fertility,* 1984, 29;104-108. The same is true for Africa as a whole where tubal factor from infections is the highest single cause of infertility.

[152]See O. GIWA-OSAGIE "ART in Developing countries with particular references to sub-Saharan Africa," in *WHO Progress in Reproductive Health Newsletter* – Issue No. 63, 2003, 22-27.

associated with urethral structure and hormonal imbalance, and 2.2% were caused by *orchitis.*[153]

It has been suggested that infections play a significant role in both male and female infertility. Secondary infertility is caused mainly by genital infections. In males, these infections may be linked to vascular injuries sustained during hernia surgeries or to sickle-cell disease.[154] In females, such infections result from STDs (especially chlamydia and gonorrhea), childbirth under unhygienic conditions, and infections during or after an abortion.[155]

The facilities for the investigation and treatment of infertility problems are inadequate or nonexistent in many parts of Nigeria. Even where they are available, many couples are ignorant of the causes of their infertility due to a dearth of scientific information and education at the national, state, and local government levels. As a result of this ignorance, the high cost of treatment, and religious fanaticism and myth, some couples do not seek or continue with fertility treatment, preferring to take their problems to spiritual healers or native doctors.[156]

---

[153]See A. NWOFOR – A. UGEZU (ed.), "The Difficulties Encountered in…, *op. cit.,* 1.

[154]See S. KUKU – D. OSEGBE "Oligo/azoospermia in Nigeria," *Archives of Andorology,* 1989, 22:233-238.

[155]Cf. I. POLLARD, *Life, Love and Children…,op. cit.,* p. 108.

[156]Cf. NZEAGWU, "Making Pregnancy a Natural Experience," in *This Day Online* of 16/11/2004 http://www.thisdayonline.com/archive/2004/10/20040410plu01.html.

CHAPTER 3

CHILDLESSNESS

In every society and culture, children are cherished; it is for this reason that we place a high value on the procreation and education of children. It follows naturally that many cultures tend to loathe any form of deliberate childlessness in marriage, except where a life-threatening medical condition exists. Our primary task in this chapter is to discuss the problems associated with childlessness, taking Nigeria as the case in point.

DISTINCTION BETWEEN VOLUNTARY AND INVOLUNTARY CHILDLESSNESS

When we speak of childlessness today, we need to make a vital distinction between voluntary and involuntary childlessness. Culturally, the former is not approved of in Nigeria, or Africa as a whole, and those who choose it are likely to be coerced and ridiculed within the traditional African cultural setting.

VOLUNTARY CHILDLESSNESS

Voluntary childlessness refers to a situation in which a couple makes a deliberate decision to not have children. Such a decision could be permanent or temporary. The former reflects a firm decision to never have children, whereas the latter involves postponing child-bearing to a later period in life. The decision to remain voluntarily childless on a permanent basis arises within the context of people's life experiences—health conditions, choice of work and career, relationships, and other social, economic, and psychological factors—and does not necessarily imply a rejection of children or a refusal to recognize their value in family and society.

MOTIVES FOR VOLUNTARY CHILDLESSNESS

People choose to remain childless for various reasons. F. Baum, in 1994 research carried out to ascertain the rationale behind women's decision to remain voluntarily childless, identified the four categories of motives as hedonistic, emotional, idealistic, and practical.[1] Hedonistic refers to the desire to preserve a particular standard of living that may be compromised by raising children, or it refers to the sheer unwillingness to invest either time or money in doing so. The emotional category comprises women who have no emotional feelings for babies or children. The idealistic category includes women who do not want to bring more children into a world they consider unsuitable; it also includes those who do not wish to contribute to overpopulation, which poses a threat to the survival of humans and their environment. Finally, the practical category refers to women who have a practical reason for being childless, such as

[1] See F. BAUM, in *Choosing not to have Children,* Vol. 2, No. 3, 1994, pp. 22-25.

the desire to pursue a career or the fear of passing on a genetic defect that could burden their offspring with intense physical and psychological suffering or even death.[2] In the context of our modern world, the main motives include the demands of parenting, economic concerns, desire for autonomy, the changing role of women, and increasing self-centredness.

Task of Parenting: Parenthood is a laborious domestic occupation that involves commitment, vigilance, responsibility, and sacrifice on the part of parents. Some voluntarily childless couples argue that if individuals and couples reflect on the stable and independent circumstances that are conducive to the holistic development of children, it becomes difficult to make a responsible decision regarding if and when to have children.[3] On this basis, Fiona McAllister and Lynda Clarke assert that these couples reject parenthood, not children.[4]

Economic Reasons: There are some people who choose to remain childless for economic reasons. To raise children requires money—they need to be educated and provided with health care and other basic needs. They feel it is not reasonable to bring forth children for whom they cannot adequately provide, although some will also do so to ensure for themselves a certain standard of living.

The Desire for Freedom, Self-Centredness, and Others: Nowadays, there is an exaggerated emphasis on freedom understood as autonomy or self-determination. Some couples deliberately decide to remain childless because of the desire for freedom from parental responsibility. For them, childlessness means to be "independent adults that are free to pursue their own interests."[5] This reflects the changing mentality of our times, which includes a new phenomenon of self-centredness on the part of some couples. They claim that marriage is fundamentally between a man and a woman and therefore partners ought to be fully available to one another. Raising children is time consuming and tends to eliminate the

---

[2] Ibid.

[3] See F. MCALLISTER – L. CLARKE, "Choosing Childlessness," in *Findings by the Family Policy Studies Centre,* 738 (July 1998).

[4] Ibid.

[5] Ibid.

couple's "private world of love and intimacy." They see freedom and additional time to spend together as direct benefits of childlessness.[6]

One of the reasons often cited in favour of marriage is that parents need the help and care of their children in their old age. Today, some voluntarily childless couples neither see any advantage here nor do they see any disadvantage in being childless. Also, women increasingly define their roles as being more than those of homemakers and wives. Hence, it is not uncommon for some career women to choose to remain childless. Their commitment to their careers makes it extremely difficult for them to cope with the responsibility of parenting.

INVOLUNTARY CHILDLESSNESS

Involuntary childlessness refers to a situation in which a couple who wishes to have children cannot have them. This state of affairs, which is often traumatic for couples, can result from medical conditions in the male or female that cause infertility. In the next section, we will extensively examine some of the problems that this condition poses to couples and individuals in society, using Nigeria as a case study.

[6] P. LUNNEBORG, *The Chosen Lives of Childfree Men*, Bergin & Garvey, Westport 1989, p. 25.

CHILDLESSNESS: NIGERIA AS A CASE STUDY

A critical study of the problems of childlessness, especially in Nigeria and Africa, shows that this condition has several adverse effects on couples.[7] Speaking on what constitutes the most traumatic aspect of childlessness, respondents cited the following: being in an unstable and fearful relationship; inability to relate to others who offer you humiliating pity; loneliness arising from the absence of a child on whom one can shower true love; fear arising from the thought that one may never have a child; fear of loneliness in one's old age without a child to provide care; third party interference (i.e., the "in-law syndrome"); and being addressed as "aunty" instead of as "mother." Those who were not yet experiencing any trauma were found to be almost 99% males from young couples who have been married for less than five years. Two factors that featured prominently in the responses were the fear of stigmatization and social pressure. Additionally, most women were afraid of the collapse of their marriages and resented interference and pressure from in-laws, especially if the woman was not responsible for the couple's infertility.

Involuntarily childless couples suffer grave social and psychological consequences in society. The condition is more devastating for women[8] than for men and often leaves women shattered emotionally. The extended family system and the communal way of life in most communities make it difficult for childless couples to go unnoticed. Nonetheless, the impact of childlessness varies from couple to couple and person to person. In this section we will examine the problems involved.

---

[7] Information in this area is from the review of questionnaires sent to some childless couples, gynaecologists and others in Nigeria as well as from books and personal interaction with some childless couples. The issue of infertility or childlessness is very sensitive as was observed in the course of this study. Perhaps, it explains why some childless people refrained from completing the questionnaires and some who volunteered information verbally did so with great difficulty. In discussing the problems of childlessness here, we shall draw from other sources, even though Nigeria is our main focus.

[8] In the recent past, in Nigeria, infertility was often blamed on the woman as was the case in the developed countries a long time ago, but scientifically infertility can exist in both men and women.

STIGMATIZATION

In a culture where infertility is abhorred and sometimes looked upon as a curse, childlessness can be a traumatic experience. This traumatic experience stems from the fact that childlessness brings social stigma and public ridicule. Describing the experience of infertile people, Marcia Inhorn refers to Scrambler's distinction between "felt" and "enacted" stigma.[9] In the first case, the one who is stigmatized internalizes how society evaluates his or her condition and consequently feels a sense of failure for not measuring up to the standard of normality. The second case involves intentional discrimination against the stigmatized.[10] Emphasizing this point, the WHO observes that for millions of couples all over the world, infertility is a personal tragedy; for a significant percentage of them, "the private agony is compounded by a social stigma, which can have serious and far-reaching consequences."[11]

In Nigeria, ongoing stigma, shame, and profound suffering characterize the experience of most childless couples. However, this tendency is not peculiar to Nigeria or Africa. It is a universal phenomenon, but the intensity may be lower in the more developed countries, where individualistic lifestyles are prevalent compared to African societies, where communal lifestyle is dominant. Resulting from this major difference are other factors such as the level of education, awareness of one's legal rights, and the need to respect other people's autonomy and privacy, all of which affect the degree of stigmatization of infertile couples. For instance, a study by two anthropologists of some infertile women in South Florida, USA, suggests that the lived experience of infertility is one of stigmatization, isolation, and alienation. According to this study, infertile American women feel that they are not understood and accepted; it seems to them

[9] See G. SCAMBLER, "Perceiving and Coping with a Stigmatizing Condition," in R. FITZPATRICK - J. HINTON *et al.* (eds.), *The Experience of Illness,* Tavistock, New York 1984, pp. 203-226. Cited in M. INHORN, *Local Babies, Global Science: Gender, Religion and In Vitro Fertilisation in Egypt,* Routledge, New York 2003, p. 244.

[10] Ibid.

[11] WORLD HEALTH ORGANIZATION, "Infertility," WHO *Progress Report., op. cit.* p. 1.

as though they have broken some accepted, if unspoken, cultural rule, and they pay for it by being classified as "other."[12]

In general, these negative feelings are consistent with those of infertile people, especially women, in Nigeria and Africa. While the man is sometimes regarded as "less than a man" by others in society, it is the woman who bears the full burden of infertility—even when she is not the infertile partner. A typical Nigerian abhors being labeled *nwanyi-iga* or *agan*, meaning "infertile one" or "barren woman."[13] The abhorrence of stigmatization and the accompanying ridicule, shame, and isolation exert serious pressure on infertile couples and on their families. Hence, there is a common tendency among childless couples to conceal their infertility. Although this is extremely difficult to conceal in the traditional African village, urbanization and the drift towards individualistic lifestyles are making it easier. It is clear that in Nigeria there is an unequal treatment in the management of infertility. While there is no serious effort to conceal female infertility, society tends to hide male infertility or sterility. The practice among some tribes, usually the less-educated ones, is to arrange for the infertile man's close relative or friend to impregnate his wife with no rights over the child to be born.[14] The issue of paternal right over the child to be born may not arise in some African cultures, which generally accept that any child that a legally married woman conceives by another man still belongs to her husband. It is common for some fertile women to take responsibility for their husband's infertility to protect them from public ridicule. When women are infertile, they try to hide it as much as possible. In rare occasions, to conceal their infertility, women fake pregnancy to later feign miscarriage, hoping to prove that they are, at least, capable of conceiving. As Inhorn observes, in some cases, women who

[12] L. WHITEFORD – L. GONZALEZ, "Stigma: The Hidden Burden of Infertility," *Social Science and Medicine* 40, 1995, 29; Cited in M. INHORN, *Local Babies, Global Science…, op. cit.*, p. 244.

[13] Owing to misconceptions about childlessness, childless couples may be subjected to ridicule and stigmatized in their communities. In a quarrel, others may call an infertile woman *nwanyi-iga* or *agan* meaning barren woman. In general, childless women and their parents find this extremely hurting.

[14] Cf. L. MAGESA, *African Religion: The Moral Traditions of Abundant Life*, Orbis Books, Maryknoll New York 1997, p. 146.

have never conceived view those who have conceived and experienced miscarriages as being more fortunate. They at least have proven that they are capable of conceiving, even if this does not solve their problem.[15]

In rural settings, childless women become victims of village gossip, and they are commonly treated as outcasts. Sometimes, they are accused of evil practices by ignorant villagers who interpret spontaneous abortion as a sign that the woman destroyed her unborn child through witchcraft. Although women bear the main burden of the negative social consequences of childlessness, evidence abounds that a man can also suffer humiliation when it is obvious that he is the infertile partner.

PRESSURE ON PARENTS OF CHILDLESS COUPLES

In Nigeria, the need to marry and have children is imperative and widespread. Many parents mount pressure on their children to marry and have children and are restless when they cannot have a child. There are various reasons for this. Sometimes, parents are put under pressure by relatives, neighbours, and the community. At other times, the pressure is self-imposed, that is, rooted in personal desires stemming from the common mentality regarding the rearing of children. Most Nigerian and African grandparents, especially grandmothers, are desirous of grandchildren from each of their children. The more the grandchildren, the happier they are. Above all, parents believe that they have the duty to save their children from being labelled "barren" and from the trauma of childlessness in a culture that loathes infertility.

The responsibility to further the family lineage falls directly on the male child. When this male child is an only son, the problem gets more complicated. Under such circumstances, his family may go to any length to ensure that he takes a second wife or engages in extra-marital affairs that would result in an offspring. In the case of childlessness, the pressure is not only on the couple concerned, but also on their respective families. When parents are pressured by the community (their relatives and friends), they end up mounting pressure on their childless children.

[15] Cf. M. INHORN, *Local Babies, Global Science…*, *op. cit.*, p. 29.

SOCIAL PRESSURE ON THE COUPLE

African marriage involves not only the couple, but also the couple's families. Besides the natural desire for parenthood, the social pressure on infertile couples to have children—represented by the "in-law syndrome" or "mother-in-law syndrome"—was identified by many respondents as one of the most traumatic aspects of childlessness.[16]

The extended family system is still strong in Nigeria, in spite of the people's exposure to Western culture. Since the success of marriage is measured, first and foremost, from the viewpoint of offspring, families and friends of the couple often expect a child to be born 9 to 12 months after their marriage. Shortly after marriage, they begin to look for visible signs of pregnancy in the woman, and they often ask questions if nothing happens. Hence, it is not unusual to find childless couples under intense pressure to have a child. In fact, family members, especially parents, see it both as a right and as a duty to intervene in matters affecting their children—even more so when the issue at stake is childlessness. Such an intervention can be positive or negative. It is positive when it takes the form of solidarity with the couple, of offering support to cope with this difficult situation and assistance in finding solutions. It becomes negative when it resorts to verbal abuse or to physical or emotional violence, which is usually directed at the woman.

Experience shows that during the first few years of marriage, the husband's family can be understanding, tolerant, caring, and even supportive. However, if the infertility persists over the years, intolerance and other negative attitudes gradually set in. During this time, the man's family may try to frustrate the woman out of the marriage by making life unbearable for her. In such instances, the mother or sister of the man often becomes the woman's albatross. Still further, there is usually a subtle or intense pressure on the man to divorce his spouse or to take another wife who can have children for him, even though he may be the infertile partner. In traditional Nigerian societies, there is a cultural prejudice in favour of men; as such, it is rare for a fertile woman to seek divorce because of her husband's infertility, while it is often easy for a fertile man to divorce his infertile wife. This is consistent with Marcia

[16] For men, the thought of being the end of the family lineage in the absence of a child to carry on the family name is extremely troubling coupled with society's attitude of viewing them as not being manly.

Inhorn's observation that such a "choice" is socially prohibited to women in African cultures.[17] Nowadays, although some enlightened women are making this choice due to the influence of modern culture, the fact remains that people generally consider it shameful for a woman to leave her matrimonial home and return to her family after marriage.

In some extreme cases, a daring mother could arrange another wife for her son and bring her into his home, with or without his consent. Should he refuse and choose to identify with his infertile wife, some family members will quickly conclude that he has been bewitched by her. In fact, it is common for a mother to move into a couple's home to harass and, at times, to forcefully eject her son's wife.[18] At other times, through negative criticism, verbal abuse, and even physical violence, she makes life difficult or unbearable for the woman, who is already burdened by her childless condition. Ironically, if the same daughter-in-law eventually conceives, she may become the pearl of her previously antagonistic mother-in-law, who then becomes protective, loving, and caring.

THREAT TO MARITAL AND INTER-FAMILY RELATIONSHIPS

We have already noted that African marriage is equally an alliance between the partners themselves and between their respective families. The desire for children is so strong that childlessness often poses a serious threat to the marital stability of the couple and of their families. Such negative impacts on the couple's marriage and inter-family relationships are examined below.

EFFECT ON THE RELATIONSHIP OF THE COUPLE

Childlessness may jeopardize the close relationship between couples and exacerbate existing problems. With infertility come frustration, coldness, negative criticism, and violence. Each spouse, and especially the woman, may constantly fear emotional or actual abandonment by the other. This was clear in the response of one woman who reported

---

[17] Cf. M. INHORN, *Local Babies, Global Science…, op. cit.*, p. 245.

[18] The tendency to think that the man owns the home is still common in Nigeria. Hence, in the face of a rift between some mothers and their sons' wives, they are quick to tell them to leave their sons' homes. Sometimes, at the death of their husbands, defenceless widows are chased out of their home by family members.

that "the fear of abandonment by one's spouse occurs with every childless couple." This fear is more commonly expressed by women who contribute to the couple's infertility. If the man is solely responsible, the woman is often encouraged by her in-laws, and even by her own family, to protect and support her husband. But if the woman is responsible for the couple's infertility, the man's family may pressure him to divorce her or take another wife who can give him children. Although infertility can sometimes strengthen a couple's relationship, this does not appear to be the experience of most Nigerian and African couples. On the contrary, a persistent childless state often ruptures a previously blissful marriage by creating tension, misunderstanding, and fear. The effect of infertility on a couple's relationship depends on a variety of factors. These factors include the different manners of coping with stress and third party interference.

Gender strongly influences behaviour; the difference between men and women is psychological as well as physical.[19] By nature they react to issues like infertility in different ways. In addition, the reaction to childlessness may vary among people of the same gender. Individuals respond differently to life's occurrences because of past conditioning, education, experience, motivations, natural resilience, or even religious faith. Where these differences between the genders and individuals are not understood and considered, the experience of infertility may damage a couple's relationship.

In general, women are more emotionally motivated than men and tend to be engrossed in their infertility crisis. This is understandable because their upbringing within the family and society prepares them to view motherhood as their primary role. This recognition of society's expectation exerts tremendous pressure on them. A woman may feel that her husband is not showing enough concern because he does not express intense emotions similar to hers; thus, she may withdraw emotionally. On the other hand, the man may feel that his wife worries too much and become easily irritated by her complaints. The negative impact of childlessness on the couple's relationship usually occurs over a period of time, increasing after a protracted and unsuccessful fertility treatment process.[20] Mutual coldness, resentment, and gradual hostility, with their

---

[19] For instance, the brain of a man is not exactly the same as that of a woman.

[20] Cf. P. MAHLSTEDT, "Psychological Issues in Infertility…, *op. cit.,* p. 463.

attendant effects, may result from this. As Deveraux and Hammerman suggest, this situation can result in poor communication and create constant arguments and tension. Additionally, it may lead to mutual or one-sided withdrawal; this worsens the experience of fertility as the spouses now live in their private misery.[21] Under such circumstances, the woman may suffer severely as she grieves the loss of her fertility and the potential loss of her emotional relationship with her partner.[22] Stressing this point, Mahlstedt maintains the following:

> In general, the potential loss of fertility is more threatening for women, whose core identity is tied in with becoming a mother. Men, whose primary identity is not dependent on fatherhood, are less affected by that potential loss. Not understanding this basic difference, women often feel unloved or abandoned when their husbands do not experience the same emotional pain during the infertility crisis.[23]

This means that men's and women's different attitudes towards an infertility crisis arise, to a large extent, from their gender identity, which is formed by stereotypes and societal conditioning during childhood. As Mazor contends, the phases in a woman's life are often defined by events related to her reproductive function. Hence, the inability to fulfil this "natural" role is a personal tragedy for a woman because society may view her as a failure.[24] Quite naturally, a woman seems to be prepared for motherhood from childhood, and thus she sees pregnancy and childbirth as the normal functions that distinguish her from a man. Moreover, many women take motherhood for granted. For instance, one respondent described infertility as "a situation one never expected." This is partly what underpins the intense stress most women undergo in comparison

---

[21] Cf. L. DEVERAUX – A. HAMMERMAN, *Infertility and Identity*, Jossey-Bass Publishers, San Francisco 1998, pp. 62-63.

[22] Ibid., p. 66, 69.

[23] P. MAHLSTEDT, "Psychological Issues in Infertility..., *op. cit.*, p. 463.

[24] See M. MAZOR, "Emotional Reactions to Infertility," in M. MAZOR – H. SIMON, *Infertility: Medical, Emotional and Social Considerations,* Human Sciences Press Inc., New York 1984, p. 30.

to their male counterparts. Although the above remark is generally true for women, it also applies to Nigerian and African men. Though a man may be unperturbed during the first few years of his infertility crisis, if the situation persists for some years and presents the possibility of lacking a biological heir, he too may become restless and desperate, especially with pressure from family and friends. Consequently, men's slowness in pursuing fertility treatments may not stem from lack of interest. As it was observed in the course of this study, Nigerian men find it humiliating to discuss their infertility crises; it erodes their confidence and makes them feel they are not manly enough.

EFFECT OF INFERTILITY ON INTER-FAMILY RELATIONSHIP

The strain of childlessness can negatively affect the relationship between a couple's families. In some extreme cases in Nigeria, when the physical and psychological damage to the woman becomes obvious and unbearable, her family may forcefully withdraw her from her matrimonial home or even end the marriage by returning the bride-wealth. In most cases, this is done with her consent, though sometimes she may be pressured into accepting this option. Should she refuse and decide to remain with her partner, her family may abandon her. There are numerous cases of parents disowning their children, especially their sons, for remaining with infertile spouses. In some rare cases, such dissenting children are ostracized from the family, meaning that other members of the family will be forbidden from visiting them.[25]

A study of the Nigerian situation shows that the more-educated couples handle their infertility crisis better. Such couples are better equipped to handle family pressure and have mutual love and friendship as fundamental constituents of their marriage. Nonetheless, childlessness remains a serious threat to every African marriage; it can lead to the breakdown of law and order in a home and to divorce, even among educated couples and those who are exposed to the Western culture. As

---

[25] Many respondents (both fertile and infertile persons) saw the external pressure from in-laws as a major factor that compounds the infertility crisis of many couples by introducing a rupture into their relationship. Some infertile women maintained that stigma, insults, ridicules, disrespect, rejection and unfair treatment by in-laws worsened their plight and endangered their marriage while men equally resented interferences by in-laws and their own family.

one female respondent remarked, "In Nigeria the childless condition always threatens every home and marriage. The in-laws and the respective families expect children from the union and when this expectation is not met, there is always tension." This view is reinforced by Giwa-Osagie when he states emphatically that childlessness causes major marital, family, and social disruption in Africa,[26] where marriage is primarily for the purpose of having children.

PSYCHOLOGICAL SUFFERING OF CHILDLESS COUPLES

The meaning we give to something to a large extent determines the seriousness with which we view it and the impact it can have on our emotional or psychological state when we lack it. It is absolutely clear that, to most infertile couples and particularly to Nigerian and African women, childlessness means more than not having a child. Respondents used the following expressions to describe the emotional stress of infertility: suffering, loneliness, unhappiness, anxiety, trauma, vacuum in marriage, and ill-fate. Some described their infertility crisis as the most difficult time of their life, and the majority of the respondents described themselves as unhappy. Additionally, women with unsupportive husbands and interfering in-laws expressed deep sentiments of bitterness and frustration. Most of them were sensitive and fragile.

The foregoing clearly shows that involuntary childlessness is characterized by suffering. But suffering is difficult to describe objectively because it is structurally subjective. Unlike physical pain, which can be localized, suffering affects the whole person. One author describes it as the "pain of the soul."[27]

Childlessness can have a serious negative effect on the psychological well-being of a couple and especially of women, who, by nature, are more emotionally motivated than men. Childless women tend to verbalize intense emotions or even cry[28] when recounting their terrible ordeals:

[26] See O. GIWA-OSAGIE, "ART in Developing Countries..., *op. cit.*, p. 25.

[27] See A. MORACZEWSKI, "The Ethics of Pain Management," in P. CATALDO – A. MORACZEWSKI (eds.), *Catholic Health Care Ethics...*, *op. cit.*, Part 14/2.

[28] Some cry in private, even when they succeed in controlling their emotions in public. This gives us an insight into the trauma of childlessness.

abandonment, loneliness, suffering in the hands of antagonistic in-laws or uncaring spouses. The emotional suffering of the woman is aggravated if she is the infertile partner and her spouse has not been understanding and supportive in the face of intense criticism and pressure from his family. This emotional or psychological aspect of childlessness makes it even more dreadful. Regarding this, Mazor maintains that the mere acknowledgement of infertility after several years of seeking a pregnancy is a tremendous blow to most infertile couples; they feel damaged, defective, and bad.[29] In fact, in Nigeria, some even wish they were dead because of the stigma, discrimination, and rejection that accompany this condition. It is not surprising, therefore, that the depth of the emotional distress experienced by infertile couples has been described as almost unimaginable—comparable only to that experienced by terminally sick patients in the final phase of life.[30]

Usually, this experience goes together with other phenomena, such as memory factors and the presence or absence of distracting stimuli.[31] Childless people who find it difficult to accept their situation are usually unhappy, despite their attempts to conceal it from the public. After several failed attempts to establish a pregnancy, they often express feelings of frustration, irritation, deep sorrow, loneliness, insecurity, bitterness, fear, anxiety, boredom, depression, and anger. Under such circumstances, they are emotionally battered and may turn their frustration inward and exhibit self-hatred. They may also project anger at their spouses and those around them at the least provocation. Some are overwhelmed by guilt from a procured abortion or a past immoral behaviour, real or imagined, and tend to see their childless condition as a punishment from God; this adds another dimension to their suffering.[32] On the other hand, those

---

[29] See M. MAZOR, "Emotional Reaction to Infertility," in K. ALPERN (ed.), *The Ethics of Reproductive…*, *op. cit.*, pp. 32-33; ID. "Emotional Reactions to Infertility," in M. MAZOR – H. SIMON, *Infertility: Medical, Emotional…*, *op. cit.*, pp. 26-27.

[30] Cf. C. TURKINGTON – M. ALPER, *Understanding Fertility and Infertility*, *op. cit.*, p. 204.

[31] Ibid.

[32] M. MAZOR, "Emotional Reactions to Infertility," in M. MAZOR – H. SIMON, *Infertility: Medical, Emotional…*, *op. cit.*, p. 28. This guilt feeling is heightened if a woman had procured an abortion in the past because as

who preserved their virginity until marriage may project anger at God, feeling that He is unjustly punishing them. Worse still, some attribute their infertility to witchcraft, to the fetish practices of their enemies, or even to a curse. Overall, there is a clear religious dimension to the experience of childlessness among many Nigerian couples. This is similar to the finding of Mazor that "some childless people try to be extra good to atone for whatever sin, real or imagined, they may feel is responsible for their predicament." In fact, many of the respondents cited their faith in God as their main source of strength during their agonizing moments, and they found spiritual direction extremely beneficial. According to some, their experience of infertility brought them closer to God and strengthened them spiritually. Now they are stronger, more prayerful, and expect a miracle. While few of the respondents married for less than five years saw their condition as temporary, believing that God would turn things around, many of those who had been married for 10 years or more did not express so much enthusiasm. Some of them found it difficult to understand why God was allowing them go through this traumatic experience.

In conclusion, it remains clear that, even in today's scientific world, religion plays a vital role in maintaining homeostasis in a person's life in the face of infertility. Faith in God provides solace to many infertile couples, keeping their hope alive. This fact partly explains why many infertile couples in Nigeria flood the churches for spiritual solutions to their problem. At other times, infertile people feel guilt, not only because of their infertility, but also because they feel they have disappointed their spouses, parents, and relatives who are deprived of children and grandchildren.

IMPACT ON SELF-CONCEPT AND IDENTITY CRISIS

Childlessness often triggers a massive identity crisis.[33] Given the ridicule and the indignity to which most childless people are subjected

---

Mazor states, she may focus on this and carry a heavy load of guilt which may or may not be related to the current problem.

[33] Cf. L. SHANNER, "Bioethics Through the Back Door: Phenomenology, Narratives and Insights into Infertility," in L. SUMMER – J. BOYLE (eds.), *Philosophical Perspectives on Bioethics,* University of Toronto Press, Toronto – Buffalo – London 1996, p. 129.

in Nigeria, many have a low sense of self-esteem. Overcome by intense feelings of shame and failure, they often feel socially inadequate, diminished, empty, and unworthy.[34] As Shanner observes, "Their self esteem and image are frequently battered in the ongoing struggle with infertility.... Any doubts about their bodies were re-activated by their inability to have children."[35] Deveraux and Hammerman contend that "it is as if their human value has been reduced, and their whole being, body and soul, has become 'infertile.' Therefore, infertility no longer becomes a medical condition, but a definition of self."[36] In fact, some of these couples begin to see themselves only as "infertile women" or "infertile men."

In Nigerian and African societies that place an exaggerated emphasis on biological parenthood, infertility is extremely degrading to both men and women, damaging their ego in a profound way. Worse still, some childless people are so battered that they begin to view themselves as failures, even when they are extremely successful in other fields of human endeavour. An infertile woman may feel that she is not a "woman," and an infertile man may feel that he is not really a "man." For example, several women in a study confessed to feeling like "neuters," not classifiable as male or female, and some men described intercourse as "shooting blanks."[37] This is because, in the minds of many people, infertility symbolizes impotency. Masculinity is usually associated with potency and virility, and womanhood is associated with fertility and motherhood. As Deveraux and Hammerman maintain, "The underlying message is that motherhood is the ultimate expression of femininity."[38] Among Nigerians, and Africans in general, a child is both a vindication of womanhood and a proof of masculinity. However, these ideas are not limited to Africa. For instance, a study by Russel Webb and Judith Daniluk in

---

[34] Cf. Ibid., p. 129.

[35] Cf. Ibid., p. 128.

[36] DEVERAUX – HAMMERMAN, *Infertility and Identity..., op. cit.,* p. 66.

[37] M. MAZOR, "Emotional Reactions to Infertility," in M. MAZOR – H. SIMON, *Infertility: Medical, Emotional..., op. cit.,* p. 27. Here, she quotes: B. MENNING, *Infertility: A Guide for the Childless Couple,* Prentice Hall, Eaglewood Cliffs, New Jersey 1977.

[38] Cf. DEVERAUX – HAMMERMAN, *Infertility and Identity, op. cit.,* p. 65-66.

the United States reveals that infertile men are subjected to profound stigmatization and that they feel a sense of personal inadequacy. Many described themselves as a failure, useless, a dud, inadequate, not a real man, garbage, a loser, defective, and unable to "give their wife a child." In Nigeria, such feelings may be more intense because some infertile couples fail to find meaning in life in the absence of a biological child. They feel profoundly diminished and ashamed, especially because parenthood is viewed as a sign of adulthood.[39]

The impact of childlessness on a couple or an individual depends to a large extent on the level of acceptance and the ability to manage life issues. If the problems associated with this condition are not properly managed, they can further impact the reproductive ability of women,[40] as well as their physical appearance and overall health. Some childless women lose their charm, appear emaciated, or age rapidly due to loss of appetite, severe stress, negative feelings, and restlessness. Although childless men appear to be able to face their situation better, they are not without such negative feelings. Some take to excessive drinking or become engrossed in work. Others tend to nag, stay out late, and become easily irritated or aggressive. In their frustration, they may resort to verbal, emotional, and even physical abuse of their spouses. For instance, some men call their infertile spouses "men" or "wood," meaning that they are incapable of conceiving. Women find these expressions derogatory and perhaps more devastating than physical violence. Childless people may feel there is no longer meaning in life, and, in extreme cases, they may contemplate suicide.[41] Making a similar observation, R. Matthews and A. Matthew assert the following:

---

[39] Cf. R. WEBB – J. DANILUK, 1999, "The End of the Line: Infertile Men's Experience of Being Unable to Produce a Child," *Men and Masculinities* 2:6-25, p.15; Cited in M. INHORN, *Local Babies Global science…, op. cit.,* p. 244.

[40] Many childless women undergo severe stress. This can lead to menstrual irregularity and indirectly impair fertility.

[41] This feeling is not unfounded as it reflects the mentality of the traditional society where all other achievements, especially riches and fame, are regarded as worthless if there is no child to inherit them and perpetuate the family name. In the case of a wealthy and highly successful man, he may be

> To the extent that the couple regard having children as a fulfilment of both their marriage and even their purpose on earth, infertility calls into question the meaning and purpose of both their marriage and their very existence.[42]

FERTILITY WORK-UP AND LOSS OF CONTROL

The diagnosis of infertility, the crisis that follows, and the subsequent treatment often result in a couple's loss of control over their bodies, privacy, time, goals, and work. As Turkington and Alper point out, the experience of infertility can be a shock to that notion of self-control.[43] Once the fertility treatment is initiated, they have to make sacrifices to complete the numerous medical tests and examinations, some of which may require long travel. Furthermore, some of the medical examinations are physically invasive, humiliating, and emotionally distressing.[44] Emphasizing the physical and emotional demands of an IVF cycle, Mastroianni Jr. cites the need for several visits to the doctor for hormone determinations and ultrasound; the need for egg-retrieval, which is not without complications; and the rare ovarian infection that can further compromise the fertility status of the patient.[45] Moreover, infertility treatment involves loss of sexual spontaneity and privacy. As Mazor asserts, "Sex is no longer a spontaneous, pleasurable activity; it is an assignment,

---

suspected of sacrificing his unborn offspring for money and success through occult practices.

[42] R. MATTHEW – A. MATHEWS, "Infertility and Involuntary Childlessness: The Transition to Nonparenthood," *Journal of Marriage and the Family,* 1986, 48, 641-649. Cited in L. SCHWARTZ, *Alternative to Infertility: Is Surrogacy the Answer?* Brunner/Mazel, Inc., New York 1991, p. 24.

[43] See C. TURKINGTON – M. ALPER, *Understanding Fertility and Infertility, op. cit.,* p. 204.

[44] Cf. Ibid. 204. Women may become so engrossed with resolving their infertility crisis to the extent that many other things suffer due to lack of attention while most men tend to get busier as a distraction technique or coping mechanism.

[45] See MASTROIANNI JR., "Reproductive Techniques," in S. POST (ed.), *Encyclopedia of Bioethics…, op. cit.,* p. 2263.

a mission with a definable goal, that is, pregnancy."[46] As patients, infertile couples must expose their bodies for medical examination and manipulations; they must reveal intimate details of their private and sexual lives and of fears surrounding their desire for a child.[47] This situation is further aggravated if they have to repeat several cycles before they can achieve conception, move from one doctor to another, or see a psychologist. All these factors compound the trauma of infertility.

Women tend to suffer more from infertility treatments than do men; they bear the greater part of the extremely invasive treatment cycles, even when they do not contribute to the couple's infertility. For instance, a female respondent described IVF, and the experience of fertility work-up in general, as emotionally strenuous and humiliating. However, it is more frustrating to women if their spouses do not seem to appreciate their efforts by showing adequate commitment to the fertility work-up. Describing the psychological stress of a fertility work-up, Lara Deveraux and Ann Hammerman write the following:

> Whereas menstrual cycles and frequency of intercourse were once a woman and her partner's private concern, after a diagnosis of infertility a client's cycles and sexual practices are often scrutinized by a number of individuals, from infertility specialist to family members.[48]

Another author describes this experience further, insisting that

> The infertility evaluation itself adds stress as past sexual behaviours and reproductive histories are explored. The partners become wrapped up [in] a whirl of appointments, decisions, and the monitoring of their bodies and sex lives. They experience an increased sense of loss of control.[49]

---

[46] M. MAZOR, "Emotional Reactions to Infertility," in M. MAZOR – H. SIMON, *Infertility: Medical, Emotional…, op. cit.,* p. 27. During fertility work-ups, couples may be required to have intercourse at specific times during the fertile period of the woman's cycle.

[47] Ibid.

[48] L. DEVERAUX – A. HAMMERMAN, *Infertility and Identity, op. cit.,* p. 60.

[49] B. COOPER-HILBERT, *Infertility and Involuntary Childlessness,* W.W. Norton & Company, Inc., New York 1998, p. 42.

During the fertility work-up, the couple's cycle, sex life, and privacy become public, and various people offer all sorts of unsolicited suggestions about how to handle their infertility.[50] From this perspective, it may be said that the cost of fertility work-up, understood in terms of finances, time, and physical and emotional discomforts, is very high. Repeated failures tend to increase this cost tremendously and may result in intense frustration or depression, because all their sufferings seem to have been in vain. In fact, a respondent reported that she felt "absolute frustration" at the end of each "failed treatment cycle," while some gave up initiating a new cycle of treatment after several trials. Ironically, while a new cycle tends to rekindle hope of success, it may also escalate the couple's fear of possible failure.

DISRUPTION OF RELATIONSHIP WITH OTHERS AND ISOLATION

The journey through childlessness is lonely and traumatizing for most Nigerian couples, and especially for women. The diagnosis of infertility for a man or woman marks the beginning of many sorrows and humiliations. Let us now examine the impact of infertility on a couple's relationship with others.

RELATIONSHIP WITH FAMILY

Infertility can lead to the loss of a cordial relationship, not just with one's spouse, but also with family members, relatives, and friends. It is not uncommon for some childless couples to become estranged from their family members. As a result of their fragility during this ordeal, they may easily feel hurt and abandoned by parents who become close to their other children who have given them grandchildren. This can result in jealousy, which may be compounded by misunderstanding or the insensitivity of the other siblings to their plight. At other times, a previously cordial relationship may be lost because families offer too much negative criticism to the infertile couple.

RELATIONSHIP WITH CHILDREN AND THEIR PARENTS

As a few respondents admitted, infertile couples can become jealous and resentful of pregnant women or parents who complain about the

[50] See L. DEVERAUX – A. HAMMERMAN, *Infertility and Identity, op. cit.*, pp. 60, 61.

burden of pregnancy or parenting. Although only a few infertile women expressed such emotions, it did not in any way affect their love or attachment to children themselves.[51] Some become extremely careful about playing with them or correcting them to avoid conflicts with their parents. Many, however, interact closely with children; they feel terrible anger when children are neglected or abused, and they scorn those who procure or promote abortion. In their pain, some even wonder why God keeps giving children to those who do not want them and deprives those who really desire them.

ISOLATION FROM OTHERS

Being childless can significantly disrupt a couple's social life. As a respondent stated, "Being childless has made me become anti-social, preferring to keep to myself always." Infertile couples show a strong tendency to isolate themselves from others. They tend to reduce their social engagements, including family gatherings. Infertile women in particular usually wish to avoid questions and discussions about pregnancies and children, which can rekindle their pains. Describing the impact of infertility, a respondent stated that it has eroded her confidence when among family members and friends, particularly those that intentionally make her feel like a failure. According to her, this has led to reduction in her participation at social and family activities. Although infertile couples tend to isolate themselves, they may also feel abandoned by family members and friends who stay away for fear of saying the wrong thing.[52]

Infertile persons can be extremely sensitive to issues and remarks about children, pregnancies, and the childless state. Certain insensitive remarks can be a source of tremendous frustration and depression. An assumed feeling that others are insensitive to their plight and the need to avoid being pitied force many of them to withdraw from friends and family. Such self-isolation may be their way of coping with their infertility, but it reveals the need for a better understanding of their psychological situation. For instance, a respondent volunteered, "I must confess I have low moments during social activities when I look at other families

[51] This information is from an informal questionnaire I sent to some childless couples.

[52] Cf. L. DEVERAUX – A. HAMMERMAN, *Infertility and Identity*, *op. cit.*, p. 58.

or when I am asked if I have any kids yet." Questions of this sort are often difficult for most infertile women to answer, and they are sometimes followed by what a respondent labelled "hurtful sympathy." In social gatherings in African settings, questions such as "How are your children?" or "How many children do you have?" are almost unavoidable when women exchange pleasantries. Oftentimes, they may be asked over and over again by different women, some of whom offer "hurtful sympathy." This further strengthens the resolve of infertile couples to avoid or reduce social activities.

Though some people offer false sympathy, many ask such questions with no previous knowledge of the other person's childlessness; they tend to offer sympathy out of concern, knowing the implications of childlessness in Nigerian society. Men, on the other hand, tend to focus on work or business when they meet at social gatherings. Describing the pain that infertile couples in the United States experience at social functions, M. Chase states the following:

> For couples who have to be around friends and relatives with babies and children, contact can be painful.... Thanksgiving with the family can be an ordeal when you have no one to sit at the kids' table, no one to brag about—how well she eats, how fast he got toilet trained, or all the new words she's saying now.[53]

In addition, commenting on the tendency of infertile couples to isolate themselves and the effect of this isolation, Beth Cooper-Hilbert maintains:

> The partners feel more alienated as their friends become pregnant; they have less in common with these friends, who are absorbed with creating their families. They believe their friends tire of hearing about their infertility ups and downs. They may feel embarrassed because they are different. This self imposed isolation and alienation may reinforce feelings of being defective, which further

[53] M. CHASE, *Waiting for Baby: One Couple's Journey Through Infertility to Adoption,* McGraw-Hill, New York 1990, p. 33.

> isolate them. They want support, and perhaps advice, but are afraid of being pitied.[54]

Since man is a social being, isolation usually carries negative consequences, such as loneliness and despondency. As expected, many childless persons suffer grievously from loneliness and emptiness, especially after several failed attempts to have a child. This situation is even worse if the communication or relationship between the spouses has been impaired.

[54] B. COOPER HILBERT, *Infertility and Involuntary Childlessness, op. cit.,* pp. 42-43.

SOME ETHICAL ISSUES ASSOCIATED WITH CHILDLESSNESS

Due to the inability to withstand the pressure, discrimination, and social rejection to which they are often subjected, some childless couples go to any length to ensure that they will have children. In their desperation to find a solution to their problem, some sacrifice many moral values. We will examine some of them here.

THE PHENOMENON OF "PREGNANCY BEFORE MARRIAGE"

Premarital sexual relationships are a worldwide phenomenon today, irrespective of race, culture, and place. In the distant past, sexuality and sexual relations were considered sacred by Nigerians. Within the moral framework of African Traditional Religion (ATR), sex in itself is good because human beings transmit life and perpetuate themselves through sex. Long before the advent of Christianity and Islam in Africa, sexuality and sexual relations were considered sacred, and any form of abuse was punished. Commenting on this, Laurent Magesa writes that "for Africans, sexuality and sexual expression are sacred and must in no circumstances be abused."[55] Following this perspective, Kisembo, Magesa, and Shorter maintain:

> If it were misused, evil surely resulted. Initiation rites prepared the adolescent for the right use of his/her sexuality, to get married and raise a family. Today, things are falling apart.... The so-called sexual liberation is spreading out rapidly from Europe and America and bring in its wake both values and dangers.[56]

In the recent past, virginity was highly prized in Nigeria and it was a moral imperative for women to marry in the state of virginity. Among some tribes, a newly married woman was given a piece of white cloth to be used during her first marital act with her husband. Later, the blood-stained cloth was returned to her family as a mark of her virginity and

[55] L. MAGESA, *African Religion..., op. cit.,* pp. 143, 144.

[56] B. KISEMBO – L. MAGESA – A. SHORTER, *African Christian Marriage,* Pauline Publications Africa, Nairobi, Kenya 1988, p. 127.

moral uprightness. Usually, this made her family proud, whereas the absence of the blood-stain brought shame and embarrassment to the whole family. Consequently, parents ensured that their children were properly brought up. But in more recent times, this value has been eroded as chastity is not stressed in society as it used to be. Ironically, some young women who insist on remaining chaste until marriage are either branded, abandoned by their intended spouses, or ridiculed as old-fashioned by their peers.

The latest trend in some parts of Nigeria is the "Pregnancy before Marriage Phenomenon," which is a form of "trial marriage." Some Catholic and Anglican dioceses have made various laws to curb it, but it still remains a common practice in some places. The underlying reason for this emerging phenomenon is simply the desire to have children. Here, we see a clash between fidelity to Christian and traditional African chastity and the desire to fulfil the cultural value and duty of begetting children. In African culture as a whole, a childless marriage is not considered a real marriage, whereas Christian marriage has the character of indissolubility even in the face of childlessness. To avoid the need to consider divorce on the basis of infertility and consequently be suspended from the sacraments, some Christian men now insist that, before the marriage can take place, their prospective spouses become pregnant as evidence that they are not infertile. This new phenomenon promotes the culture of cohabitation before marriage.

The situation is further aggravated by some parents who make it a *sine qua non* for giving consent to their son's marriage, even when the parties concerned do not insist on it. Whereas the Catholic Church requires only the consent of two mature adults (male and female), two witnesses, and a Church minister for a marriage to be valid, in Nigerian customs, the consent of parents is necessary. Normally, no intending couple, with the exception of some daring ones, would contract a marriage without parental consent, as this may jeopardize their relationship with their respective families. Sometimes, it could lead to their being isolated, ostracized, or disowned by their parents and to being denied certain benefits that are due to them in the family. This trend of "no pregnancy, no marriage" in Nigerian society is well depicted in the film *Woman in Red*, directed by Lancelot Oduwa Imaseun. Addressing his son, Chief Odogwu declares emphatically

> I hope she [his son's fiancée] is pregnant. My principle is that whoever my son will marry must be pregnant before the marriage.... You must be sure that the lady you want to marry can have children for you. You have to guarantee that she is fruitful.[57]

This issue of "pregnancy before marriage" poses a serious ethical problem. Not only does it involve social acceptance of premarital sex, it is also very reductive of women and constitutes an assault on their dignity. It treats them as objects and creates room for abuse, since infertility can only be established after one year of regular unprotected sex. This poses a serious moral problem and may have grave consequences for marriage, which ordinarily should be entered into freely and unconditionally.[58]

EXTRA-MARITAL SEXUAL RELATIONSHIPS, OR ADULTERY

Adultery is widely accepted to be unethical. In the past, adultery was considered a very serious sin, not just against one's spouse, but against the clan, the ancestors, and God, all of which were involved in

[57] *Woman in Red* is a home video produced in Nigeria. Many of the current happenings in the Nigerian society are depicted more in Nigerian films, newspapers and magazines than in books.

[58] For instance, if the ability to conceive or have a child is made a condition for marriage and a woman actually conceives only to have a miscarriage or a still birth after the marriage, and subsequently experiences secondary infertility, then what happens to the marriage? Will her spouse not be justified in seeking annulment on that basis since being able to have a child was the condition for marriage from the outset? Furthermore, what happens to the lady if the marriage does not take place eventually, for instance, if the man changes his mind or dies as has been the case with some women in the past? Trial marriage is an assault on the dignity of women, especially as their consent is never completely free. However, it is regrettable that many Nigerian women do not think about their own dignity in this area given some decisions they take. If things must change, women must take their destiny with their own hands and be prepared to shun such degrading marriages which tend to reduce their worth to their reproductive ability. On their part, parents should see weddings involving pregnant brides as a personal indictment of their failure to educate their children morally although we cannot make a generalization of every single case.

every marriage. Female adultery in particular was taboo and was severely punished for fear that it would bring calamity on the whole community. In some communities, an adulterous woman was required to make a public confession, walk naked in public, and perhaps be banished from the community. Although punishment may not reach such extreme measures at the present time, female adultery is still viewed as grave misconduct by the vast majority of people. Besides the fact that it could mark the end of a marriage, it attracts all kinds of punishments in different traditional communities, some of which expose the woman and her family to public ridicule.

In spite of the severe cultural punishments connected with adultery, condemnation by the various religions, and the risks of life-threatening STDs, some desperate women who suspect their spouses to be infertile still resort to it, hoping to have children in order to save their marriages. Some mothers even lure their childless daughters into this practice, while in other circumstances women are influenced by their colleagues. This fact is well-depicted in the film *Private Sin*, by Rob Emeka Eze and Emem Isong. Here, the mother of Faith, a pastor's wife, advises her daughter to engage in an extra-marital affair in order to have a child for her husband, whom she thought to be the infertile partner.[59] There are also some cases in which males resort to adultery to resolve the problem of childlessness. In the United States, as Mazor remarks, "there have been reports of increased incidence of promiscuity and extra-marital affairs in an effort to 'prove' one's masculinity or femininity."[60] Such practice raises an ethical problem because the second man or woman becomes only a means to an end; this is a very reductive way of treating a person who is worthy of respect and dignity.

[59] No doubt, some desperate fertile women whose spouses may be infertile engage in extra-marital affairs without their knowledge just to have children. But then, many fertile women are known to have refused such offers, preferring to stand by their infertile spouses and focusing only on potential solutions they consider ethically permissible.

[60] M. MAZOR, "Emotional Reactions to Infertility," in M. MAZOR – H. SIMON, *Infertility: Medical, Emotional…, op. cit.*, p. 27. Here she makes reference to: H. WALKER, "Sexual Problems and Infertility." *Psychosomatics* 19(8), Aug. 1978, 477-484.

ABUSE OF WOMANHOOD

Male adultery for the purpose of having children is a more common phenomenon. Usually, the man secretly takes a second wife or impregnates another woman just to have a child. His infertile wife may even recommend this action, in which case she accepts the woman as a second wife. In some very rare and extreme cases, a childless couple may deceptively arrange for the fertile male partner to bring another woman into their home under the pretext of marriage; as soon as she gives birth to one or two children, she is thrown out of the house. Apart from the issue of adultery, this is a serious abuse of womanhood. Every woman has an intrinsic dignity and is worthy of respect and protection; she cannot be reduced to a means to an end, no matter how noble the end is.

RESORT TO FETISH PRACTICES

In Nigeria, infertile couples or their families may seek spiritual help in churches and mosques or consult some traditional healers. Some of them may exclude medical treatment and patronize sorcerers, witch doctors, or native doctors (*babalawo* or *dibia*) to resolve their infertility crises.[61] Nzeagwu asserts that "spiritualists and native doctors are smiling to the bank on account of a large army of patrons that consult them."[62] In addition, he asserts that "a childless couple can do anything, just anything, wise or foolish, ethical or unethical, moral or immoral to have children."[63]

---

[61] In traditional African communities, and even amongst urbanized Africans, there is a certain belief or fear that certain mystical powers or spiritual forces can influence the events in daily life. Among other things, they can cause infertility through their negative spiritual influences. Consequently, some patronize these native doctors who are believed to possess some spiritual powers to appease them. However, the main moral issue here is that, these witch doctors may recommend rituals and sacrifices, some of which may be injurious to others. At other times, they may blame their inability to conceive on another person (a friend, a neighbour or even a family member), thereby causing a rift.

[62] NZEAGWU, "Making Pregnancy a Natural Experience," in *This Day Online…*, *op. cit.*, p. 1.

[63] Ibid.

CHILD STEALING AND SELLING: TREATING A CHILD AS A COMMODITY

When some women can no longer bear the shame and agony of childlessness, they fake pregnancy and later try to steal a child. Although this is rare, it does happen. In fact, there have been instances of child-stealing in the maternity wards of some clinics and even in family homes. A good example of such an occurrence is the celebrated "Miracle Child" case in Lagos, which led to the discovery of some cases of child-stealing and racketeering.[64] This poses a serious ethical problem: children have an inherent dignity, and it is never morally permissible to treat a child as a commodity.

[64] About eight years ago, *News Line*, a weekly television programme aired by the Nigerian Television Authority (NTA Channel 10), repeatedly relayed the story of a battle to determine the real parents of a baby. The story began with the appearance of a sixty-five year old woman, Wurola Abayomi, who claimed to have given birth to a "miracle child" at Oluwaseyi Clinic and Maternity Home run by one nurse, Esther Kubari. A renowned gynaecologist in Lagos, Dr. Bello Osagie, described the story as incredible. Later, two other women, Folashade Adeyemi and Kikelomo Odukoya, appeared on television to lay claim to the same child. Their story was exactly the same: each of them had delivered a baby at the same maternity home on different days, but Esther Kubari told them that their babies died without showing them their corpses. But when the story of the miracle baby delivered at the same maternity home was relayed by NTA, each of them suspected foul-play and appeared on television separately to make claims. A DNA test revealed that one of them, Kikelomo Odukoya, was actually the biological mother of the child. Both Wurola Abayomi and Esther Kubari, who were involved in stealing and selling babies, were arrested and charged to court. In another case, a couple, Ibe and Ngozi Okonkwo, reported the disappearance of their ten-day-old baby at their home in Abuja on 25 December, 2001. A woman Ngozi claimed to have met earlier at a clinic where she went to immunize her baby, visited her home on the fateful day and was believed to have disappeared with the baby.

CHAPTER 4

THE ARTIFICIAL REPRODUCTIVE TECHNOLOGIES

Human beings, through the faculty of reason, have always found ways to intervene in nature. With the rapid advances in science and technology in recent times, scientists have acquired incredible powers to control physical and biological processes, including reproduction. The turning point in the history of human reproduction occurred in 1978 when Louise Brown was born following *in vitro* fertilisation—an event that made headlines all over the world. Since then, scientists have developed a variety of reproductive techniques known as Artificial or Assisted Reproductive Technologies (ART),[1] leading to thousands of pregnancies and births worldwide.

1 Most authors use "artificial" and "assisted" reproductive technologies interchangeably. Without going into semantics here, they represent the same reality in their minds. But further clarification on the use of the two terms will be revisited.

MEANING AND GOAL OF ARTIFICIAL REPRODUCTIVE TECHNOLOGIES

For many authors, ART refers to any fertility treatment that brings sperm in direct contact with eggs that are surgically retrieved from the ovaries.[2] In other words, they exclude treatments, such as artificial insemination, that involve only the handling of the sperm. Other authors, however, include these treatments as techniques of assisted conception. Consequently, we can define assisted reproductive technology as "any treatment or procedure for assisting reproduction, which includes the handling of human eggs, sperm or embryos."[3] The goal of ART, and of any other fertility treatment, is not merely to achieve conception, but to establish an uncomplicated pregnancy that will lead to the birth of a healthy baby.

---

2 See C. TURKINGTON – M. ALPER, *Understanding Fertility and Infertility, op. cit.*, p. 39.

3 NATIONAL ACADEMY OF SCIENCES – NATIONAL ACADEMY OF ENGINEERING – INSTITUTE OF MEDICINE – NATIONAL RESEARCH COUNCIL, *Scientific and Medical Aspects of Human Reproductive Cloning*, National Academy Press, Washington, D.C. 2002, p. 61.

TYPES OF ARTIFICIAL REPRODUCTIVE TECHNOLOGIES

Different techniques have been designed to circumvent the problem of infertility, which prevents couples from having children through normal sexual intercourse. They range from the seemingly simple procedure of artificial insemination to the more complex and strenuous procedure of *in vitro* fertilisation, which has opened the door to other high-tech procedures and made it possible for scientists to manipulate human embryos in the laboratory. These techniques, which vary in their complexity and in their ethical problems, can be grouped under two broad headings: artificial insemination and artificial fertilisation. In the former, fertilisation occurs *in vivo* (inside the womb), while in the latter it occurs outside the womb.

ASSISTED INSEMINATION (AI)

Assisted insemination, also known as artificial insemination,[4] is the oldest and most widely used assisted reproductive technique. The first use resulting in a pregnancy was in 1790 by the Scottish anatomist and surgeon John Hunter, who inseminated a woman with her husband's sperm.[5] AI covers a wide range of techniques that involve placing sperm directly into the female reproductive tract in the absence of sexual intercourse.[6]

Three common forms of AI are intra-uterine insemination (IUI), intra-cervical insemination, and intra-vaginal insemination. Among these three, IUI is the most common technique. It is a simple and painless procedure in which a semen specimen is treated with special media and

---

4 Cf. L. SPEROFF – R. GLASS – N. KASE (eds.), *Clinical Gynecologic...*, *op. cit.*, p. 1025; See also C. TURKINGTON – M. ALPER, *Understanding Fertility and Infertility, op. cit.*, pp. 44-45.

5 L. WALTERS, "Reproductive Technologies and Genetics," in R. VEATCH, *Medical Ethics, Second Edition,* Jones and Bartley Publishers, Sudbury, Massachusetts 1989, p. 213. Here, the author states that the technique was demonstrated first in toads in 1779 by Larazo Spallanzani, an Italian priest and physiologist. Cited G. COREA, *The Mother Machine: From Artificial Insemination to Artificial Wombs,* Harper & Row, New York 1985, p. 35.

6 C. TURKINGTON – M. ALPER, *Understanding Fertility and Infertility, op. cit.*, p. 44.

then injected through a catheter into the woman's uterus, thus bypassing the cervical mucus. The clinical indication for it arises when the sperm cannot penetrate the cervical mucus, and postcoital tests reveal that good mucus is absent of sperm or contains dead and immotile sperm. It is also indicated in cases where the mucus is repeatedly poor and in couples with sexual dysfunction.[7] The procedure may be performed during a woman's natural cycle or following a stimulation of her ovaries that increases the chance of success by making more eggs available. Although IUI is a simple and safe procedure with no need for general anaesthesia, there are risks of infections, transmission of venereal diseases, multiple pregnancy, and ovarian hyperstimulation syndrome (OHSS). A success rate between 10% and 20% per cycle is often cited if the man has normal sperm count and the woman has healthy tubes.

ASSISTED INSEMINATION BY HUSBAND (AIH)

Sperm for AI is obtained from the man through masturbation or sexual intercourse with a plastic condom. Mastroianni Jr. contends that *coitus interruptus* is not recommended because the first portion of the ejaculate, which contains most of the active and motile sperm, may be lost in the process.[8] In cases involving the obstruction of the vas deferens, sperm could be obtained surgically from the epididymis, which is the storage depot for sperm.[9] When it is obtained through masturbation, semen may be obtained several times to increase the chances of conception. Usually, laboratory techniques are used to separate, treat, and concentrate the most active spermatozoa. Some scientists recommend introducing the sperm into the uterus 12 hours before ovulation because fertilisation usually occurs 12 to 24 hours after ovulation. If conception occurs, pregnancy should develop normally.

---

[7] L. SPEROFF – R. GLASS – N. KASE (eds.), *Clinical Gynecologic…, op. cit.*, p. 1025.

[8] L. MASTROIANNI JR., "Reproduction Technologies: Introduction," in S. POST (ed.), *Encyclopaedia of Bioethics…, op. cit.*, p. 2261. *Coitus interruptus* means the withdrawal of the penis before ejaculation.

[9] Ibid.

INDICATIONS FOR AIH

AIH is indicated when a man cannot ejaculate viable sperm inside the vagina of his fertile wife during normal intercourse. For some reason, a man may be unable to ejaculate during coitus but can do so through masturbation or the use of vibratory stimuli.[10] Mastroianni Jr. explains that the man's inability to ejaculate in the vagina may be due to premature ejaculation. Likewise, certain penile abnormalities can result in retrograde or misdirected ejaculation. Other possible causes that interfere with normal intercourse are erectile dysfunction, congenital or acquired vaginal abnormalities, and certain psychological problems on the part of the male or the female.[11] Additional factors include diabetes, spinal cord injury, trauma, and drug side-effects.

AIH is required when a man adds anti-sperm antibodies to his own sperm, which need to be removed to enhance their fertilising capacity; it is also indicated in cases of deficient or poor quality sperm that require treatment to increase their chances of fertilising an egg. AIH can be used when a couple's fertility is at risk because of radiotherapy, chemotherapy, or vasectomy. In this case, the sperm is obtained and frozen to maintain its quality for future use in reproduction. Cervical mucus infertility may also require the use of AIH. If a woman's cervical mucus is very poor or hostile to her husband's sperm, IUI is typically used to achieve conception because it bypasses the cervical mucus. Finally, AIH may be required in some cases of unexplained infertility.[12]

ADVANTAGE AND SUCCESS RATE

The main advantage of assisted insemination is that it is a simple procedure that does not involve the many risks of *in vitro* fertilisation. The success rate is between 10% and 20% per treatment cycle if the man has a normal sperm count and the woman has healthy fallopian tubes.[13]

---

[10] L. SPEROFF – R. GLASS – N. KASE (eds.), *Clinical Gynecologic…, op. cit.*, p. 1025.

[11] Cf. L. MASTROIANNI JR., "Reproductive Technologies: Introduction," in S. POST (ed.), *Encyclopaedia of Bioethics…, op. cit.*, p. 2261.

[12] O. GIWA–OSAGIE, "Assisted Reproductive Technology…, *op. cit.*, p. 3.

[13] C. TURKINGTON – M. ALPER, *Understanding Fertility and Infertility, op. cit.*, p. 44.

ARTIFICIAL INSEMINATION BY DONOR (AID)

The only difference between AID and AIH is the use of a donor. In this case, semen is obtained from an anonymous donor who is usually paid, or it is purchased from a licensed sperm bank. Usually the sperm is characterized to indicate the donor's race, blood group, skin colour, height, educational background, and occupation; this enables the physician or the prospective recipients to choose the characteristics they desire, as some prefer to choose characteristics that match those of their partners. To reduce the chances of intermarriage among a donor's offspring, a limit is often set regarding the number of pregnancies that he can establish.[14] In general, the medical details of the donor are obtained and recorded; the whole procedure is marked by confidentiality.

INDICATIONS FOR AID

Artificial insemination by a donor is required when the male partner cannot produce any sperm, when his sperm count is too low for effective pooling, or when his sperm has an impaired ability to fertilise a healthy egg. It is also used when he has antibodies that are incompatible with the woman, or when he has a serious hereditary disorder, such as haemophilia or Huntington's disease.[15] Sometimes, it is used by unmarried women who wish to conceive without having sex or by lesbian couples who desire a baby.[16] Additionally, it is utilized in surrogacy arrangements, in which case the semen obtained from a donor is used to inseminate a woman who will give up the baby at birth.

SCREENING OF THE DONOR'S SEMEN

In AID, the sperm donor is usually anonymous, but in some cases the recipient may prefer to use the semen of a close relative or friend. As a standard practice, his family medical history is recorded and he is screened for genetic disorders, serum hepatitis B and C, antibodies to the

---

[14] Ibid., pp. 44-45.

[15] L. MASTROIANNI JR., "Reproduction Technologies: Introduction," in W. REICH (ed.), *Encyclopaedia of Bioethics…, op. cit.,* p. 2208.

[16] Cf. B. ANDOLSEN, "Marriage and Other Domestic Partnerships," in W. REICH (ed.), *Encyclopedia of Bioethics…, op. cit.,* p. 641.

AIDS virus, STDs, and other communicable diseases.[17] This screening is performed initially and repeated after six months to avoid transmitting a disease to the woman and the future child.[18] The following example demonstrates the necessity of the repeated screening: The antibodies to AIDS may not be detected in the blood of an infected person in the first six months when the virus is in the sero-conversion stage. During this period, an HIV test may not detect that the person is positive, making it absolutely necessary to repeat the test before the person's semen is used for insemination. This precaution significantly reduces the risk of disease transmission, but the risk is not completely eliminated because errors can occur.

IN VITRO FERTILISATION

The most widely publicized and celebrated ART method is *in vitro* fertilisation (IVF). *In vitro* literally means "in glass;" as such, *in vitro* fertilisation is the Latin term for the union of sperm and egg in a glass petri dish.[19] In the standard IVF protocol, embryos are created in the laboratory and subsequently transferred into the recipient's uterus. This procedure could be homologous, in which case the woman's eggs are fertilised in the laboratory with her husband's semen, or it could be heterologous, in which case eggs harvested from a donor are fertilised and implanted into the woman's uterus. We will now discuss this in greater detail.

In vitro fertilisation and egg transfer (IVF-ET) is an artificial reproductive technique whereby "test tube babies" are produced. The first recorded uses of IVF technology that resulted in live births were accomplished with rabbits in 1959 and with laboratory mice in 1968.[20] Today, the standard IVF procedure involves the fertilisation of one or more eggs

[17] C. TURKINGTON – M. ALPER, *Understanding Fertility and Infertility, op. cit.*, p. 45.

[18] Cf. Ibid., p. 45.

[19] L. CHARLESWORTH, *The Couple's Guide to In Vitro Fertilization, op. cit.*, p. 3. This is because in the beginning, fertilisation used to take place in a glass lab dish. Now plastic ones are used.

[20] C. TURKINGTON – M. ALPER, *Understanding Fertility and Infertility, op. cit.*, p. 39.

outside the womb and the subsequent transfer of the fertilised eggs into the uterus. The first successful use of this technique to achieve a live human birth occurred in the United Kingdom. Here, the world's first "test tube baby," Louise Brown, was born to James and Lesley Brown in Greater Manchester in July 1978. Her birth was the culmination of extensive research that was credited to an embryologist, Dr. Robert Edwards, and to Dr. Patrick Steptoe, who had experimented with IVF for over 10 years and recorded about 80 failed attempts prior to Louise's birth. At present, over 25,000 babies have been born worldwide using this procedure.

INDICATIONS FOR IVF-ET

Initially, IVF-ET was used exclusively to achieve a pregnancy in women with blocked, damaged, or absent fallopian tubes. Because of recent improvements in IVF success rates, it is increasingly being applied to other cases of infertility, such as male factor infertility and unexplained infertility.[21] For instance, it is used for cases of oligoospermia, endometriosis, and immunological factor infertility.[22]

THE STANDARD IVF PROCEDURE

Before initiating an IVF cycle, couples meet with a physician to decide on an appropriate course of treatment. They are required to perform general tests, which include semen analysis, tests for HIV, and presence of STDs in the reproductive tract. Also, the medications vary from couple to couple to suit their peculiar circumstances and medical conditions.

In the early years of IVF, the normal practice was to use the natural cycle of the woman and transfer a single embryo into her uterus. This was the case with Lesley Brown, whose tubes had been surgically removed. No fertility drugs were used to stimulate her ovaries—the birth of Louise Brown resulted from a single egg she produced through normal ovulation. Today, the natural cycle has been abandoned because of the

---

21 L. SPEROFF – R. GLASS – N. KASE (eds.), *Clinical Gynecologic…, op. cit.*, p. 2209.

22 C. TURKINGTON – M. ALPER, *Understanding Fertility and Infertility, op. cit.*, p. 44.

low success rate, which is less than 5%.[23] Instead, doctors use a more complex, risky, and delicate procedure requiring artificial stimulation of the woman's ovaries.

The standard IVF procedure can be divided into four different phases: the stimulation of the ovaries, egg retrieval, fertilisation, and the transfer of embryos into the uterus.

Ovarian Stimulation and Monitoring: Under normal circumstances, the ovary releases one mature egg in the middle of each cycle. A typical IVF procedure begins by temporarily shutting down the woman's natural cycle with medications called GnRH agonists, which are administered for about two weeks starting one week before her anticipated period.[24] At the start of her cycle, her ovaries are stimulated with hormonal drugs such as Pergonal or Gonal F.[25] This ovarian stimulation triggers the development and subsequent retrieval of multiple healthy and mature eggs; it also controls the timing of the woman's cycle to ensure that the eggs are retrieved before she ovulates normally.[26] The overall goal is to enhance the chances of fertilisation and, ultimately, the IVF success rate.[27]

Following the injection of the fertility drugs, the physician monitors the development of the follicles with transvaginal ultrasound examinations and with daily blood tests that measure the oestradiol hormone

---

[23] S. BAYER – M. ALPER – A. PENZIAS, *The Boston IVF Handbook of…, op. cit.*, p. 80.

[24] C. TURKINGTON – M. ALPER, *Understanding Fertility and Infertility, op. cit.*, p. 41. These hormonal drugs are administered daily to suppress the natural hormones of the woman or to shut down her natural cycle, which allows the reproductive endocrinologist to have greater control over the IVF treatment cycle.

[25] Ibid., pp. 29-35. Some of these drugs are also used to induce ovulation, to correct ovulatory disorders, to increase egg production and to correct luteal phase deficiency. However, there are circumstances in which superovulation cannot be employed. For instance, in the case of a woman with breast cancer, which is estrogen receptor positive.

[26] L. CHARLESWORTH, *The Couple's Guide to In Vitro Fertilization, op. cit.*, p. 5. Such drugs reduce the risk of unexpected ovulation prior to egg retrieval.

[27] Cf. C. TURKINGTON – M. ALPER, *Understanding Fertility and Infertility, op. cit.*, p. 41.

level.[28] This enables the physician to monitor the patient's response to stimulation and prevent over-stimulation and under-stimulation. Usually, she is placed on daily dosage for 8 to 12 days.[29] If the reproductive endocrinologist is satisfied with the progress of the cycle and the number of follicles that are available, he gives the patient a final injection of human Chorionic Gonadotropin Hormone (hCG). This causes further development of the follicles and ensures that the eggs mature on schedule for retrieval, since a minimum number of follicles must develop to make retrieval worthwhile.[30] Also, this drug triggers ovulation to occur within the next 36 hours.[31]

Egg Retrieval: Eggs develop inside fluid-filled cysts of the follicles located in the ovaries. In the IVF procedure, egg retrieval is usually timed to take place 34 to 37 hours after the hCG injection. Eggs are retrieved before the natural ovulation occurs to avoid the cancellation of the cycle, which would make it impossible to retrieve all the other mature eggs. A fresh semen sample is usually obtained[32] while the egg retrieval is being performed. This period is often very stressful for men, and some are unable to produce a fresh semen sample. Because of this, a back-up semen sample is often collected a few days earlier and preserved. This is used as an alternative when the man fails to produce a fresh sample. It is important that the man does not lose any part of the sample. To ensure high sperm concentration, the couple is usually advised to abstain from sexual intercourse for at least two days before insemination. The woman may be required to refrain from eating solid food after midnight.

[28] Oestradiol is a hormone produced by the growing follicles and the level normally increases as they develop.

[29] C. TURKINGTON – M. ALPER, *Understanding Fertility and Infertility, op. cit.*, pp. 31-32.

[30] L. KAPLAN– C. KAPLAN, "Natural Reproduction…, *op. cit.*, p. 24.

[31] Cf. C. TURKINGTON – M. ALPER, *Understanding Fertility and Infertility, op. cit.*, pp. 41, 61.

[32] To produce the semen sample, a man has to masturbate either by watching a sexually arousing video clip or through other means.

The eggs are retrieved in two ways. During the early years of IVF, physicians retrieved eggs through laparoscopy,[33] which employs a long, thin fibre optic tube to view the inner part of the body. When this is used, the woman is placed under general anaesthesia. An incision is made in her abdomen through which the laparoscope is inserted and guided to the ovary. Next, a second incision is made, and a long, hollow double-aspirating needle is inserted to puncture the follicle and suck out the fluid and mature eggs.[34] Laparoscopy offers some diagnostic and therapeutic benefits; notably, it enables the physician to evaluate and correct anatomical conditions that may be contributing to the couple's infertility.[35]

Nowadays, a non-surgical ultrasound-guided aspirating needle is more effective[36] because of improvements in ultrasound imaging; this procedure involves inserting a needle guided by ultrasound through the woman's vagina to retrieve the eggs. This simplifies and reduces the risks of IVF because it requires only local anaesthesia. The number of follicles that develop after the stimulation of the ovaries varies from person to person and from one treatment cycle to the next. The average number of eggs recovered is five,[37] but some have reported harvesting as many as 50 eggs at a time.[38] The retrieval procedure lasts for 10 to 15 minutes, and the patient can go home after two hours of recovery.

Examination, Fertilisation, and Incubation: The retrieved follicles contain fluids that are immediately transferred to an IVF laboratory where a powerful microscope is used to identify the eggs. The malformed or damaged eggs are discarded, and the healthy ones are washed immediately

---

[33] G. SHER – V. DAVIS – J. STOESS, *In Vitro Fertilization: The Art of Making Babies, Updated Edition,* Facts on File, Inc., New York 1998, p. 69.

[34] Cf. L. SPERROF – R: GLASS – N: KASE (eds.), C*linical Gynecologic…, op. cit.,* p. 2209.

[35] G. SHER – V. DAVIS – J. STOESS, *In Vitro Fertilization…,op. cit.,* p. 69.

[36] L. MASTROIANNI JR., "Reproduction Technologies: Introduction," in S. POST (ed.) *Encyclopaedia of Bioethics…, op. cit.,* p. 2209.

[37] CHARLESWORTH, *The Couple's Guide to In Vitro Fertilization, op. cit.,* p. 8.

[38] G. SHEY – V. DAVIS – J. STOESS, *In Vitro Fertilization…, op. cit.,* p. 63.

and placed in petri dishes containing a nutrient solution.[39] Four to six hours after retrieval, the embryologist mixes the treated sperm[40] from the male partner or donor with the eggs, adding about 100,000 sperm to each of them. Subsequently, he incubates the eggs under controlled laboratory conditions.[41] The special incubator acts as a substitute for the natural conditions of the fallopian tube. Following insemination, the eggs are incubated for approximately 24 hours in a nutrient solution designed to enhance their fertilisability. After this time, the physician examines each egg with a high-powered microscope, looking for tentative evidence of fertilisation. The formation of the male and female pronuclei is evidence that fertilisation has been successful, whereas the presence of more than two pronuclei indicates a condition of polyspermy. If fertilisation occurs, the fertilised eggs are removed and placed in an incubator for a few days to allow the cells to divide. Meanwhile, progesterone injection is administered to the woman to prepare her uterine lining for implantation.

Embryo Culture and Transfer: On day three, when the embryos have two to eight cells, the embryologist selects the embryos with an "optimal chance" of implanting; he then transfers them into the woman's uterus by inserting a long catheter, under ultrasound guidance, through her vagina and cervix. This procedure takes about one hour and does not require anaesthesia. In the past, it was common to transfer four or more embryos to increase the chances of implantation, but today the guidelines on IVF usually limit the number to two or three to reduce the risk of multiple pregnancies. These guidelines differ from country to country, however. In Australia and France, not more than three embryos can be

---

[39] Cf. C. TURKINGTON – M. ALPER, *Understanding Fertility and Infertility, op. cit.*, p. 42.

[40] L. SPEROFF – M. FRITZ, *Clinical Gynecologic…, op. cit.*, p. 238. Cited J. OVERSTREET J. GOULD D. KATZ, "In vitro capacitation of human spermatozoa after passage through a column of cervical mucus," *FertiSteril* 34:604, 1980; See also G. SHER – V. DAVIS – J. STOESS, *In Vitro Fertilization…, op. cit.*, pp. 71-72. About 100,000 motile sperm are added to each. In IVF procedure, capacitation of sperm is artificially induced through the incubation of sperm in a defined medium for several hours and the time required for this is approximately two hours.

[41] L. MASTROIANNI JR., "Reproduction Technologies: Introduction," in S. POST (ed.) *Encyclopedia of Bioethics…, op. cit.*, p. 2209.

transferred, whereas countries like England and Italy have reduced the number to two. Taking into consideration the local laws, the couple and the physician choose the number of embryos to be transferred and the fate of the extra embryos; they then sign a consent form to that effect. Presently, in Nigeria, there are no official guidelines on this, although the Nigeria Fertility Society proposes that only two embryos be transferred. Some authors state that if a single embryo is transferred into the woman's uterus, there is a 9% probability of achieving a pregnancy. The probability increases to 18% if two embryos are transferred, 29% if three are transferred, and 32% if four are transferred.[42] Normally, fewer embryos are transferred to younger women and more to older women.

Nowadays, some embryologists culture the embryos to the blastocyst stage,[43] in which they contain 100 cells; this increases the chances of conception, but it also requires the use of sequential-culture media systems. On day five, not more than two embryos are transferred into the uterus. The disadvantage of culturing embryos to this stage is that it destroys some viable embryos that may have implanted if they were transferred earlier—no *in vitro* culture system is as good as the fallopian tube itself. The primary advantages are the following: the implantation rate at the blastocyst stage is higher, increasing the chances of pregnancy; it is easier to determine the best embryos for transfer because the more viable embryos grow more quickly; and it reduces the risk of multiple pregnancy since only two blastocysts are usually transferred.[44]

The physician usually prescribes daily hormonal therapy after the transfer of the embryos. The woman begins the daily injection of progesterone to prepare her uterine lining and create optimal conditions for implantation. To achieve this, physicians often target a thickness of a

---

[42] R. PINON JR., *Biology of Human Reproduction, op. cit.*, p. 417.

[43] Cf. C. TURKINGTON – M. ALPER, *Understanding Fertility and Infertility, op. cit.*, p. 43. In the past, the culture media could only sustain growth for about two or three days, but with improved technology some new culture solutions rich in nutrients are now available, allowing embryos to be cultured to blastocyst stage in the laboratory.

[44] Cf. S. BAYER – M. ALPER – A. PENZIAS, *The Boston IVF Handbook of…*, pp. 87-88.

millimetre or more.[45] About 12 to 14 days after the transfer, a blood test is performed to ascertain if implantation occurred. The detection of hCG, a hormone produced by an implanted embryo, is considered a clear sign of pregnancy. Ultrasound can detect pregnancy 18 days after the transfer and can also determine whether it is a single or multiple pregnancy. The surplus embryos may be frozen in liquid nitrogen for future use, donated anonymously to other infertile couples, used for research, allowed to die, or intentionally destroyed. They also may be adopted by women or couples who wish to prevent their destruction on moral grounds. Usually, cases of multiple pregnancy are resolved by selective abortion.

SUCCESS RATE AND PROBLEMS OF IVF-ET

IVF is a complex, expensive, labour-intensive, stressful procedure. Initially, in the United States, each attempt cost $10,000 or more,[46] but now it ranges from $5,000 to $7,000 per treatment cycle.[47] However, success in terms of conception and live birth cannot be guaranteed in one cycle or even in several cycles.[48] In about 10% of the cases, an IVF cycle will be cancelled because of several possible complications, including the following: the woman responds poorly to stimulation with fertility drugs and produces no follicles or poor-quality follicles; the physician is unable to reach the follicles to retrieve them; and natural ovulation occurs unexpectedly before egg retrieval. If the IVF cycle is cancelled, the woman will rest for a few months to allow natural cycles to take place before a new cycle will begin. It is clear that the failure of a cycle, requiring a repeat of the entire procedure, can be for the couple a source of profound psychological distress, frustration, and depression.

At present, IVF-ET cannot improve the rate of live birth in natural procreation. The success rate (live birth per cycle) is about 18% to 25%

[45] Cf. L. CHARLES WORTH, *The Couple's Guide to In Vitro Fertilization, op. cit.*, p. 176.

[46] L. KAPLAN–C. KAPLAN, "Natural Reproduction…, *op. cit.*, p. 26.

[47] S. BAYER – M. ALPER – A. PENZIAS, *The Boston IVF Handbook of…, op. cit.*, p. 2.

[48] One of the greatest problems presented by the IVF treatment is that there is no certainty of success.

once embryos are successfully transferred into the uterus;[49] the success rate will depend on the skill and experience of the clinicians,[50] the characteristics of the couple, the age of the woman, the quality of the man's sperm, and the cause of infertility. The most serious factor that can affect the success rate of an IVF cycle is the quality of a woman's egg, which diminishes with age. Embryos may also be lost during transfer if they cannot pass through a narrowed or scarred cervical canal. Human error and equipment failure can also occur. IVF can fulfil a diagnostic role: if healthy eggs are harvested and none of them is fertilised, this could indicate that the couple has a fertility problem that is yet to be diagnosed.[51]

THE RISK OF IVF-ET

The IVF procedure carries several risks. Such risks are usually mild, but they can sometimes be severe. The following sections describe the various risks.

Risks to Mother and Oocyte Donor: The woman bears the major burdens and risks of the IVF protocol because almost all the procedures take place in her body. The procedure of egg retrieval can cause ovarian infection and even permanent sterility.[52] Injury to abdominal and pelvic organs can also occur. Pelvic infections and abdominal perforation can result from transvaginal retrieval, and the use of laparoscopy can cause haemorrhage, intestinal perforation, and infections.

Hormonal drugs used in stimulating the ovaries can cause Ovarian Hyperstimulation Syndrome (OHSS), a condition in which the ovaries produce too many eggs. This can cause the ovaries to enlarge, allowing fluid to collect in the abdomen. Severe cases of OHSS can result in blood clots, kidney damage, fluid build-up in the abdomen, and chest and ovarian twisting. A hyperstimulated ovary can twist and cut off its own blood supply; when this happens, emergency surgery is required to untwist

---

[49] See C. TURKINGTON – M. ALPER, *Understanding Fertility and Infertility, op. cit.*, p. 42.

[50] R. PINON JR., *Biology of Human Reproduction, op. cit.*, p. 418.

[51] G. SHER – V. DAVIS – J. STOESS, *In Vitro Fertilization ..., op. cit.*, p. 72.

[52] W. TURECK *et al.*, "Perioperative Complication Arising After Transvaginal Oocyte Retrieval," *Obstetrics and Gynaecology*, 81(4) (1993) 590-593.

it. This condition can also affect the woman's overall health, expend the couple's financial resources, and lead to frustration.[53] The condition occurs in 1% to 5% of cycles among women taking fertility drugs, but it could be higher in women with polycystic ovarian syndrome.[54] Further, fertility drugs can cause the woman's ovaries to rupture[55] and are associated with depression. According to Turkington and Alper, they "trigger hormonal changes that can cause depression by interfering with estrogen (a natural antidepressant)."[56] Likewise, hyper-stimulation is correlated with genetic defects such as neural tube defect.[57]

Some authors link fertility drugs to ovarian cancer[58]—it is on this basis that some people reject IVF.[59] The data linking ovarian stimulation to ovarian cancer are controversial, especially because the vast majority of studies fail to establish any significant link between the two.[60] Instead, it has been suggested that the increased risk of cancer results from continuous stimulation of the ovaries without the establishment of a pregnancy.[61] Turkington and Alper contend that ovarian cancer is more

---

[53] Cf. L. MASTROIANNI JR., "Reproduction Technologies: Introduction," in W. REICH (ed.), *Encyclopaedia of Bioethics…, op. cit.*, p. 2212.

[54] See C. TURKINGTON – M. ALPER, *Understanding Fertility and Infertility, op. cit.*, p. 37.

[55] T. SHANNON, *An Introduction to Bioethics,* Paulist Press, New York/N.J. 1997, p. 60.

[56] C. TURKINGTON – M. ALPER, *Understanding Fertility and Infertility, op. cit.*, pp. 37-38.

[57] Cf. I. POLLARD, *Life, Love and Children…, op. cit.*, p. 120.

[58] A. JONSEN – R. VEATCH – L. WALTERS (eds.), *Source Book in Bioethics: A Documentary History,* Georgetown University Press, Washington D.C. 1998, p. 94.

[59] See NUALA SCARISBRICK, "Health: Why I Oppose IVF," In *BBC News World Edition, op. cit.*, p. 3. Nuala Scarisbrick argues that there is anecdotal evidence, citing the case of magazine editor Liz Tilberi, who blamed repeated IVF cycles for her fatal ovarian cancer.

[60] C. TURKINGTON – M. ALPER, *Understanding Fertility and Infertility, op. cit.*, p. 38.

[61] A. WISOT – D. MELDRUM, *Conceptions and Misconceptions, Second Edition,* Hartley and Marks Inc., WA 2004, p. 21. Childbearing reduces the risk of ovarian cancer.

likely to be related to the number of times a woman ovulates; it is therefore connected with infertility because pregnancy suppresses ovulation and lactation delays its return after childbirth. However, most experts recommend caution regarding the frequency and duration of fertility drug use.[62] Finally, laparoscopy carries the morbidity and mortality risks associated with general anaesthesia.[63]

Risks to Mother and Foetus: Under normal circumstances, the embryo implants along the uterine wall, but sometimes it implants outside the uterus. This condition is known as ectopic pregnancy. IVF carries an increased risk of ectopic pregnancy—3% to 5.5% of IVF pregnancies compared to 1% to 2% of natural pregnancies.[64] Ectopic pregnancy can occur in the ovary, abdomen, or fimbriae, but the most common site is the fallopian tube. Generally, such a pregnancy never reaches full term because the growth of the foetus is seriously restricted. It also carries serious health consequences for the mother. Rupture of the fallopian tube wall can lead to bleeding; if this is not properly managed, it can be fatal to the woman. This condition and the necessary corrective surgery can further compromise the woman's fertility.

IVF poses a dramatic increase in the risk of multiple pregnancy—from 1% of cases in natural conception to about 20% of cases in IVF. This is due to the administration of fertility drugs, such as gonadotropins, and to the transfer of multiple embryos[65] into the woman's uterus. A pregnancy is said to be multiple if it involves more than one foetus at the same time, such as in the case of twins, triplets, quadruplets, and so forth. A multiple pregnancy carries risks of morbidity and mortality for the mother.[66] Besides its well-known impact on a woman's general

---

[62] C. TURKINGTON – M. ALPER, *Understanding Fertility and Infertility, op. cit.*, p. 38.

[63] T. SHANNON, *An Introduction to Bioethics, op. cit.*, p. 60.

[64] Cf. C. TURKINGTON – M. ALPER, *Understanding Fertility and Infertility, op. cit.*, p. 38.

[65] See C. TURKINGTON – M. ALPER, *Understanding Fertility and Infertility, op. cit.*, p. 38.

[66] NATIONAL ACADEMY OF SCIENCES – NATIONAL ACADEMY OF ENGINEERING – INSTITUTE OF MEDICINE – NATIONAL RESEARCH COUNCIL, *Scientific and Medical Aspects of…, op. cit.*, p. 62.

health and reproductive system,[67] it causes additional discomfort during pregnancy and delivery.[68] Furthermore, it increases the risk of numerous complications for the children, including pregnancy loss, premature delivery, birth defects, physical problems, mental retardation, blindness, and stillbirth.[69] Premature delivery increases the social cost[70] due to an increased use of the newborn intensive care unit.[71] Although many of the premature babies are saved, according to Christine Ammer, "Combined prenatal and neonatal mortality is four times higher than with single births."[72]

Multiple pregnancies may require selective abortion of some of the embryos through a technique known as foetal reduction; this gives one or two of the embryos a better chance of surviving. This is usually done before the 12th week of pregnancy. It can be achieved by injecting "a lethal drug into one or more of the foetuses through the mother's abdomen guided by ultrasound."[73] The most common injection is of potassium chloride into the heart of each of the targeted foetuses.[74] Worse still, the procedure can lead to the miscarriage of all the foetuses. IVF also

---

[67] C. AMMER, *The New A to Z of Women's Health...*, *op. cit.*, pp. 269-270.

[68] See C. TURKINGTON – M. ALPER, *Understanding Fertility and Infertility*, *op. cit.*, p. 54. Multiple pregnancies carry an increased risk of pregnancy-induced high blood pressure, prolonged labour, complicated delivery, diabetes and haemorrhage.

[69] Ibid.

[70] See Ibid., p. 34.

[71] See. R. JONES, *Human Reproductive Biology*, *op. cit.*, p. 234. According to Jones, the organs of premature newborns are not fully developed and this may reduce the chance for survival of these infants. Being "premature" is measured by the weight rather than age. If development of the infant has reached 38 weeks, 99% may survive, but only about 59% will survive at 25 weeks. However, he adds that about 85% of premature babies will face some developmental problems as they grow up.

[72] C. AMMER, *The New A to Z of Women's Health...*, *op. cit.*, p. 270.

[73] Ibid.

[74] See C. TURKINGTON – M. ALPER, *Understanding Fertility and Infertility*, *op. cit.*, p. 55.

increases the risk of spontaneous abortion, which is estimated at 18%[75] of IVF pregnancies.

Risks to Embryo, Foetus, or Offspring: The quality of the sperm that fertilise the ovum *in vitro* may differ from the quality of the sperm that fertilise in the fallopian tube because the female reproductive tract selects against abnormal sperm.[76] The quantity of sperm that simultaneously reach the ovum *in vitro* may compromise the natural impediments to fertilisation by multiple sperm, resulting in more *polyploid* embryos.[77] Such embryos usually do not survive. Finally, there is the risk of the embryo not implanting because of poor synchronization of the cycle or a defective embryo.

VARIATIONS OF THE IVF PROCEDURE

With the successful use of IVF technology, there has been a series of breakthroughs that have improved the ability of infertile couples to have children. Most of these use the standard IVF protocol. The principal breakthroughs are described below.

FREEZING AND STORING OF SPERM

In general, the term "cryopreservation" covers a wide range of practices, such as the freezing and storing of embryos, sperm, eggs, and even parts of the ovaries.[78] The freezing and storing of semen was first used to establish a pregnancy in 1953[79] and is still recommended for ART procedures involving masturbation. Such frozen semen samples are used as substitutes when a man cannot produce fresh semen during an ART procedure. It is also employed if a man is exhibiting problems with sperm production or is about to experience a treatment or occupation that may impede his sperm production. Semen samples collected from donors are

---

[75] L. ROMANO, "Infertilità..., *op. cit.,* n. 3.

[76] A. JONSEN – R. VEATCH – L. WALTERS (eds.), *Source Book in Bioethics..., op. cit.,* p. 94.

[77] Ibid.

[78] Cf. C. TURKINGTON – M. ALPER, *Understanding Fertility and Infertility, op. cit.,* p. 50.

[79] Cf. L. MASTROIANNI JR., "Reproductive Technologies: Introduction," in W. REICH (ed.), *Encyclopedia...,op. cit.,* p. 2208-2209.

frozen in sperm banks for use by those who require sperm donation to achieve a pregnancy. The response of spermatozoa to cryopreservation is unpredictable and varies among individuals. While some semen samples respond well to freezing, others do not. Overall, the pregnancy rate with frozen semen is low, making a freshly ejaculated sample preferable.

CRYOPRESERVATION OF EMBRYOS

Cryopreservation is able to preserve embryos that are not used in a particular IVF treatment cycle. This procedure of freezing and storing embryos began in the early 1980s, with the first human birth occurring in Australia in 1984. In this procedure, physicians try to retrieve and fertilise as many eggs as possible, using IVF technology. The best two or three resulting embryos are transferred into the woman, while the remaining potentially viable embryos are quickly frozen and preserved in liquid nitrogen. Embryos can be preserved from the one-cell stage to the blastocyst stage. The goal of embryo preservation is to avoid repeating the strenuous, expensive, and risky IVF egg retrieval procedure in the event that implantation or a live birth does not occur. When they are required, the frozen embryos are thawed and transferred into the uterus. If the couple does not need them, they may be donated to other IVF couples, used for research, or destroyed.

INDICATIONS FOR CRYOPRESERVATION

Cryopreservation of embryos for subsequent transfer is used if a woman is at risk of any of the complications associated with ovarian stimulation, such as OHSS. It is equally indicated if the physician has previously encountered difficulties achieving fertilisation.

ADVANTAGES OF CRYOPRESERVATION

Cryopreservation of embryos reduces the physical, psychological, and financial costs of a subsequent ART procedure in the event that the current treatment cycle fails or the couple decides to have another child. It eliminates the need for ovarian stimulation, egg retrieval, fertilisation, and, in some cases, for a donor. While a typical IVF cycle costs $5,000 to $7,000, implantation of already-created embryos only costs about $1,200.[80] It also eliminates the problem associated with the inability to achieve fertilisation, leaving the physicians to contend with implanta-

[80] Ibid., p. 51.

tion and the maintenance of a potential pregnancy. Finally, cryopreservation prevents the destruction of potentially viable embryos, which is considered its main advantage because such embryos can be offered to other infertile couples who need them.

RISKS AND SUCCESS RATE

Cryopreserved embryos remain viable for a long time; about 50% of them can be thawed successfully and used in a natural cycle, with about 18% of them resulting in pregnancies.[81] A major risk of this technology is that the process of freezing and thawing embryos may affect their viability. The technique may also produce mutations,[82] but not much is known about its long-term effects on children resulting from it. Current knowledge indicates that it has no adverse effects on the foetus.[83]

OVARIAN TISSUE FREEZING

Ovarian tissue freezing allows the egg to be preserved for future fertilisation. In this case, a woman may freeze her gamete to guarantee more successful pregnancies and healthier children in the future if she is about to undergo a medical procedure that could affect her fertility.

GAMETE INTRA-FALLOPIAN TUBE TRANSFER (GIFT)

GIFT was developed in 1984 as a variation on standard IVF. It was first successfully used to establish a pregnancy in San Antonio, Texas, by Dr. Ricardo Asch.[84] The technology involves the transfer of freshly recovered eggs and sperm into the fallopian tube; unlike conventional IVF, fertilisation occurs *in vivo*, that is, inside the fallopian tube.[85]

---

[81] Ibid.

[82] A. JONSEN – R. VEATCH – L. WALTERS (eds.), *Source Book in Bioethics…, op. cit.*, p. 94.

[83] L. MASTROIANNI JR., "Reproductive Technologies: Introduction," in S. POST (ed.), *Encyclopedia of Bioethics…, op. cit.*, p. 2264.

[84] A. WISOT – D. MELDRUM, *Conceptions and Misconception…, op. cit.*, p. 12.

[85] Given this fact, we cannot say it is an IVF technique.

PROCEDURE FOR GIFT

The ovaries are stimulated and eggs are retrieved by ultrasound-guided needle aspiration under light sedation. The eggs are examined under a microscope to ensure that they are mature, and then they are carefully cultured in a special nutrient solution. Next, they are placed in a special catheter with prepared sperm and transferred into the fallopian tube for fertilisation to occur naturally. The transfer of the gametes into the tube is performed with laparoscopy under general anaesthesia.

INDICATIONS FOR GIFT

GIFT is not applicable to every form of infertility because it can only be used by women who have at least one functioning fallopian tube. It is employed in the treatment of couples with unexplained infertility and of women with extra-tubal diseases, such as pelvic adhesions or minimal endometriosis.[86] GIFT is also used by those who do not wish to contravene the tenets of their religion. For instance, some Roman Catholics, who oppose *in vitro* fertilisation, use GIFT to ensure that fertilisation occurs inside the womb. Finally, GIFT is useful for couples with cervical factor and immunological factor infertility and for couples that could not conceive through standard IVF.

SUCCESS RATE AND RISKS OF GIFT

A success rate of about 28% deliveries per retrieval is reported for GIFT,[87] with some authors citing figures between 30% and 35%.[88] Mastroianni Jr. adds that in its early days, GIFT had a higher success rate than standard IVF, but standard IVF is now more successful in most centres.[89] The major advantage of GIFT is that fertilisation occurs in the natural site—the fallopian tube.

---

[86] Cf. L. MASTROIANNI JR., "Reproductive Technologies: Introduction," in W. REICH (ed.), *Encyclopaedia of Bioethics...*, *op. cit.*, p. 2211.

[87] C. TURKINGTON – M. ALPER, *Understanding Fertility and Infertility, op. cit.*, p. 48; See also R. PINON JR, *Biology of Human Reproduction, op. cit.*, p. 419. Pinon cites 28.5%. The discrepancies may be a result of other factors, such as the skill of the physician, the quality of the gametes and so on.

[88] Cf. L. MASTROIANNI JR., "Reproductive Technologies: Introduction," in W. REICH (ed.), *Encyclopaedia of Bioethics...*, *op. cit.*, p. 2211.

[89] L. MASTROIANNI JR., "Reproductive Technologies: Introduction," in S. POST (ed.), *Encyclopedia of Bioethics ...*, *op. cit.*, p. 2265.

ZYGOTE INTRA-FALLOPIAN TRANSFER (ZIFT)

ZIFT is an ART method that combines the standard IVF procedure of egg retrieval with the GIFT procedure of gamete transfer. Unlike GIFT, fertilisation occurs *in vitro,* and the resulting zygote is inserted immediately in the fallopian tube with the hope that implantation will occur. The transfer, which requires laparoscopy, occurs before the zygote begins to divide.[90]

ZIFT is used if a man has severe male factor infertility or if the physician has experienced difficulty confirming fertilisation with other procedures. Like GIFT, it can only be used if the woman has at least one functioning tube. It involves all the risks of IVF, including operation risks, since the transfer of the zygote is usually performed with a laparoscope, which is inserted into the woman's abdomen to place the embryos in the fallopian tube. This is why it is considered more invasive than IVF, which is increasingly performed without surgery. A success rate of 24.4% is cited for ZIFT.[91]

SURROGACY PRACTICE

Surrogacy is a method in which an embryo created *in vitro* is transferred to a woman who is expected to give up the baby after birth. A surrogate is a woman who agrees to bear a child on behalf of an infertile couple or individual. This decision can result from altruistic or commercial motives, because the surrogate mother may be paid for her services. Some authors distinguish between two types of surrogacy. Genetic or partial surrogacy involves inseminating a surrogate with sperm from the partner of the infertile woman or from a donor. Gestational or total surrogacy involves a surrogate who provides the gestational component for a child that will not be genetically related to her.[92] The woman is referred to as surrogate mother, placental mother, or gestational mother.

---

[90] Cf. A. WISOT – D. MELDRUM, *Conceptions and Misconceptions…, op. cit.,* p. 13. The rationale behind this is that placing the fertilized egg in its natural environment in the fallopian tube instead of the uterus might enhance the chances of success.

[91] Cf. C. TURKINGTON – M. ALPER, *Understanding Fertility and Infertility, op. cit.,* p. 46.

[92] Cf. I. POLLARD, *Life, Love and Children…, op. cit.,* pp. 123-124.

The surrogate mother carries the pregnancy, and she may or may not provide the genetic component.

TYPES OF PARENTHOOD IN SURROGACY

In surrogacy, several types of parenthood are possible. In one type, eggs are obtained from the woman and are fertilised with her husband's spermatozoa. The resulting embryos are then transferred into the uterus of the gestational mother, who may be a relative, a friend, or someone contracted to carry the pregnancy. In this case, the offspring is genetically related to the man and his wife and has no direct genetic relationship to the gestational mother. A more complex type involves the use of a surrogate mother who actually donates the eggs, thus contributing half of the chromosomal make-up of the child. In this case, the spermatozoa of the man are used to fertilise the eggs donated by the gestational mother. A third type of gestational parenthood involves a surrogate who donates the egg and another man who donates the sperm. In this case, the child will not be genetically related to the couple.

Reflecting on the various types of parenthood that are possible in surrogacy, Shannon states that the new technical capabilities have radically redefined parenthood. For the woman, we have seven possible types of motherhood: the genetic mother, who is the source of the egg; the gestational mother, who carries the pregnancy; the nurturing mother, who raises the child; the genetic-gestational mother, who is the source of the egg and carries the pregnancy but does not raise the child; the genetic-nurturing mother, who is the source of the egg and raises the child without carrying the pregnancy; the gestational-nurturing mother, who does not provide the egg but carries the pregnancy and raises the child; and the whole mother, who is the source of the egg, carries the pregnancy, and raises the child. For the man, there are three types of fatherhood: the genetic father, who is merely the source of the sperm; the nurturing father, who raises the child; and the whole father, who provides the sperm and raises the child.[93]

THE PROCEDURE

The procedure for surrogacy requires the selection and screening of potential donors. Usually, if egg donation is required, the medical history

---

[93] T. SHANNON, *An Introduction to Bioethics, op. cit.* pp. 61-62.

and the characteristics of the prospective donors are recorded. An essential aspect of surrogacy procedures is the signing of the consent form, which indicates that both the surrogate and the couple truly understand and agree to the terms of the arrangement. To ensure that the prospective surrogate meets the criteria for IVF-surrogacy, she is examined medically and psychologically.[94] The procedure follows the standard IVF sequence of ovarian stimulation, egg retrieval, and transfer, but the resulting embryo is transferred into the uterus of the surrogate mother, who may or may not have supplied the eggs. If implantation occurs, pregnancy should develop normally, but the surrogate gives up the baby at birth. The eggs used in this procedure can be excess eggs from IVF patients, eggs from women undergoing sterilization, eggs donated by a relative or friend, or eggs harvested from younger women[95] during a donor programme.

The procedure is much more complicated if the gestational mother is different from the donor of the eggs, because this requires a coordination of their menstrual cycles.[96] An alternative approach is to fertilise the donor's oocytes and preserve the resultant embryos; this avoids repeating the entire process if the first attempt fails.

INDICATIONS FOR SURROGACY

Surrogacy is indicated in women with functioning ovaries but with congenital or surgical absence of the uterus. It is also indicated for women who cannot carry a pregnancy to term because of a weak or non-functional uterus.

The presence of some life-threatening medical conditions that are aggravated by pregnancy, such as heart problems, diabetes, and high blood pressure,[97] may require a woman to use surrogacy. It may also be

---

[94] Importantly, she is examined for Rhesus antibodies, diabetes and the like, while her uterus is examined with ultrasound. Also, there is effort to ensure that she does not have an unhealthy lifestyle that can jeopardize the health of the foetus or affect the future child, such as smoking, drinking and drug use.

[95] See L. MASTROIANNI JR., "Reproductive Technologies: Introduction," in W. REICH (ed.), *Encyclopedia of Bioethics …, op. cit.,* p. 2212. Such women are often paid.

[96] See Ibid., p. 2212.

[97] Ordinarily, many of these conditions can be effectively managed with special medications, but they may be compounded and become life-threatening

recommended for women with a history of repeated miscarriages. Surrogacy may also be required to avoid transferring a genetic disease to one's offspring. In this case, the sperm from the woman's partner is used to inseminate another woman who will give up the child at birth.

Surrogacy allows for the use of eggs from donors; as such, other clinical indications for the procedure are premature menopause and the inability of the woman to produce genetically normal eggs.[98] Finally, women who do not wish to interrupt their careers, actresses, and homosexual couples can use surrogacy to have children.

COST AND SUCCESS RATE

Surrogacy is a very expensive procedure. It involves both the cost of an IVF cycle and the additional payments made to the surrogate mother and the agent. A pregnancy rate of 35% to 50% of egg donation cycles is reported, with 15% to 20% ending in miscarriage.[99] Surrogacy carries all the risks of IVF in addition to other risks, including psychological problems on the part of a surrogate mother, especially if she is also the genetic mother of the child.

INTRA-CYTOPLASMIC SPERM INJECTION (ICSI)

ICSI represents one of the most significant breakthroughs in the history of ART. It is a micromanipulation technique that can be applied to human sperm, oocytes, and embryos to facilitate fertilisation or implantation. More precisely, it is a micro-insemination procedure in which a single sperm is injected directly into a single mature egg through a small glass needle[100] with the help of a robotic machine called a micromanipulator. It was developed by Belgian reproductive specialists and was first successfully used to establish a pregnancy in 1993 following repeated testing in animals since 1966.[101]

with pregnancy.

[98] L. MASTROIANNI JR., "Reproductive Technologies: Introduction," in W. REICH (ed.), *Encyclopedia of Bioethics ..., op. cit.*, p. 2212.

[99] C. TURKINGTON – M. ALPER, *Understanding Fertility and Infertility, op. cit.*, p. 53.

[100] Ibid., p. 48.

[101] R. PINON JR., *Biology of Human Reproduction, op. cit.*, p. 420

ICSI PROCEDURE

ICSI is based on the standard IVF procedure. Following ovarian stimulation and egg retrieval, the oocytes are prepared in the laboratory. Under a powerful microscope, the cumulus cells and the *corona radiata* cells that surround them are removed to ascertain the stage of their maturation. The presence of the first polar body indicates that an oocyte has completed metaphase II and can therefore be used for ICSI. The eggs are placed in a droplet of medium, and, using a high-powered microscope, the embryologist immobilizes a single sperm (washed and prepared to enhance fertilisation capacity) by compressing the tail and then placing it in an injection pipette.[102] The pipette pierces the zonapellucida and *oolemma*, and he injects a single spermatozoon directly into the *ooplasm* of the mature eggs using a micro needle, instead of allowing fertilisation to occur in the petri dish as with IVF.[103] The procedure takes less than 10 minutes. ICSI is a delicate procedure that requires quality equipment and expertise on the part of the embryologist. The procedure theoretically requires only one viable sperm to achieve fertilisation; once the eggs are fertilised, the resulting embryos are inserted into the uterus after three days.

INDICATIONS FOR ICSI

ICSI is indicated when the male has extremely low sperm count, decreased sperm motility, or less than 4% normally formed sperm. Also, it is used for men with a very high level of anti-sperm antibodies in their semen samples.[104] Couples who have failed to achieve conception or who are highly unlikely to achieve it with standard IVF can benefit from ICSI;

---

[102] C. TURKINGTON – M. ALPER, *Understanding Fertility and Infertility, op. cit.*, p. 48. The embryologist aspirates a single spermatozoon into an injection micropipette. Holding each egg with a second pipette, he micro-injects a single sperm into each egg.

[103] L. SPERROF – M. FRITZ, *Clinical Gynecologic…, op. cit.*, p. 1236. The procedure involves perforating the membrane of the egg with glass pipette before inserting a single spermatozoon.

[104] See C. TURKINGTON – M. ALPER, *Understanding Fertility and Infertility, op. cit.*, p. 48. It is also used when a man cannot produce sperm or good quality sperm and his previously frozen sperm is limited in number and quality or if he does not want AID.

however, the technique is not usually successful if failure to achieve fertilisation is due to poor egg quality.

A couple who had a low yield of eggs following ovarian stimulation and egg retrieval can use ICSI to maximize their chances of conception, because only one spermatozoon is needed to fertilise an egg. In addition, ICSI is indicated when there is need to surgically retrieve spermatozoa from the epididymis or testis, such as in cases of azoospermia resulting from irreparable vasectomy or abnormal ejaculatory ducts.[105]

ADVANTAGE OF ICSI

Unlike most of the other techniques, ICSI requires only one viable spermatozoon to achieve fertilisation; viability is not impaired even if there are no motile sperm. As a result, ICSI makes it possible to establish pregnancies that would never have otherwise occurred due to severe deficiencies in the sperm.[106] This also means it can help couples conceive with their own gametes, rather than resort to donor's sperm or to adoption. Additionally, ICSI eliminates the incidence of polyspermy because only a single spermatozoon is injected into the oocyte.[107]

SUCCESS RATE OF ICSI

A pregnancy rate of 50% to 70% has been cited for ICSI,[108] but most ART centres report a success rate of 15% to 35% deliveries per egg retrieval. Others put the fertilisation rate per egg at 70% despite poor sperm quality, and they cite a pregnancy rate of about 50%. More than 10,000 babies have been born worldwide using ICSI, and many practitioners claim that IVF/ICSI with poor sperm quality offers fertilisation and pregnancy rates similar to what standard IVF offers only to those with normal sperm quality.[109]

---

[105] Ibid. This can be achieved through techniques of microsurgical epididymal sperm aspiration (MESA) or testicular sperm aspiration (TESA).

[106] Cf. L. MASTROIANNI JR., "Reproductive Technologies: Introduction," in S. POST (ed.), *Encyclopedia…*, *op. cit.*, p. 2265.

[107] Cf. G. PALERMO – H. JORIS *et al.*, "Pregnancies after Intracytoplasmic Injection of a Single Spermatozoon into an Oocyte," *Lancet*, 340:17, 1992.

[108] L. SPERROF – A. FRITZ, *Clinical Gynecologic…*, *op. cit.*, p.1236.

[109] See C. TURKINGTON – M. ALPER, *Understanding Fertility and Infertility*, *op. cit.*, p. 49.

RISKS OF ICSI

ICSI involves all the risks of the standard IVF procedure, but it is more invasive than standard IVF because it bypasses the natural barriers to fertilisation. There is a higher incidence of chromosomal abnormalities in children born through ICSI—the rate is 0.2% in the general population and 0.8% following ICSI.[110] The technique also increases the risk of multifoetal pregnancies. Although no significant genetic risk has been reported so far, potential effects on offspring resulting from ICSI cannot be determined with certainty because it has a relatively short history.

ASSISTED ZONA HATCHING (AZH)

Once fertilisation is accomplished in any ART procedure that relies on IVF, implantation of the embryo poses a major challenge to the embryologist. During the transport from the fallopian tube to the uterus in natural reproduction, the cells of the implanting embryo are held together by the zona pellucida (ZP). As Pinon explains, the movement through the tube at this time follows a specific procedure that allows the ZP to degenerate only after the embryo has reached the uterus. Prior to implantation, the embryo must first "hatch" from the ZP, but if the wall of the ZP is too thick, it may fail to hatch, meaning that implantation will not occur.[111]

To resolve the serious challenge posed by implantation in artificial reproduction, scientists have designed a technique known as Assisted Zona Hatching (AZH). This micro-manipulation technique facilitates hatching and implantation and thus increases the delivery rate. Under a powerful microscope, the physician uses a micro-needle to artificially thin the embryo or to make a small cross-shaped opening in the ZP.[112] Once hatching is accomplished, the embryo is transferred into the uterine cavity. The common methods of AZH utilize a special chemical, a laser beam, or mechanical techniques.[113]

---

[110] S. BAYER – M. ALPER – A. PENZIAS, *The Boston IVF Handbook…, op. cit.*, p. 86.

[111] R. PINON JR., *Biology of Human Reproduction, op. cit.*, pp. 288–289.

[112] Y. VERLINSKY – A. KULIEV, *Atlas of Pre-implantation Genetic Diagnosis, Second Edition,* Taylor & Frances, London 2005, p. 18.

[113] C. TURKINGTON – M. ALPER, *Understanding Fertility and Infertility, op. cit.*, p. 49.

INDICATIONS FOR AZH AND RISKS

AZH is indicated when women have a history of repeated implantation failure or when the embryos from IVF have a thick ZP that makes hatching difficult or impossible. Also, it can improve chances of implantation in ART procedures involving older women, because implantation is less likely to occur naturally in women over age 38, who may have high FSH levels.[114]

Since the ZP serves as the embryo's protective shell during its movement to the site of implantation, AZH may expose it to infections; to prevent this, physicians usually administer antibiotics to the woman.

MICROSURGICAL EPIDIDYMAL SPERM ASPIRATION (MESA) AND TESTICULAR SPERM ASPIRATION (TESA)

If a man cannot produce sperm normally, it can be retrieved surgically from the epididymis, vas deferens, or testes. Physicians accomplish this using MESA and TESA. The former involves the surgical aspiration of sperm from the epididymis, while the latter involves the extraction of sperm from the testicles. In both procedures, sperm retrieval is performed under local or general anaesthesia.

INDICATION FOR MESA AND TESA

These techniques are indicated if a man's testes are not producing sperm or if he has obstructive azoospermia. In the latter case, the testicles produce normal sperm, but it cannot be ejaculated due to blockage of the epididymis or vas deferens, leading to complete absence of sperm in his semen specimen. Similarly, congenital absence of the vas deferens or a history of failed vasectomy reversal may require the use of these techniques.

SUBZONAL INSERTION (SUZI)

SUZI is an ART procedure that involves the micromanipulation of a mature oocyte to mechanically insert a spermatozoon through the ZP into the space between the zona and the oocyte.[115] This facilitates the penetration of the sperm into the oocyte and thereby increases the chances of fertilisation.

---

[114] Ibid.

[115] See L. MASTROIANNI JR., "Reproductive Technologies: Introduction," in W. REICH (ed.), *Encyclopedia of Bioethics…, op. cit.,* p. 2211.

EGG DONATION

Egg donation is an ART procedure that involves harvesting eggs from carefully selected donors. The purpose is to ensure that sufficient eggs are available for infertile couples. The first successful use of this method to achieve a pregnancy was in Australia in 1984.[116] Usually, prospective donors should be less than 35 years of age. Prior to selection, they undergo physical and psychological examinations and are screened for infections, STDs, genetic diseases, and drug abuse. Each successful candidate is matched to a recipient couple according to the characteristics they desire.

Most egg donations are anonymous to assure confidentiality, but some couples prefer donations from family members or friends. Generally, the legal aspect of this procedure involves the signing of a consent form, which ensures that both the donor and the recipients understand the issues involved and will respect each other's rights. Donations may be made by women who are undergoing sterilization or by IVF patients who have surplus eggs. The eggs may also come from an altruistic donor or an egg harvesting programme, which provides financial compensation to the donors. For instance, in the United States, donors are paid from $1,000 to $5,000, and the agent also receives from $1,000 to $5,000.[117]

THE PROCEDURE FOR EGG DONATION

Egg donation requires the conventional IVF egg retrieval procedure. In addition, it involves synchronizing the cycles of both the donor and the recipient. Usually, as the donor undergoes ovarian stimulation, oestrogen is administered to the recipient. On the night of the egg retrieval and fertilisation, the recipient is placed on daily progesterone injection to prepare her endometrium for implantation and maintenance of the pregnancy.[118]

[116]C. TURKINGTON – M. ALPER, *Understanding Fertility and Infertility, op. cit.*, p. 52-56.

[117]C. TURKINGTON – M. ALPER, *Understanding Fertility and Infertility, op. cit.*, p. 52-56.

[118]Ibid., p. 53.

INDICATIONS FOR EGG DONATION

The need to resort to egg donation arises when a woman cannot produce eggs of her own, as in the case of women whose infertility arises from premature ovarian failure. It is also used for women whose ovaries have been removed due to disease, for those who do not respond well to ovarian stimulation, and for those who have hormonal problems that interfere with egg production. Because eggs lose fertilisation capacity as women age, some older women may require egg donation to conceive. A fertile woman with a genetic defect may have recourse to it to avoid transmitting the disease to her offspring,[119]and women who have undergone several IVF cycles and failed to achieve pregnancy due to poor egg quality may use egg donation as a last resort.

EMBRYO ADOPTION

Some couples who undergo ART procedures requiring egg retrieval produce surplus eggs that are fertilised and cryopreserved for future use. Sometimes, successful IVF couples no longer require the cryopreserved embryos, and they can choose to destroy them or to donate them to research. Some find these options morally unacceptable, and the resulting attempts to remedy the situation gave rise to embryo donation. This involves anonymously donating one's spare embryos to other IVF couples and reserving no rights over the child that may result.

[119]Cf. J. HARRIS – S. HOLM (eds.), *The Future of Human Reproduction,* Clarendon Press, Oxford New York 1998, p. 6.

CHAPTER 5

ARTIFICIAL REPRODUCTIVE TECHNOLOGIES: THE NIGERIAN SITUATION

ART AND THE NIGERIAN EXPERIENCE

As we discussed in chapter two, the incidence of infertility is quite high in Nigeria. In response this situation, a number of private ART clinics have been set up to provide fertility services to affected couples. Such services have been available in Nigeria since the early 1980s;[1] however, the first IVF pregnancies were not achieved until 1984, and the first live birth did not occur until 1989.

The recent growth of ART in Nigeria was made possible by the technical collaboration between ART units in Nigeria and more established units in the United Kingdom, Denmark, and South Africa.[2] Initially, foreign experts handled the ART procedures in some centres, but today, indigenous reproductive endocrinologists and embryologists have completely taken over this role. Indigenous practitioners continue to work in collaboration with their foreign counterparts, who come at regular intervals to perform treatment cycles and to carry out quality checks. Some of the centres continue to train their staff overseas or to bring in experts to train people in Nigeria.

In spite of the apparent growth in Nigerian ART services, such services are still not widespread. This is related to a number of factors, including the lack of awareness of the availability of the services, the high cost of treatment, and the sociocultural and religious beliefs of the people.

AVAILABILITY OF ART SERVICES

At present, there are only 12 privately owned centres that provide ART services in Nigeria[3]—considering that about 12 million Nigerians are infertile, practitioners consider this largely inadequate. However, the Nigeria Fertility Society (NFS) claims that many more centres are being

---

[1] O. GIWA-OSAGIE *et al.*, "Clinical Profile, Assessment for IVF and the Outcome of IVF in Lagos," 12th World Congress of Fertility and Sterility, 1986, Abstracts, p. 737.

[2] O. GIWA-OSAGIE, "ART in Developing Countries…, *op. cit.,* p. 24.

[3] NIGERIA FERTILITY SOCIETY, Communiqué from the first…, *op. cit.,* p. 1. In reality, there are five ART centres because the others are their subsidiaries.

developed.[4] To compound the problem, these clinics are located in only four major cities out of the 36 States in Nigeria: five in Lagos, three in Abuja, three in Port Harcourt, and one in Aba. Ironically, some of these centres are underutilized. Commenting on this point, Giwa-Osagie asserts that only a few ART centres in sub-Saharan Africa perform enough ART cycles to keep them busy;[5] in the case of Nigeria, he identifies the problem with a lack of participation in the public sector. According to him, this lack of public funding has seriously hindered the availability of ART because setting up an efficient ART centre is capital intensive.[6] Currently, the services provided by most of the units include AIH, AID, IVF, GIFT, ZIFT, Sperm/Oocyte donation, Embryo Donation, Egg-sharing, TESA, MESA, AZH, Cryopreservation, Surrogacy, and the Microsort Sex Selection Technique.

ACCESSIBILITY TO ART

ART procedures are expensive and are largely inaccessible in Nigeria,[7] even though by1989 five hospitals had already acquired the capacity to deliver IVF services.[8] The cost of ART treatment poses a major challenge in Nigeria and precludes an equitable access to services, even though it is only one-sixth to one-third the cost of similar services in the United States and Europe.[9] The cost of IVF treatment ranges from$1,200 to $4,000,

---

[4] Ibid.

[5] O. GIWA-OSAGIE, "Assisted Reproduction Technology or Medically Assisted Conception," A paper delivered in the Department of Obstetrics and Gynecology, College of Medicine, University of Lagos Teaching Hospital, Lagos, March 2004, pp. 6, 15.

[6] Ibid.

[7] O. GIWA-OSAGIE - B. KAYODE, "A Rational Approach to Increasing Access to ART Procedures in Low Resource Countries: Meeting the Challenges of a Public Health and Human Rights Issues," A lecture delivered at the Department of Obstetrics and Gynaecology, University of Lagos, Nigeria, April 2003, pp. 1-2.

[8] See S. AKINTOYE - F. ANENE, "Five Hospitals Acquire Capability…, *op. cit.*, p. 3.

[9] O. GIWA-OSAGIE - B. KAYODE, "A Rational Approach…, *op. cit.*, pp. 1-2.

while the monthly minimum wage in Nigeria is between \$52 and \$60.[10] A large number of infertile couples may be earning less than \$150 dollars per month, and many others may be unemployed.[11] Consequently, many potential ART patients lack the financial resources to undergo treatment, especially considering the fact that success is not assured in one treatment cycle or even in several cycles. In the early years of ART in Nigeria, the existing centres could only perform a few cycles of IVF per year. For instance, from 1999 to 2000, only 50 to 160 cycles were performed in most of the centres. To make the ART services more accessible and to attract potential customers in a competitive market, some centres resort to advertisement and various financial arrangements. For example, the Bridge Clinic in Lagos offers a three-treatment cycle for \$6,000, with a provision to refund any excess payment if pregnancy is achieved within one or two cycles.[12] The NFS continues to explore ways to make the services more accessible and to promote equity in ART delivery without compromising the quality of the services. Some potential solutions are to address the infrastructural decay in Nigeria, to promote collaboration among the various centres for egg-sharing, and to reduce the incidence of multiple pregnancy—and the attendant costs—by transferring only one or two embryos per cycle. The NFS stressed the need to use a low ovulation induction regime for ovarian stimulation and to arrange a pooled procurement of drugs and equipment to reduce costs.[13]

CHALLENGES FOR ART IN NIGERIA

ART equipment, such as freezing systems, sonographic machines, and incubators, requires a steady supply of electricity to function; unfortunately, the power supply in Nigeria is seriously unstable. As a result, ART units must often rely on expensive backup generators. In addition, Nigeria is besieged by other serious infrastructural problems that add

[10] O. GIWA-OSAGIE, "ART in Developing Countries..., *op. cit.,* p. 26. This means that the fertility clinics in Nigeria charge between 156,000 and 520,000 Naira, depending on the particular treatment in question.

[11] As such, many of them resort to spiritual help to resolve their infertility problems.

[12] R. AJAYI, "Nigerian..., *op. cit.,* p. 1.

[13] NIGERIA FERTILITY SOCIETY, "Communiqué from the first..., *op. cit.,* p. 3.

to the numerous challenges faced by ART practitioners. Giwa-Osagie alludes to this when he states that "difficulties often present in assuring the ideal conditions of infrastructure, including water, light and the quality of medical gases for embryo incubations."[14] There is no certainty that these problems will be addressed by the government in the near future, meaning that ART services will continue to be limited.

SUCCESS RATE AND REPORTING SYSTEM

Statistics show that AIH, AID, and standard IVF treatments are the most widely practiced ART methods in Nigeria, with the greater success rates achieved with AIH and AID.[15] IVF pregnancy and live birth rates in Nigerian units are still low compared to figures reported in the developed countries. Giwa-Osagie reports a pregnancy rate of 20% to 42% per embryo transfer and a success rate of "take-home babies" from 10% to 16%.[16]

An important factor affecting the success rate of ART in Nigeria is the relatively high age of couples presenting for fertility treatment. On this, Giwa-Osagie and Kayode maintain that the average age of women who present for ART in some Nigerian centres could be as high as 46 years; this occurs because some couples use ART as a last resort following their failures with other orthodox and unorthodox therapies.[17] Another factor is the refusal of older couples to resort to egg donation on religious, moral, or cultural grounds.[18] Also, the practitioners may not have the same expertise as do their counterparts in the more developed countries.

Modern medical practice should provide the patient with all the scientific information that will help him choose the appropriate treatment. In the area of ART, such information should include the success rate of each technique. In the more established centres in Europe and the United States, well-documented facts are accessible to prospective

[14] O. GIWA-OSAGIE, "ART in Developing Countries..., *op. cit.*, p. 15.

[15] O. GIWA-OSAGIE, "ART in Developing Countries ..., *op. cit.*, pp. 23-25.

[16] O. GIWA-OSAGIE, "Assisted Reproduction..., *op. cit.*, p. 25; ID., "ART in Developing Countries..., *op. cit.*, pp. 23-25. Most centres perform ART in batches and some perform less than 100 cycles per annum.

[17] O. GIWA-OSAGIE - B. KAYODE, "A Rational Approach..., *op. cit.*, p. 5;

[18] Ibid. As these authors claim, only the older couples can afford IVF in Nigeria.

users so they can choose the appropriate treatment. But in Nigeria, Giwa-Osagie and Kayode assert that there is no uniform system of reporting results:

> A review of how ART centers report their results is confusing.... It is desirable that results should be stated by type of ART and terms of pregnancies per stimulation cycle, pregnancies per embryo transfer. The take home baby rate per stimulation cycle as well as rate per embryo transfer are useful statistics.[19]

This situation is disturbing, especially considering the fact that currently there is no way to verify the success rates reported by some of these centres, and there is only minimal information available to the general public.

REGULATION OF ART IN NIGERIA

At present, there are no laws or guidelines regulating the practice of ART in Nigeria, even though the techniques are not morally neutral. Some centres have their own ethics committee, but there is no National Ethics Committee to monitor and review the activities of practitioners and prevent abuses. Commenting on this situation in sub-Saharan Africa, Giwa-Osagie states the following:

> In all the countries surveyed, there is no state regulation of ART. ART practitioners in the sub region, however, stated that they have a voluntary adherence to guidelines set by the American Society of Reproductive Medicine, the British Human Fertilization and Embryology Authority or the equivalent body in France or Germany. Because of the interaction and collaboration of Africa, Australia and America, the African centers voluntarily abide with accepted guidelines from those countries.... Most of the countries do not have national ethics committees.[20]

---

[19] O. GIWA-OSAGIE -B. KAYODE, "Rational Approach..., *op. cit.,* p. 6.

[20] O. GIWA-OSAGIE, "ART in Developing Countries... , *op. cit.,* p. 25. The countries referred to in this survey include Nigeria, Ghana, Cameroon, Togo, Senegal, Benin Republic, Zimbabwe, Kenya and Sierra Leone.

The absence of clear national regulations leaves most clinical decision-making to ART providers and their patients, a situation that is open to abuses and malpractice. However, the NFS is currently studying this problem with the intention of making legal recommendations to the National Assembly.

SOCIOCULTURAL FACTORS THAT PROMOTE WIDE ACCEPTANCE OF ART IN NIGERIA AND AFRICA

ART is relatively new in Nigeria, but it is gradually spreading across the country. Some condemn the majority of the techniques, while others are favourable to them. Our aim in this section is to discuss the sociocultural factors that will promote a wide acceptance of ART in Nigeria.

FACTORS THAT PROMOTE THE SPREAD OF ART

There are several social and cultural factors that can promote a wide acceptance of ART in Nigeria. These range from the importance of children in marriage to the desire for personal immortality.

As a prelude to the discussion of the factors that will foster acceptance of ART in Nigeria, we will review the different types of marriage practiced in this part of the world. This will give us a better insight into the African mentality that underpins the intense desire to marry and have children.

The forms of marriage in Africa are monogamy, polygamy, levirate, ghost, and woman marriages—the main goal of each one is to have children. Monogamy is the practice of being married to only one person at a time. Polygamy involves being married to two or more persons at the same time. In the past, in Nigeria and most African societies, the dominant form of marriage was monogamy, although polygamy was nonetheless practiced in many communities. Levirate marriage is the practice in which a man inherits his dead brother's widow as a wife; in most cases, the consent of the woman is required. This is common in some African regions, such as the eastern part of Nigeria.[21]

Woman marriage should not be confused with same-sex marriage, which is prevalent in popular culture only among westernized people; it is taboo in virtually all traditional African societies. In some parts of Nigeria and sub-Saharan Africa, it is an acceptable practice for a woman to marry the widow of her deceased (childless) brother and permit a relative to cohabit with her. The children from such a union belong to the so-called "husband" of the woman, ensuring that the deceased man has an offspring. The practice of what is termed "ghost marriage" exists in

[21] C. OBI, "Marriage Among the Igbo of Nigeria," in *ATR Special Topics,* See http://www. africaworld.net/afrel/igbo-marriage.htm, p. 7.

some parts of Africa. In this case, if a man dies without children, his clan or community will marry a woman on his behalf to beget children for him and so ensure that his name or lineage does not go into extinction. In other places, if he dies without a male child, one of his daughters is expected to remain in his house and cohabit with a man to beget a male child on behalf of her father. This child will inherit the property of the deceased man and continue his lineage.[22]

As we noted earlier, in traditional African thought, marriage is not merely a contract between a man and a woman; it is also an alliance between their families and relatives, which explains why the consent of parents is essential.[23] It is a fact that the marriage bond does not necessarily cease with the death of one's partner,[24] and any child born in the latter union belongs to the deceased man. This strong desire to have offspring that perpetuate one's name and lineage is what underpins these different forms of marriage.

PRIMARY PURPOSE OF MARRIAGE IN NIGERIA AND AFRICA

In Nigeria, marriage and child-bearing are essential and highly recommended for all members of society.[25] As Mbiti states, they are considered sacred or ethical duties that every normal person must fulfil.[26] As with biblical Jewish culture, infertility is abhorred and childlessness carries a stigma. As one practitioner in Lagos, Nzeagwu, declares, "It would

---

[22] Ibid., p. 7.

[23] J. ATADO, *African Marriage Customs and Church Law: A Case Study of the Igbos,* Modern Printers Limited, Kano, Nigeria 1998, pp. 102-103.

[24] A. SHORTER, *African Culture, An Overview,* Paulines Publications Africa, Nairobi Kenya 2001, p. 89; See also J. MBITI, *Introduction to African Religion, op. cit.,* p. 108.

[25] M. GETUL, "The Evolution of the Family in Africa," in TANGAZA OCCASSIONAL PAPERS/NO. 3, *Theology of the Church as Family of God,* Paulines Publications Africa, Nairobi 1997, p. 44; See also I. IGWEGBE, *The Meaning of the Beginning,* Snaap Press, Enugu 2002, p. 27.

[26] J. MBITI, *Introduction to African Religion, op. cit.,* p. 104; See also A. SHORTER, *African Culture: An Overview, op. cit.,* p. 91. In reality, the need to resolve the problem of childlessness is the reason for some polygamous marriages.

be an abomination for a Nigerian to decide not to have children."[27] As this implies, childlessness is sometimes viewed as a curse;[28] it is extremely stressful for a couple and can damage or destroy their marriage. This is simply because, in Nigeria and Africa as a whole, the primary purpose of marriage is to have children.[29,30] Tangwa asserts that "in African culture, children are highly valued; so highly valued that procreation is considered the main purpose of marriage. In Africa, marriage for mere companionship is rare, if not completely non-existent."[31] The process leading to marriage in a traditional African setting is long and complex; usually, both families conduct extensive pre-marriage investigations[32] to ensure permanence once the union is contracted. The potential absence of children is a serious impediment to a proposed marriage. In fact, when cases of infertility are associated with a particular family, any marriage proposal to a member of that family is ruled out; if the infertility is discovered during the pre-marriage investigations, it may automatically mark the end of that investigation.

[27] NZEAGWU, "Making Pregnancy a Natural Experience..., *op. cit.,* p. 1.

[28] NIGERIA FERTILITY SOCIETY, The Communique of the first..., *op. cit.,* p. 1.

[29] The unitive aspect of marriage does not receive equal emphasis as the procreative aspect. The whole essence of marriage is to cooperate with God to bring a new life into existence for the continuation of the family lineage and human race.

[30] WORLD HEALTH ORGANIZATION, "Assisted Reproduction in Developing Countries–Facing Up to the Issues," *op. cit.,* p. 4; See also J. MBITI, *Introduction to African Religion, op. cit.,* pp. 112-114.

[31] G. TANGWA, "Some African Reflections on Biomedical and Environmental Ethics," in K. WIREDU (ed.), *A Companion to African Philosophy,* Blackwell Publishing Ltd., Oxford 2004, p. 391.

[32] Today, things are changing as a result of the interaction with the West and many young people arrange their own marriages and tend to ignore certain things.

STRONG EMPHASIS ON CHILDREN IN NIGERIA AND AFRICA

Children occupy an extremely important place in traditional African culture[33] and thought. In Nigeria in particular, fertility is seen as a treasure and as a sign of God's favour and the blessing of the ancestors. Marriage and procreation are a unity that cannot be separated in the mind of most Nigerians. In most cultural areas of Africa, marriage is only consummated when a child is born, and it is never complete or successful in the absence of children. The implication is that a childless marriage ceases to be meaningful in the eyes of the people.[34] According to Jonathan Kasule, head of the Department of Obstetrics and Gynaecology at the University of Zimbabwe, "The success of marriage in Africa depends on a woman's ability to have children."[35] Commenting on this, John Mbiti asserts the following:

> In some African societies, marriage is not fully consummated until the wife has given birth. For this reason, there is general abhorrence of barrenness in most African societies. Unhappy is the woman who fails to get children for, whatever qualities she might possess, her failure to bear children is worse than committing genocide: she has become the dead end of human life, not only for the genealogical line but also for herself.[36]

[33] B. IDOWU, *African Traditional Religion: A Definition,* SCM Press, London 1973, p. 104. The phrase "African culture" refers to the way of life of Africans in general and the meaning we give to things. However, different African tribes have their own cultures such that in Nigeria alone, we can speak of Yoruba culture, Igbo culture and so on. Even in the same tribe, there exist certain sub-cultures and practices, but in general, as Bolaji Idowu too observes, the great similarities of the cultural and religious beliefs and practices of Africans seem to make the phrase "African culture" appropriate to a large extent.

[34] Despite the influences of the more liberal Western culture, a very significant number of Nigerians still do not find any meaning in a childless marriage.

[35] S. MATETAKUFA, "Infertility is not just a problem in the West," published in http://www.newint.org/issue303/infertility.html (17/3/2005). In this article, Kusule was quoted by Sue Njanji Matetakufa, a Zimbabwean journalist with special interest in women and health.

[36] J. MBITI, *African Religions and Philosophy, op. cit.,* p. 110.

Only after a woman gives birth does she acquire a new status and respect among her husband's people. Until then, her place in the family is not really guaranteed; with the birth of a child, the bond of marriage between the spouses and their families is fully sealed. This cultural factor will naturally increase the desire for ART among infertile couples, especially when a woman wishes to protect her marriage. The NFS contends that the isolation of infertile couples is a cultural reality that justifies the practice of ART in Nigeria; for the 12 million infertile individuals in Nigeria, this isolation makes effective infertility treatment a priority—and many cases of infertility in Nigeria are only treatable through ART.[37]

FAMILY LINEAGE AND PERSONAL IMMORTALITY

It is essential to note that the various forms of marriage in Nigeria were not aimed at sexual pleasure or promiscuity,[38] contrary to popular belief outside the culture. Apart from minor motives such as economic value and community recognition,[39] they were primarily intended to foster life.[40] The fundamental reason for such marriages was the desire for children based on the people's belief in personal immortality. This is clear in John Mbiti's statement:

> He who has many descendants has the strongest possible manifestation of "immortality," he is "reborn" in the multitude of his descendants, and there are many who remember him after he has died physically and entered

[37] NIGERIA FERTILITY SOCIETY, The Communique of the first..., *op. cit.,* p. 1. Children are so important in Africa to the extent that childlessness is seen as a curse to the family and community.

[38] L. MAGESA, *African Religion..., op. cit.,* p. 137. As Laurenti Magesa asserts, polygamous unions for reasons of concupiscence on the part of African males was not sanctioned by African religion.

[39] Many of the people were farmers and needed more wives and children to assist in farm work and in some communities a man with a large family was considered very successful, a fact that conferred a kind of recognition or social status on him in society.

[40] C. OBI, "Marriage Among the Igbo of Nigeria..., *op. cit.,* p. 7.

> his "personal immortality," such a man has the attitude that "the more we are, the bigger I am."[41]

The different forms of marriage exhibit a strong emphasis on the transmission of life, which is rooted in the desire of Africans to preserve their family lineage and guarantee their personal immortality. In the African world-view, ancestors continue to live in the physical realm as long as their living descendants continue to remember them, but they completely die if there is no one to remember and honour them with libation or physical drinking offerings. Thus, infertility is a tragedy that does not only imply the full death of one's ancestors, but also spells doom for the childless individual who will have no one to remember him and pour out libation to him.[42] Mbiti asserts that a person who has no descendants "in effect quenches the fire of life, and becomes forever dead since his line of physical continuation is blocked if he does not get married and bear children." For this reason, parents forbid their children to remain single and are restless if they cannot have children. Even today, despite the influence of Christianity, Islam, and Western culture, the desire to bear children that will assure personal immortality remains deep and strong. According to Obi, among the Igbo of south eastern Nigeria, "marriage is deemed indispensable and this is because it is necessary for the continuation of the family descent,"[43] such that a childless marriage is regarded by the vast majority of the people as *Chioojo,* or "bad-luck," which will eventually lead to a conflict between the couple. Regarding the wider implication of infertility in African tradition, Bujo states that the idea of fertility is not a private matter restricted to the infertile individual alone. Rather, it extends to his entire fellowship, which comprises the living, the living-dead, and the yet-to-be-born. In African thought pattern, each person

---

[41] J. MBITI, *African Religions and Philosophy, op. cit.,* p. 142.

[42] P. PARIS, *The Spirituality of the African Peoples,* Fortress Press, Minneapolis 1995, p. 84. Some forms of marriages described earlier are meant to ensure that there will be children to remember the dead.

[43] C. OBI, "Marriage Among the Igbo of Nigeria..., *op. cit.,* p. 1. In Africa, parents pray unceasingly for their children to bear children and as Obi states, if you ask an ordinary Igbo man or woman why he or she desires to marry, the spontaneous answer will be: "I want to marry in order to beget my own children." However, this is not limited to the Igbo, but it is a universal phenomenon in Nigeria and Africa.

who generates a child "narrates the biography of his ancestors and writes his own autobiography." Every child that is born represents both the yet-to-be-born and the ancestors; the child keeps alive the memory of the ancestor and symbolizes the continuity of the lineage in its future generations.[44] He concludes, "When so much weight is attached to the birth of a child, it follows that the worst death is to die childless."[45] Concurring, Kabore describes it as the "most abominable death."[46] Thus, the transmission of life, which assures personal immortality and the continuation of the family lineage, is the single most important factor that determines the success of a marriage. Consequently, infertility poses the ultimate challenge to the survival of marriage and the welfare of couples. As Mbiti writes,

> The bearing of children is central to marriage, and no efforts are spared to ensure that there are children in each marriage; otherwise, the couple fails to become a family. In effect, the family never dies; only its members do. If, for example, the husband is impotent, his "brother" (in the wider sense of kinship ties) will (must) sleep with his wife so that she will bear him children. If the wife is barren, her husband will marry another wife, who will be expected to bear children for both wives.[47]

In Nigeria and most parts of Africa, infertility has far-reaching implications; the travails of a childless couple are multifaceted, which makes coping extremely challenging. The exaggerated emphasis on children for personal immortality[48] produces the suffering, shame,

---

[44] B. BUJO, *Foundations of an African Ethic,* Paulines Publication Africa, Nairobi Kenya 2003, p. 58.

[45] Ibid.

[46] E. KABORE, "Identity and Status of the Human Embryo in African Traditional Societies," in J. CORREA - E. SGRECCIA (eds.), *Identity and Statue of the Human Embryo,* Proceedings of the Third Assembly of the Pontifical Academy for Life, Vatican City, February 14-16, 1997, p. 431.

[47] J. MBITI, "African Religion," in W. REICH, *Bioethics: Sex…, op. cit.,* p. 65. However, this is not applicable to some sub-cultures in Nigeria and Africa.

[48] For instance, a childless man is often overwhelmed by the thought of being the end of the genetic line of his family especially if he is an only son and

stigma, and rejection that characterize childlessness in the community. This is, therefore, the principal factor that will foster a wide acceptance of ART in Nigeria and Africa.[49]

PREFERENCE FOR MALE CHILDREN

Because of the patriarchal system, which is prevalent in most African societies, the woman does not enjoy the same social status as the man. It is for this reason that there exists a preference for male children,[50] who are considered more important than female children. Among some ethnic groups, a male child enjoys the right of inheritance to his father's property even while his mother is still living; as such, a woman is never really secure in her matrimonial home until she has given birth to a male child. Even after a couple has female children, the desire to have a male child is almost as strong as if they did not have any children.[51] Consequently, if the techniques of sex selection become affordable in Nigeria, they will be extremely attractive to couples—especially to the men—who are seeking male children. Because family genealogy is traced through the male, the absence of a male child to carry on the family name is to reach a cul-de-sac in the ancestral lineage, a reality that most Nigerian men dread. Additionally, a male child is often preferred for a number of practical reasons. A male child appears to be an asset from a financial standpoint. In the past, when farming was the mainstay of the people, male children (being physically stronger) were more useful on the farm; even now, most men are the breadwinners in their families.

Many African parents believe that a woman will eventually marry into another family, regardless of her relationship with her natural family.

---

besides, he feels he has failed himself and his family.

[49] G. TANGWA, "Some African Reflections on Biomedical…, *op. cit.,* p. 391. Reaching the same conclusion, Godfrey Tangwa maintains that there will be great interest in ART in Africa among infertile couples because of the high premium the culture places on procreation.

[50] I. IGWEGBE, *The Meaning of the Beginning, op. cit.,* p. 27. This preference for a child of a particular sex is a universal phenomenon, but the reasons vary from place to place.

[51] G. WANJOHI, "African Marriage, Past and Present," in *WAJIBU: A Journal of Social and Religious Concern,* Vol. 14, No. 1, 1999, p. 1.

Furthermore, a male child has the right of inheritance to ancestral property in most Nigerian and African cultures, and he has a traditional duty to provide for his parents in their old age. Nevertheless, male children are primarily preferred because they are a symbol of the continuity of life in the family or clan. According to G. J. Wanjohi, it is especially this last factor that makes African marriage an unavoidable duty.[52]

OTHER FACTORS IN FAVOUR OF ART

Long before the introduction of ART, some African communities, such as certain subcultures among the Yoruba of Nigeria, practiced a form of altruistic surrogacy—the distinction being that adultery was adopted as the means of achieving conception. Similarly, in some subcultures among the Igbo of Nigeria, a man may secretly help his infertile friend or relative to impregnate his wife, but this practice is neither common nor culturally sanctioned.[53] Quite naturally, these subcultures will readily accept the techniques of altruistic surrogacy and artificial insemination, provided they are shrouded in secrecy to prevent stigmatization of the couple and the prospective child.

[52] Ibid.

[53] Such an arrangement must be kept secret. If it is known, both the infertile man and the resulting child will be subjects of ridicule in the community.

FACTORS THAT INHIBIT THE SPREAD OF ART

Despite the potential for a wide acceptance of ART in Nigeria, there are some sociocultural and religious factors that militate against the spread of some of the techniques. The key factor is the belief that it is an "unnatural" way to procreate. Although ART has existed in Nigeria for some years now, it is relatively unfamiliar to Nigerians, and society still views it with suspicion. Ordinarily, Nigerians consider a child to be a gift from God that results from sexual intercourse between a man and a woman. Consequently, many find laboratory conception to be absurd or even abominable; however, others are starting to embrace the various techniques because of their practical benefits or their potential for preventing stigmatization.[54] The vast majority of Nigerian couples who use ART do so secretly to elude such stigmatization. Describing a similar finding in her study of ART in Egypt, Inhorn writes,

> IVF in Egypt performs a kind of "double stigmatization," whereby the very treatment designed to overcome an already stigmatizing health condition leads to an additional layer of stigma, secrecy, and suffering.[55]

Another factor that may impede the wide acceptance of ART is the religious attitude of many Nigerians. The tendency of some infertile couples to seek spiritual help—as a replacement for or supplement to medical assistance—may arise from religiosity or ignorance of the causes of infertility. Richardson Ajayi, an ART practitioner, remarks, "Religion has a very strong hold on the people and most throng the churches with the belief that God will eventually cause them to achieve pregnancy." Similarly, Nzeagwu states that Church programmes aimed at helping childless couples to conceive are always filled to capacity.[56] This tendency can also result from the belief that some illnesses have underlying spiritual causes and can only be treated in a spiritual way. It is not unusual for some childless people to attribute their infertility to the witchcraft or

---

[54] R. AJAYI, "Nigeria…, *op. cit.* p. 1.

[55] M. INHORN, *Local Babies, Global Science…, op. cit.,* p. 243.

[56] R. AJAYI, "Nigeria…, *op. cit.,* p. 1; See also NZEAGWU, "Making Pregnancy a Natural Experience…, *op. cit.,* p. 1.

sorcery of their enemies.[57] Additionally, many adherents of religions that prohibit ART procedures are unwilling to use them.

In spite of the sociocultural and religious attitudes that militate against ART, some infertile people in Nigeria will do almost anything to have children; this includes using ART, provided the techniques are affordable and confidentiality can be guaranteed. In this light, an important question arises: Is what is scientifically feasible and pragmatic therefore morally permissible? Is science or technology morally neutral? This will be our focus in the next chapter as we examine the ethical implications of ART.

[57] D. WESTERLUND, "Spiritual Beings as Agents of Illness," in J. OLUPONA (ed.), *African Spirituality..., op. cit.*, pp. 168-169.

CHAPTER 6

ART: RELATED TECHNIQUES

The modern era can be described as the golden age of genetics. The discovery in 1953 of the genetic code, which is one of the most remarkable discoveries in the history of science, has led to many breakthroughs. Today, our world is witnessing tremendous advances in biotechnology and genetic engineering of plants, animals, and human beings, with potential benefits for agriculture, pharmaceuticals, and medicine.[1] Genetic testing in human beings can be performed at several stages of life. Prior to conception, it is achieved through the analysis of the first polar body; prior to implantation, Preimplantation Genetic Diagnosis (PGD) is used; prior to birth, various techniques of prenatal diagnosis are available. It can also be performed after birth and during adulthood, such as when one is considering marriage, is about to enter a particular occupation, or is likely to be at high risk of developing a particular genetic disorder.[2] In this chapter, we are only interested in PGD, sex selection techniques, and human genetic enhancement technology.

---

1 R. LUCAS LUCAS, *Bioetica Per Tutti, op. cit.,* p. 91. Plants and animals can be engineered genetically to produce more food, proteins, milk with valuable medicinal properties (such as vaccines and antibiotics).

2 Neonatal genetic testing involves obtaining an insignificant amount of body fluid or tissue for genetic analysis and in most cases, it is not harmful.

PREIMPLANTATION GENETIC DIAGNOSIS (PGD)

PGD, an aspect of human genetic engineering, is now an established method of ART that is used in conjunction with IVF and ICSI.[3] As Robert Song asserts, it represents a culmination of the developments in the field of artificial reproduction and genetics.[4] PGD is a technique used to determine genetic defects of *in vitro* embryos before they are implanted into a woman.[5] Although Yury Verlinsky and Richard Gardner started working on the concept about 53 years ago, the technology was not developed until 1990;[6] it was first successfully used for a couple at risk of having a child with cystic fibrosis.[7]

The procedure, which is still in the experimental stage, is seen as an alternative to prenatal diagnosis and selective abortion using techniques such as amniocentesis, chorionic villi sampling (CVS), embryoscopy, and ultrasound. Before PGD was developed, prenatal diagnosis was used to detect if a developing embryo had a genetic defect that could cause profound physical suffering, mental retardation, or death. At present, there is little that can be done to remedy such cases, leaving parents with the decision to accept the future child with its defects or to procure an abortion. A serious ethical problem in this situation is that positive indications of a genetic disorder frequently lead to selective abortion; PGD was developed to prevent this problem before conception occurs.

BACKGROUND TO PGD: GENETIC DEFECTS AND THE CAUSES

Most human beings are born healthy, but a few are born with defects. In chapter two, we noted that even though many human embryos are

---

3 Y. VERLINSKY – A. KULIEV, *Atlas of Preimplantation Genetic Diagnosis, Second Edition,* Taylor & Francis, London 2005, p. 2. These authors describe PGD as an integral component of ART and genetic services.

4 R. SONG, *Human Genetics…, op. cit.,* p. 21.

5 B. STEINBOCK, "Perimplantation Genetic Diagnosis and Embryo Selection," in J. BURLEY – J. HARRIS (eds.), *A Companion to Genetics,* Blackwell Publishing Ltd., Malden, MA 2004, p. 175.

6 Y. VERLINSKY – A. KULIEV, *Atlas of Preimplantation…, op. cit.,* p. xiii.

7 S. BAYER – M. ALPER – A. PENZIAS, *The Boston IVF Handbook of…, op. cit.,* p. 88.

conceived with defects, they either do not implant or they are aborted spontaneously. The cause of a birth defector known as a congenital anomaly[8] is categorized as a genetic factor,[9] an environmental factor,[10] or multi-factorial inheritance, which is a combination of the first two. In this section, we are interested in genetic factors, which are the primary objects of PGD.

Genetic disorders can arise from mutations in the gene or chromosome of the cells of the human body. About one-third of all birth defects, and an estimated 85% of those with known causes, are caused by genetic factors.[11] These arise mainly from chromosomal aberrations, single-gene defects, and multi-factorial or polygenic disorders.

CHROMOSOMAL ABERRATIONS OR ABNORMALITIES

Chromosome mutation involves a change in a chromosome; this change may be in number, in large-scale loss or gain of DNA, or in large-scale rearrangement of segments of DNA within or between chromosomes.[12] Chromosomal abnormalities can be either structural or numerical. Usually, it is the gene that undergoes mutation, but sometimes this change can cause chromosomal abnormalities. It is estimated that one out of every 100 newborns presents with this condition.[13]

---

8 K. MOORE – T. PERSAUD, *The Developing Human…, op. cit.,* pp. 158-159. Teratology studies the causes, mechanisms and patterns of abnormal development. About 50–60% of congenital anomalies in humans are unknown.

9 P. FLAMAN, *Genetic Engineering: Christian Values and Catholic Traditions,* Paulist Press, New York 2002, p. 34. Current estimates by scientists suggest that there are about 4,000 human diseases that are hereditary or related to genetic factors.

10 C. AMMER, *The New A to Z of Women's Health…, op. cit.,* p. 47. Environmental factors are factors outside the embryo itself that can cause anomalies in it during gestation and delivery, such as high dosage of radiation, exposure to harmful chemical agents, alcohol consumption, drugs, smoking, virus infections and all kinds of chronic diseases and damages that occur during labour and delivery.

11 Ibid.

12 R. PINON JR., *Biology of Human Reproduction, op. cit.,* p. 42.

13 R. JONES, *Human Reproductive Biology, op. cit.,* p. 178. More than 90% of affected embryos are spontaneously aborted.

The normal chromosome complement of a human being is 46, that is, 22 pairs of autosomes and a pair of sex chromosomes that are maternally and paternally derived. If a change occurs in any of these pairs, chromosomal abnormality in the child will result. Numerical aberrations of chromosomes often arise from nondisjunction during spermatogenesis or oogenesis;[14] these aberrations include *aneuploidy, polyploidy*, and *tetraploidy.* Aneuploidy refers to the presence of an abnormal number of chromosomes in an embryo. It is said to be *monosomy* in the case of a shortage, in which an individual has only 45 chromosomes instead of the normal 46, implying that one of the parental gametes had 22 chromosomes instead of 23. An example is monosomy X, meaning a missing X chromosome arising from an error in gametogenesis. On the other hand, it is *trisomy* if an individual has excess chromosomes, such as 47 chromosomes, meaning that he has three of a particular kind instead of the normal two;[15] this is the case with Down syndrome, which is caused by trisomy 21.[16] This condition arises when a gamete containing 24 chromosomes fuses with a normal gamete containing 23 chromosomes.

Most chromosomal abnormalities are correlated with advanced maternal age. They cause a wide range of diseases, such as severe retardation, brain damage, liver and heart problems, stillbirth, and death during infancy. In fact, most embryos affected by them are spontaneously aborted.[17] This first category of chromosomal defects is generally associated with the autosomes, but there are others that affect only the sex chromosomes, leading to "ambiguities of sex differentiation" in the child. An example is Turner syndrome, which is correlated with advanced paternal age.[18] Polyploidy refers to a condition in which more than one

---

[14] Y. VERLINSKY – A. KULIEV, *Atlas of Preimplantation..., op. cit.*, pp. 38-40; See R. ANGEL, "First Meiotic Division Nondisjunction in Human Oocytes," *Am J Human Genet,* 1997, 65:23-32. More precisely, such changes often occur during the complex process of meiosis during spermatogenesis or oogenesis.

[15] K. MOORE – T. PERSAUD, *The Developing Human..., op. cit.*, p. 162; C. AMMER, *The New A to Z of Women's Health, op. cit.*, p. 47.

[16] Ibid. Others include trisomies 13, 18 and so on.

[17] Ibid.

[18] Ibid.

spermatozoon fertilises an oocyte. It can sometimes result from the failure of the second polar body to disjoin from the oocyte during the second meiotic division, but it usually ensues from *dispermy*, that is, when two spermatozoa fertilise an oocyte almost simultaneously.[19] Tetraploidy refers to the doubling of the normal 46–chromosome complement in an embryo to 92 chromosomes, which seems to occur during the first mitotic division after fertilisation.[20]

In contrast, the majority of structural chromosomal abnormalities occur when a chromosome breaks and the consequent attempt to reconstitute itself results in an abnormal combination. According to Moore and Persuad, this may be caused by various environmental factors, such as radiation, viruses, drugs, and chemicals.[21] They maintain that the only two structural chromosomal abnormalities that a child can possibly inherit from its parents are "structural rearrangements" known as inversion and translocation. While the former refers to a type of chromosomal aberration involving the reversal of a segment of a chromosome,[22] the latter occurs when a piece of one chromosome is transferred to a non-homologous chromosome.[23] If a chromosome breaks and part of it is lost, we call this deletion.

GENE MUTATION: SINGLE-GENE DEFECTS

Every biological species has a specified number of chromosomes in its cells; these are composed of genes, which contain the information

---

[19] K. MOORE – T. PERSAUD, *The Developing Human…, op. cit.,* p. 165. Triploidy, as in the case of an embryo with 69 chromosomes, is the most common type of *polyploidy*.

[20] Ibid., pp. 166-168.

[21] Ibid., p. 166.

[22] Ibid., p. 162.

[23] Ibid., pp. 166-168. Moore and Persuad explain that translocation could be reciprocal, in which case two non-homologous chromosomes exchange their broken pieces. An individual who carries a translocation between chromosomes 21 and 14 have a normal phenotype and is said to carry a balanced translocation. It is vital to note that a translocation does not necessarily cause abnormal development and it does not follow that a person carrying it will suffer from the genetic disease. Instead, he or she may be at risk of transmitting it to his or her offspring since such carriers have a tendency to produce gametes with abnormal translocation chromosome.

for the elaboration of every protein.[24] As Roy, Williams, and Dickens explain, genes contain two chains of nucleotides "intertwined in the form of a double helix," and they comprise "long molecules of DNA composed of four units known as adenine (A), thymine (T), cytosine (C), and guanine (G) known as nucleotides."[25] In the mid-1960s, extensive research by many scientists established DNA as the "basic chemical logic of life."[26] The underlying logic is well-articulated in this statement:

> That logic can be summarized in four interlinked steps, somewhat as follows: The properties of living organisms result from the proteins they contain, and the human organism contains 30,000 proteins; the proteins are determined by the sequence of the amino acids of which they are constituted; the amino acid sequence, in turn, is governed by the order of the nucleotides in messenger RNA; and that order is determined by the sequence of nucleotides in the DNA of the genes.[27]

This implies that any irregularity in the sequence of nucleotides at the DNA level can cause a genetic disorder. Mutations are changes in DNA that cause gene disorder,[28] indicating that genetic disorders can result from mutations in a single gene, in several genes, or in the chromosome. At present, scientists have catalogued over 4,000 such disorders; among these, the single-gene or "monogenic" disorders account for 7% to 8% of incurable congenital diseases.[29] The genes in the human body

---

[24] R. LUCAS LUCAS, *Bioetica per Tutti, op. cit.*, pp. 83-84, 86.

[25] D. ROY – J. WILLIAMS – B. DICKENS, *Bioethics in Canada, op. cit.*, pp. 441-442. Cited in P. FLAMAN, *Genetic Engineering…, op. cit.*, p. 3; R. LUCAS LUCAS, *Bioetica per Tutti, op. cit.*, pp. 83-84. Some scientists made this finding in the early 1950s. Genes are lined up on chromosomes contained in every cell of the body.

[26] P. FLAMAN, *Genetic Engineering…, op. cit.*, p. 3.

[27] D. ROY – J. WILLIAMS – B. DICKENS, *Bioethics in Canada, op. cit.*, p. 442. Cited in P. FLAMAN, *Genetic Engineering…, op. cit.*, p. 3.

[28] M. SELLER, "Genes, Genetics and the Human Genome: Some Personal Reflection," in C. DEANE-DRUMMOND (ed.), *Brave New World?* T&T Clark Ltd., New York, p. 31.

[29] R. PINON JR., *Biology of Human Reproduction, op. cit.*, p. 335.

are lined up on the chromosomes and occur in pairs.[30] A single gene defect arises from a mutation in one of a pair of genes. Gene mutations are random changes in the nucleotide sequence in DNA;[31] many of these involve the substitution of a single nucleotide, while others are additions or deletions of a small number of nucleotides.[32] Such mutations produce a loss or change in the normal function of a particular gene. Any permanent, transmittable change in the sequence of the DNA[33] can be inherited at birth. Stressing this point, Pinon states that most changes in the nucleotide sequence of a gene's DNA will alter the amino acid sequence in the protein encoded by that gene, leading to protein disorder; the mutant protein may not function at all or may only fulfil part of its normal functions. This, in turn, compromises vital functions of the tissues or cells and leads to potentially serious consequences for health and well-being.[34] The current belief is that most gene mutations are transmitted to offspring by men rather than women. This is because all of a woman's eggs are produced before birth, meaning they have no need to undergo further meiosis. In contrast, the germ cells that produce sperm continue to undergo meiosis throughout a man's life, which increases the chances of gene mutations as a man advances in age.[35]

---

[30] C. AMMER, *The New A to Z of Women's Health, op. cit.*, p. 173. The human body contains 46 chromosomes, which occur in pairs (22 pairs of autosomes and a pair of sex chromosomes). Each pair contains genes that govern the same trait, but they are not necessarily identical. For instance, in a plant, one of the paired chromosomes may have a gene for blue flower while the other has a gene for white.

[31] Ibid., p. 48; R. PINON JR., *Biology of Human Reproduction, op. cit.*, pp. 42-44.

[32] R. PINON JR., *Biology of Human Reproduction, op. cit.*, p. 42. D. ROY – J. WILLIAMS – B. DICKENS, *Bioethics in Canada,* Prentice Hall Canada Inc., Scarborough, Ontario 1994, pp. 441-442; Cited in P. FLAMAN, *Genetic Engineering…, op. cit.*, p. 3.

[33] K. MOORE – T. PERSUAD, *The Developing Human…, op. cit.*, p. 168.

[34] R. PINON JR., *Biology of Human Reproduction, op. cit.*, p. 42.

[35] C. AMMER, *The New A to Z of Women's Health, op. cit.*, p. 48.

TYPES OF SINGLE-GENE MUTATIONS

The different expressions of a single gene are known as *alleles*. The normal or wild-type allele encodes the protein that properly carries out a normal function in the body. Mutations produce different alleles. This mutant gene either causes the loss of the gene's proper function or encodes proteins that disrupt the gene's proper function. The effect of such a disruption can range from minor to severe, depending on the site of the mutation. However, it is crucial to note that merely possessing a genetic factor does not necessarily mean that a person will suffer from the associated disease. Instead, it may only indicate that the person has an inherited predisposition to it. In general, single-gene mutations can be either dominant or recessive.

Recessive Gene Defect: Some defective genes are recessive. Each chromosome in our cells is composed of two homologs. The mutant allele may affect one or both homologs. If only one of the homologs of the autosomal genes or of the female sex chromosome XX carries the mutant allele, the normal allele can hide the loss of function in the defective allele. This type of mutation is termed recessive because a person with recessive traits has one normal and one abnormal allele. Most mutant genes are recessive and can be masked by the normal gene such that they are not expressed. Unlike dominant genes, recessive genes will not be expressed in the offspring; however, if both parents carry this recessive gene, each one of their children will have a 25% chance of inheriting it.[36] An example of this is sickle-cell anaemia, which is common in sub-Saharan Africa. If the recessive gene is X-linked, meaning it affects only the X-female sex chromosome, there is a 50% chance of transmitting it

---

[36] M. FEINMAN, "Preimplantation Genetic Diagnosis (PGD)," in *The Fertility Network,* in http://www.fertilitynetwork.com/articles/articles-pgd.htm. Single gene disorders could carry either recessive traits or dominant traits. On average, if both parents with recessive traits (such as cystic fibrosis) procreate, about 50% of their offspring will inherit a copy of the abnormal *allele* and 25% will have two copies of the abnormal allele, meaning that they will be affected by the disease. On the contrary, one copy of the abnormal *allele* is enough to cause the disease in those with the dominant traits and their offspring have a 50% chance to inherit the gene and, therefore, the disease.

to male offspring, who carry only one X sex chromosome.[37] Thus, male offspring are inherently more vulnerable to X-linked disorders. As Christine Ammer explains,

> Genes for certain traits other than sex are located on the X chromosome. When a male offspring inherits such a trait on his X chromosome, there may be no matching gene on the Y chromosome to effect a possible repair. So, that trait will invariably be shown. A female offspring, on the other hand, has two X chromosomes, so even if she inherits such a trait it may be masked by another, more dominant gene for the same trait on the other X chromosome. For this reason certain characteristics, called sex-linked or X-linked characteristics, appear far more often in men than in women; among them are red-green color blindness and the blood-clotting disorder hemophilia.[38]

Dominant Gene Mutation: Genetic diseases can also be dominant, as is the case with Huntington's disease. Dominant mutation occurs with the synthesis of a mutant protein that distorts or interferes with the function of the normal protein. Dominant mutation is a serious condition—those affected by it often do not survive. In marked contrast to recessive gene mutations, if one of the parents has a dominant gene mutation, each child has a 50% chance of inheriting the disorder.[39]

MULTIFACTORIAL OR POLYGENIC DISORDERS

A multifactorial or polygenic disorder refers to a gene defect that is related to more than one gene; these account for about 25% of congenital diseases such as neural tube defects, congenital heart disease, diabetes,

---

[37] C. AMMER, *The New A to Z of Women's Health…, op. cit.,* pp. 173-174. Examples of the X-linked diseases include haemophilia and Duchenne Muscular Dystrophy.

[38] Ibid.

[39] Ibid., p. 48. Dominance or recessive refers to individual phenotypes within a genotype. For instance, the sickle cell is a genotype, but sickle cell *anaemia* is merely a phenotype (a recessive trait) associated with it. At present, scientists have identified as many as about 1,200 dominant-gene disorders.

and schizophrenia.[40] These disorders usually result from interactions between the pairs of genes and from environmental factors.[41]

DISTINCTION BETWEEN SOMATIC AND GERMINAL MUTATIONS

In chapter one, we stated that the two types of cells in the human body are somatic cells and germ cells. Mutation can occur in both types of cells, but with differing effects. Somatic mutations occur only in the bodily cells and therefore can only affect the person who experienced the mutation.[42] In contrast, mutations that occur in the germ cells can be transmitted through the gametes to one's children. Such disorders are hereditary and, consequently, much more serious.

PROCEDURE FOR PGD

PGD involves testing the DNA of the cell contained in a polar body or blastomere for chromosomal abnormalities or single-gene defects.[43] The overall goal is to have a healthy child; to this end, PGD employs three main procedures: polar body biopsy, cleavage stage biopsy, and blastocyst stage biopsy. The Polymerase Chain Reaction (PCR) technique is used for single-gene defects, while Fluorescent in Situ Hybridization (FISH) analysis is used for chromosomal aberrations, such as aneuploidies. The two general approaches to PGD are the analysis of the genetic material from the maternal gametes and the testing of a cell removed from an early embryo or blastocyst. As a general practice, only embryos that are free of genetic diseases are implanted into the woman's uterus. We will attempt to describe the procedure briefly.

POLAR BODY BIOPSY (PBB1 AND PBB2)

First polar body biopsy (PBB1) and second polar body biopsy (PBB2) are PGD methods that analyse the DNA from the first polar body, which is extruded by the egg during ovulation, and from the second polar body, which is extruded after penetration by the sperm. If the testing is intended to identity chromosomal abnormalities or to establish gender

---

40 R. PINON JR., *Biology of Human Reproduction, op. cit.*, pp. 335-336.

41 C. AMMER, *The New A to Z of Women's Health..., op. cit.*, p. 48.

42 R. PINON JR., *Biology of Human Reproduction, op. cit.*, pp. 43-44.

43 Y. VERLINSKY – A. KULIEV, *Atlas of Preimplantation..., op. cit.*, p. 15.

for X-linked diseases, the genetic material is removed from the first and second polar bodies and examined at the chromosomal level.[44] In PBB, the zona pellucida of the oocyte is cut open and a micropipette is inserted to aspirate the polar body through a gentle suction, making it possible for its genetic material to be analysed. Both polar bodies can be removed simultaneously, but if the PGD is for single-gene defects, they have to be removed separately to prevent DNA contamination. Using polar bodies for PGD is advantageous because they do not have any biological significance for the development of the embryo.[45] However, there are also some limitations. It is a cumbersome and labour-intensive procedure; furthermore, the results of the analysis are not certain because errors can occur during the cleavage divisions of the embryo. Also, PBB cannot detect mutations of paternal origin because the sperm is not examined.[46]

CLEAVAGE STAGE BIOPSY

The most common clinically used biopsy is blastomere or cleavage stage embryo biopsy. The procedure involves creating embryos outside the womb through IVF or ICSI and then incubating them in the laboratory for about three days. At the 6- to 10-cell stage of early embryonic development, one or two[47] blastomeres can be removed with a micropipette[48] for analysis with FISH or PCR, depending on the nature of the genetic disorder being investigated.[49] A micro needle is used to make a V-shaped or square-shaped hole in the ZP to allow the micro-pipette

---

[44] Ibid., p. 29. Although PGD was initially introduced for pre-existing genetic conditions, the most common uses for PGD worldwide are: testing for aneuploidies and establishing sex for embryos to avoid X-linked diseases.

[45] L. SPERROF – M. FRITZ, *Clinical Gynecologic…, op. cit.,* p. 1239.

[46] R. ANGELL, "Possible Pitfalls in Preimplantation Diagnosis of Chromosomal Disorders Based on Polar Body Analysis," *Hum Reprod*, 9:181, 1994. Cited in L. SPERROF – M. FRITZ, *Clinical Gynecologic…, op. cit.,* p. 1239.

[47] C. LEWIS – T. PINEL *et al.*, "Controlling Misdiagnosis Errors in Preimplantation Genetic Diagnosis: A Comprehensive Model Encompassing Extrinsic and Intrinsic Sources of Error," *Hum Reprod,* 16:43, 2001.

[48] Y. VELINSKY – A. KULIEV, *Atlas of Preimplantation…, op. cit.,* p. 21.

[49] L. SPERROF – M. FRITZ, *Clinical Gynecologic…, op. cit.,* p. 1239. FISH is used when the standard IVF procedure is used for genetic analysis, while PCR analysis is utilized in procedures involving ICSI.

enough room to retrieve the blastomeres. Then a micropipette is inserted to slowly aspirate the blastomeres into the pipette without breaking or disrupting the embryo. Although a single cell may be used for analysis, removal of two cells is generally recommended. Since about 50% of cleavage stage embryos present with mosaicism, removal of two cells may improve the diagnostic accuracy of PGD. This practice does not affect the viability of the embryo[50] as the remaining blastomeres can develop into a normal child. The 8-cell stage is considered optimal for embryo biopsy, because after this time the cells begin to compact.[51] Two major advantages of blastomere biopsy[52] are the ability to test both paternal and maternal genetic materials and the ability to differentiate between normal, carrier, and disease status.[53]

BLASTOCYST STAGE BIOPSY

Blastocyst biopsy is performed five to six days after fertilisation, when the embryo has about 100 cells; this reduces the potential for damage to occur from the removal of one or two cells for PGD.[54] Although it is not yet used clinically in many ART centres, blastocyst biopsy provides the potential benefit of confirming the results from polar body and blastomere diagnosis.[55] However, a major disadvantage of culturing the embryo to this stage is that it leaves insufficient time for proper analysis of the cells before transfer.

---

[50] Y. VELINSKY – A. KULIEV, *Atlas of Preimplantation..., op. cit.,* p. 21. These authors state that follow-up studies suggest that the removal of one or two blastomeres at this stage has no adverse effect on the embryo or children resulting from the technique.

[51] G. NIKAS – A. AO *et al.*, "Compaction and Surface Polarity in the Human Embryo *in vitro*," *BiolReprod*, 55:32, 1996. The adhesion of the membranes of the cells to one another usually makes biopsy more difficult at this stage of early embryonic development.

[52] Y. VERLINSKY – A. KULIEV, *Atlas of Preimplantation..., op. cit.,* p. 29.

[53] M. FEINMAN, "Preimplantation Genetic Diagnosis (PGD)..., *op. cit.*

[54] S. CARSON – W. GENTRY *et al.*, "Trophectoderm Microbiopsy in Murine Blastocysts: Comparison of Four Methods," *J. Assist Reprod Genet*, 10:427, 1993. Blastocyst biopsy is also known as trophectoderm biopsy.

[55] Y. VERLINSKY – A. KULIEV, *Atlas of Preimplantation..., op. cit.,* p. 22.

TECHNIQUES FOR DIFFERENT DISORDERS

As discussed previously, PCR is used to detect single-gene disorders, while FISH or PCR can be used to detect chromosomal abnormalities and X-linked disorders.

PCR FOR SINGLE-GENE DISORDER

Polymerase Chain Reaction (PCR) is used to detect single-gene disorders; specific probes exist for each disorder. The test involves obtaining genetic material either from polar bodies or blastomeres and examining it at the level of DNA sequence.[56] PGD for single-gene disorders requires the ICSI technique in order to avoid cell contamination during polar body removal or during embryo biopsy.[57] If both polar bodies are used, they are removed separately to avoid DNA contamination, which can lead to misdiagnosis.[58] This misdiagnosis is caused by a technical problem or by the phenomenon of preferential amplification, also known as allele dropout (ADO), which can cause an abnormal gene to go undetected, making an embryo appear normal when it actually carries a genetic disorder.[59]

FISH OR PCR FOR CHROMOSOMAL ABERRATIONS AND X-LINKED DISORDERS

FISH is used to detect chromosomal aberrations[60] and to determine the sex of an embryo in sex-linked disorders. Of the 46 human chromosomes, the only nine that can be screened at present are 13, 14, 15, 16, 18, 21, 22, and the two sex chromosomes X and Y. In FISH analysis, labelled fluorescent probes bind to the chromosomes being investigated

---

[56] Ibid., pp. 50, 54-56; See also M. FEINMAN, "Preimplantation Genetic Diagnosis (PGD)..., *op. cit.,* pp. 1-2. PCR allows a single gene or DNA to be copied more than a billion times in a matter of hours. DNA strands are cut into smaller pieces by the action of enzymes and are allowed to recombine again. The presence of abnormal genes causes them to align differently, making it possible to detect them. At present, it is mostly used to examine a single-gene defect called cystic fibrosis (CF).

[57] Ibid., pp. 19-20. ICSI is performed under control of inverted microscope.

[58] Ibid., pp. 8, 18.

[59] M. FEINMAN, "Preimplantation Genetic Diagnosis (PGD)..., *op. cit.,* pp. 1-2.

[60] Y. VERLINSKY – A. KULIEV, *Atlas of Preimplantation..., op. cit.,* p. 1.

and are then visible under a fluorescent microscope. This allows about five chromosomes to be examined together.[61] Currently, most PGD procedures for single-gene disorders are performed by determining gender for X-linked diseases, using either the PCR or FISH techniques.[62] As Verlinsky and Kuliev suggest, an alternative would be to limit diagnosis for X-linked disorders to polar body analysis; this would identify mutations arising from the female, which is appropriate because mutations involved in X-linked diseases are usually of maternal origin.[63]

THE INDICATIONS FOR PGD

Because most chromosomal aberrations in embryos are of maternal origin and because their likelihood increases with age, PGD is indicated in women over 35 years of age. It is also required when a couple is carrying structural (genetic) abnormalities, such as balanced translocations. Although this disease may not be expressed in female offspring who inherit an identical balanced translocation, a male offspring may inherit unbalanced translocations that will be expressed with severe consequences.

The presence of a previous child affected by a genetic disease, such as an X-linked disorder, a chromosomal abnormality, or a single-gene disorder, may be an indication for PGD. Additionally, it is indicated in a couple with a known history of genetic disease in the family,[64] with past exposure to large doses of ionizing radiation or mutagenic chemicals, or with the desire to avoid transmitting a particular genetic disease to their offspring.

---

[61] M. FEINMAN, "Preimplantation Genetic Diagnosis (PGD)..., *op. cit.*

[62] EUROPEAN SOCIETY OF HUMAN REPRODUCTION AND EMBRYOLOGY, "Preimplantation Genetic Diagnosis," Consortium Data Collection III, May 2002, *Hum Reprod,* 2002; 17, 233-246. Technically, it is easier to identify female embryos using FISH or DNA analysis.

[63] Y. VERLINSKY – A. KULIEV, *Atlas of Preimplantation..., op. cit.,* p. 56. In this way, further testing of the embryos after testing the polar bodies will not be required and the pre-selected oocytes can then be implanted irrespective of their gender or any contribution from the father.

[64] L. MASTROIANNI JR., "Reproductive Technologies: Introduction," in W. REICH (ed.), *Encyclopedia of Bioethics..., op. cit.,* p. 2211.

PGD is used by a couple who cannot conceive with IVF despite good sperm quality and by couples whose infertility is caused by severe defect in sperm production. It is also indicated in women with a history of miscarriage, stillbirth, or babies who die shortly after birth.

THE USES OF PGD

PGD is mainly therapeutic because it was originally designed and used to detect and prevent genetic diseases in embryos. Following PGD, only unaffected embryos with optimal potential for implantation and development are transferred into the woman's uterus; this helps to ensure the birth of a healthy baby.[65] The X-linked diseases, such as haemophilia, are only expressed in males, and PGD is used to prevent them by sexing the child to be female. In other words, once the sex of each embryo is determined, only female embryos are transferred into the woman's uterus. The use of PGD for gender selection to avoid a disease is considered therapeutic.

Since 1996, PGD has been used to detect balanced translocations in couples,[66] which increase the risk of miscarriage and chromosomal abnormalities. A couple is said to have a balanced translocation if both of them carry a recessive gene or one of them carries a dominant trait that will be expressed in their offspring and passed on from one generation to the next.[67] PGD can detect such a balanced translocation. If they are healthy, such information allows them to proceed with pregnancy without anxiety; if not, depending on their health status or the level of the risks, they can sex their child to avoid X-linked disorders, resort to egg donation, or avoid having children altogether. Due to the use of

[65] A. KULIEV – Y. VERLINSKY, "Thirteen Years Experience of Preimplantation Genetic Diagnosis," *Reprod Biomed Online,* 2002; 4:183.

[66] M. FEINMAN, "Preimplantation Genetic Diagnosis…, *op. cit.;* See also S. MUNNE, "Preimplantation Genetic Diagnosis of Numerical and Structural Chromosome Abnormalities," *Reprod Biomed Online,* 2002; 4:183. Although such couples are healthy, they have a highly increased incidence of spontaneous abortions or miscarriages.

[67] Ibid.

PGD, a four-fold reduction in the rate of spontaneous abortion has been reported for couples carrying translocations.[68]

As we stated previously, the risk of chromosomal abnormalities in embryos is high in humans and increases with age. About 90% of such embryos abort spontaneously. PGD for chromosomal aberrations, such as aneuploidy testing with FISH, is used to improve the efficiency of ART for women who are over age 35 and for other poor-prognosis IVF patients.[69] This is because PGD reduces the risk of spontaneous abortion in a dramatic way, namely, by allowing only unaffected embryos to be transferred into the woman. For instance, a 23.2% clinical pregnancy rate is cited for IVF–PGD for patients with maternal age of 38.5 years and using 2.3 embryos per transfer; this compares to 15.2% pregnancy rate for 2.9 embryos per transfer for IVF patients of the same age when PGD was not used.[70] This also demonstrates that PGD can reduce the number of transferred embryos and thereby reduce the risk of multiple pregnancy.

Human Leukocyte Antigen (HLA) typing during PGD was introduced in 2000; in addition to preventing genetic disorders, it offers a treatment opportunity to the older siblings of the future child who suffer from a congenital or acquired bone marrow disease.[71] In this case, the prospective child can be a stem cell donor to his sick sibling and possibly save his life. To achieve this feat, HLA-matched unaffected embryos were created and implanted into the woman, and at the time of delivery, the physician collected cord blood for stem cell transplantation, leading to complete cure in a sibling with *fanconi anaemia*.[72]

---

68 Ibid.

69 Y. VERLINSKY – A. KULIEV, *Atlas of Preimplantation…, op. cit.*, pp. 29, 67. More than half of the oocytes and embryos produced by poor-prognosis IVF patients have been found to be chromosomally abnormal, while at least, half of their chromosomally normal embryos have *mosaicism*.

70 Ibid., p. 39.

71 Y. VERLINSKY – S. RECHITSKY – W. SCHOOLCRAFT *et al.*, "Preimplantation Diagnosis for Fanconi Anemia Combined with HLA Matching," *J Am Med Assoc*, 2001; 285:3130-3133; See also Y. VERLINSKY– A. KULIEV, *Atlas of Preimplantation…, op. cit.*, p. 60.

72 Ibid.

The scientific information offered by PGD better equips the physician to counsel patients who do not produce normal embryos; such patients are advised to avoid wasting time and resources on standard IVF and to consider egg or embryo donation. Finally, PGD can be used to pre-select the gender of a future child for non-therapeutic purposes, such as family balancing.

THE LIMITATIONS OF PGD

PGD is still in its experimental stage and carries certain limitations. It is an invasive and cumbersome procedure[73] that requires IVF or ICSI and therefore involves all the associated risks, stress, and uncertainty of these procedures. In addition, the technique cannot detect certain genetic conditions that are detectable by traditional prenatal diagnosis, such as spina bifida and anencephaly;[74] this means that abortion may still be desired if prenatal diagnosis[75] reveals a genetic disorder that PGD did not detect.[76] Such misdiagnosis may arise from DNA contamination.

PGD does not guarantee that an offspring will not be affected by a genetic disease for which a test has been performed. This is due to the problem of mosaicism, which presents the ultimate challenge to the accuracy of PGD. In embryo biopsy, one or two cells that are removed and analysed may not reveal the exact genetic health status of each of the embryo's remaining cells. For instance, as Verlinsky and Kuliev maintain, accumulated studies show that about half of all cleaving embryos are mosaic.[77] Likewise, mosaicism can lead to misdiagnosis at the blastocyst stage biopsy because the inner cell mass of the embryo can carry

---

[73] PGD is a labour-intensive procedure. Polar body biopsy requires the removal of the first and second polar bodies, while blastomere and blastocyst biopsies require the removal of one or two blastomeres from the early embryo for analysis.

[74] B. STEINBOCK "Preimplantation Genetic..., *op. cit.*, p. 176-177.

[75] L. SPERROFF – M. FRITZ, *Clinical Gynecologic...*, *op. cit.*, p. 1239. Speaking on certain limitations of PGD, Leon Speroff and Marc Fritz assert that since the current methods are subject to several sources of potential error, conventional prenatal diagnosis is recommended to confirm the accuracy of PGD.

[76] B. STEINBOCK, "Preimplantation Genetic..., *op. cit.*, p. 177.

[77] Y. VERLINSKY – A. KULIEV, *Atlas of Preimplantation...*, *op. cit.*, p. 30.

abnormal cells; this is contrary to the initial prediction that such cells derive exclusively from the *trophectoderm.*[78] Such an error may cause viable embryos to be discarded and affected embryos to be implanted, leading to the birth of an unhealthy child.

At present, the techniques of PGD cannot test all 24 chromosomes that can cause a genetic disorder, and it cannot detect some rearrangements, such as chromosome insertion and inversion;[79] thus there is a limit to the number of genetic diseases the technology can detect and prevent. Certain single-gene diseases, such as cystic fibrosis, have both mild and severe forms. PGD analysis may not give a clear prognosis of how severely affected the future child would be, causing the embryo to be discarded.[80] In addition to the fact that it is a cumbersome and expensive technique, the success rate of IVF-PGD is simply not high enough. While IVF-PGD costs about $20,000 to screen for a single disease,[81] a pregnancy rate of about 20% is cited when it is used to test for single-gene disorders, and about 26% is cited when testing for aneuploidies.[82]

[78] S. EVSIKOV – Y. VERLINSKY, "Mosaicism in Inner Cell Mass of Human Blastocysts," *Hum. Reprod,* 1998; 13: 3151-3155.

[79] V. JOBANPUTRA – A. SOBRINO *et al,* "Multiplex Interphase FISH as a Screen for Common Aneuploidies in Spontaneous Miscarriages," *Hum Reprod,* 2002, 17: 1166; See Y. VERLINSKY– A. KULIEV, *Atlas of Preimplantation..., op. cit.,* p. 43. At present, scientists cannot test an embryo for every single chromosome or single-gene factor. According to these authors, "complete *karyotyping* is not even realistic in the near future."

[80] P. FLAMAN, *Genetic Engineering..., op. cit.,* p. 42.

[81] Ibid., p. 42.

[82] M. FEINMAN, "Preimplantation Genetic Diagnosis (PGD)..., *op. cit.*

SEX SELECTION AND ARTIFICIAL REPRODUCTION

Staggering advances in genetics and reproductive medicine have made it scientifically feasible for couples to choose the sex of their future children. Sex selection can be defined as "a medical process in which a couple chooses the sex of their unborn child."[83] The attempt by couples to influence the sex of their unborn child is not a new phenomenon. In fact, Turkington and Alper trace it to the ancient civilizations of China, Egypt, and Greece, in which several myths described what a couple could do, preconceptionally and during gestation, to influence the sex of their child.[84]

According to John McMillan, "Sex selection techniques usually refer to methods that can be used to help ensure that children are of a specific sex."[85] Preconception, preimplantation, and prenatal techniques are currently employed to achieve this feat.

SEX SELECTION WITH PRENATAL DIAGNOSIS

The earliest method of sex selection was infanticide, which was practiced in many places. A child of the undesired sex was killed after birth because there was no way to determine the sex of the child *in utero*. Since the 1950s, science and technology have been used to pursue this goal. Prenatal diagnosis, which originally was intended to detect genetic disease, was also applied to sex selection.[86] The procedure involves

---

[83] C. TURKINGTON – M. ALPER, *Understanding Fertility and Infertility, op. cit.*, p. 139.

[84] Ibid., p. 139; B. LEROY, "Reproduction, Ethics, Sex Selection," in T. MURRAY – M. MEHLMAN, *Encyclopedia of Ethical, Legal and Policy Issues in Biotechnology, Vol. 2,* John Wiley and Sons Inc., New York 2000, p. 969. Some of the things believed to influence the sex of an unborn child include the diet of the woman, the position of the couple during intercourse, the time of intercourse and similar.

[85] J. MCMILLAN, "Reproductive Technologies: Sex Selection," in S. POST (ed).), *Encyclopedia of Bioethics…, op. cit.*, p. 2267.

[86] J. MCMILLAN, "Reproductive Technologies: Sex Selection," in S. POST (ed.), *Encyclopedia of Bioethics…, op. cit.*, p. 2267. With the development of ultrasound in the 1970s, it became possible to know the sex of a child *in utero* and to proceed to abortion if it was not of the desired sex.

invasive and non-invasive techniques, such as amniocentesis, chorionic villi sampling, and ultrasound; these are able to determine the sex of the foetus, allowing the parents to proceed with abortion if its sex is not what the couple desires. The limited accuracy of these techniques poses a problem, however. Some may produce false-positives or false-negatives, and many of the invasive techniques are associated with risks of abortion and malformation in otherwise normal embryos.[87]

SEX SELECTION WITH SPERM SORTING TECHNIQUES

The Y-chromosome–bearing sperm supplied by the male during coitus determines the sex of the child. The fundamental procedure of the preconception techniques is to separate the X-bearing sperm from the Y-bearing sperm and inseminate the woman with the sperm that corresponds to the desired sex.[88] In general, sperm sorting techniques involve obtaining semen through masturbation and then separating the Y- and X-carrying sperm in the laboratory. Here, we will briefly discuss the preconception techniques currently available in the reproductive market, even though some of them are not considered scientific.

RONALD ERICSSON'S METHOD

The sperm sorting technique developed by Ronald Ericsson separates the Y-sperm and the X-sperm on the basis of their movement: the Y-sperm is lighter and faster than the X-sperm. Ericsson's technique attempts to sort them by placing them in a test-tube containing albumen and allowing them to swim to the bottom. The Y-sperm reach the bottom of the tube faster and can be separated to a certain degree from the X-sperm.[89] The main limitation of this technique is that it may be impossible to completely separate the X- and Y-sperm, meaning that certainty is not assured. In spite of the 70% success rate that is sometimes reported, some do not consider this method scientific and reliable.

---

87 P. FLAMAN, *Genetic Engineering…, op. cit.*, p. 35-36.

88 If they desire a boy, the Y-chromosome carrying sperm are used to fertilise the ovum and if they desire a girl, the X-chromosome carrying sperm are used.

89 R. JONES, *Human Reproductive Biology, op. cit.*, p.176.

THE LANDRUM SHETTLES METHOD

The Landrum Shettles technique of sex selection uses the timing of intercourse. The basic idea is that, since the X-sperm live longer than the Y-sperm, the fertilising capability of the X-sperm lasts longer.[90] On this basis, Shettles insists that to enhance the chances of having a boy, a couple should abstain from intercourse until the time of the woman's ovulation, because abstinence increases the number of Y-sperm in the ejaculate.[91] If they wish to increase their chances of having a female child, they should time their intercourse to take place about three days before ovulation, since the X-sperm generally live longer.[92] Despite the 80% success rate cited in some books,[93] the scientific correctness and reliability of the technique is controversial, especially as recent studies fail to establish any relationship between the timing of intercourse and the sex ratio of males to females.[94] With this, we will now shift our attention to the two scientifically acknowledged and verifiable techniques of sex selection: the Microsort technique and IVF-PGD.

THE MICROSORT TECHNIQUE OF SEX SELECTION

It is a scientific fact that there is a difference between the DNA of the X-sperm and the DNA of the Y-sperm. The latter contains less genetic material and is slightly smaller, lighter, and faster than the former, making it possible for scientists to separate them. Thus, using a flow cytometre,[95] the Microsort technique attempts to control the sex of a child by separating the Y- and X-sperm according to their size[96] and then inseminating the woman artificially with the sperm of the desired sex.

---

90 B. LEROY, "Reproduction, Ethics, Sex Selection..., *op. cit.*, p. 969.

91 R. JONES, *Human Reproductive Biology, op. cit.*, p. 177.

92 Ibid.

93 P. FLAMAN, *Genetic Engineering..., op. cit.*, p. 68.

94 R. JONES, *Human Reproductive Biology, op. cit.*, p. 177; See also B. JICK, (1999) "Gender Selection: The Latest Techniques for Choosing the Sex of Your Child," in http://www.parenthood wb.com/parent_cfmfiles/pros.cfm/839. (13/4/2006).

95 P. FLAMAN, *Genetic Engineering..., op. cit.*, p. 67.

96 C. TURKINGTON – M. ALPER, *Understanding Fertility and Infertility, op. cit.*, p. 139.

The procedure is not cumbersome: A woman with a normal cycle is told to monitor her cycle with an ovulation predictor kit; before ovulation occurs, the couple visits the Microsort laboratory where a fresh semen sample is obtained from her partner. Following this, the scientist stains the X- and Y-sperm with a fluorescent dye, which illuminates them when they are exposed to laser light. The slightly bigger X-sperm soak more dye than the Y-sperm and are better illuminated during such exposure, making it possible for the scientist to separate them by steering them into different receptacles. Then the woman is inseminated with the sperm of the desired sex. The insemination may be repeated the following day to increase the chance of success. The Microsort technology is compatible with the standard IVF protocol, allowing the physician to use the sperm of the desired sex to fertilise the woman's eggs in the laboratory.

The clinical trials with Microsort technique for family balancing began in 1995 in the United States; despite the fact that the technique is still at the experimental stage, a success rate of 75% to 80% is reported for male babies and a rate of about 85% is reported for female babies.[97] The cost of the technique for each separation and insemination is about $2,500.[98] Its major advantages are that it is non-invasive, less expensive, and less psychologically demanding compared to IVF-PGD with prenatal diagnosis and selective abortion. The first Microsort baby (a girl) was born in 1995 to a woman who had lost two brothers and two sons to the X-linked genetic disorder *hydrocephalus,* which is a fatal swelling of the brain that occurs only in male children.[99] This implies that the technique can serve therapeutic and non-therapeutic purposes as can the highly invasive PGD procedure.

---

[97] J. MC MILLAN, "Reproductive Technologies: Sex Selection," in S. POST (ed), *Encyclopedia of Bioethics…, op. cit.,* p. 2268.

[98] C. TURKINGTON – M. ALPER, *Understanding Fertility and Infertility, op. cit.,* p. 139.

[99] L. BELKIN, "Getting the Girl," in *New York Times Magazine*, July 25, 1999.

SEX SELECTION WITH IVF-PGD

Sex selection can be performed with IVF-PGD. The procedure requires ovarian stimulation,[100] egg retrieval, and the creation of embryos outside the womb using standard IVF technology; at approximately the eight-cell stage, one or two of the totipotent embryo cells are removed and analysed to determine their chromosomal makeup, which makes it possible to detect the sex of the embryo.[101] To select the sex of the future child, only embryos of the desired gender are transferred into the mother's uterus. Although sex selection with IVF-PGD, using FISH or PCR, is an invasive procedure, its greatest advantages are its accuracy and reliability. The success rate is almost 100%.[102] The technique carries all the risks of IVF and PGD, and though it does not require the termination of a pregnancy, it does involve discarding embryos of the undesired sex or donating them to research or to other IVF patients.[103]

WHY SEX SELECTION?

Couples perform sex selection for a variety of reasons ranging from medical problems to social problems. Sex selection for non-therapeutic purposes is prohibited in many countries, such as Australia. In the United Kingdom, licensed centres are prohibited from performing it, while non-licensed centres can perform it through sperm sorting and artificial insemination. In the United States, sex selection for both medical and non-medical purposes is currently performed. In Nigeria, there is no law on sex selection or ART as a whole.

---

[100] Fertility drugs are not usually used in sex selection procedures involving fertile couples, but it is required in infertile couples undergoing ART, who wish to select the sex of their child.

[101] Information about the sex of the embryos from the cleavage stage blastomere biopsy can be obtained in twenty-four hours. At this 8-cell stage, the cells of the embryo are still *totipotent*, meaning that each of them has the potential to develop into a child.

[102] J. MCMILLAN, "Reproductive Technologies: Sex Selection," in S. POST (ed), *Encyclopedia of Bioethics…, op. cit.*, p. 2267.

[103] C. AMMER, *The New A to Z of Women's Health…, op. cit.*, p. 352. Since the X and the Y sperm have equal chances to fertilise the egg, only half of the original embryos will be of the desired sex with a potential for transfer and possible live birth.

Couples use PGD for sex selection principally to avoid transmitting genetic diseases to their offspring. Regarding non-therapeutic sex selection, a couple may use PGD or the Microsort technique to balance or control the number of male and female children in the family. This course is often chosen by those who have a family history of having children of a particular gender, or if the analysis of the percentage of X- and Y-sperm in the man's total sperm production reveals few viable sperm of the desired sex and many viable sperm of the undesired sex.[104] Also, couples may use these techniques if they want a male child for social reasons, such as to continue the family lineage or to select a boy in a country like China where a couple is allowed to have only one child.

[104] J. ROBERTSON, (2001), "Preconception Gender Selection," *American Journal of Bioethics,* 1 (1):2-9.

GENETIC DESIGN AND ENHANCEMENT

Human genetic engineering was originally developed for therapeutic purposes, but the science abounds with possibilities for non-therapeutic use. One such use for genetic engineering is human enhancement that will one day create super-humans or designer babies. The goal of human genetic enhancement design is not to prevent or treat any known genetic disease, but rather to modify some of an individual's genes to improve his physical or psychological abilities.[105] According to Resnik, this biotechnology is a method "for transferring genes to human germ cells such as sperm, ova and zygotes or to human germ tissues such as the testes and ovaries."[106]

CATEGORIES OF ENHANCEMENTS

Robert Wachbroit identifies three categories of possible applications of human enhancement using biotechnology. These include therapeutic, "intra-normal," and "proper" enhancements. An enhancement is therapeutic if it seeks to prevent, ameliorate, or treat a particular medical condition. Intra-normal enhancement raises a particular trait in an individual from a point within the normal range to a higher point within the same normal range.[107] Human genetic enhancement "proper" refers to the modification of the human genome to produce super-humans or designer babies;[108] this requires the modification of certain traits at a "fundamental biological level."[109] Even though some commenta-

[105] D. RESNIK, "Genetic Engineering, Human," in S. POST (ed.), *Encyclopedia of Bioethics…, op. cit.,* p. 961. He maintains that the development of recombinant DNA technology in the 1970s has paved the way for possible enhancement of certain traits in the person in the future.

[106] Ibid., p. 962. According to Resnik, the procedure would attempt to transfer a gene into the DNA present in the chromosomes in the cell nucleus.

[107] R. WACHBROIT, "Human, Enhancement Uses of Biotechnology," in T. MURRAY – M. MEHLMAN, *Encyclopedia of Ethical…, op. cit.,* p. 550. The basic idea here is that there is a certain range that is normal for human beings and another that may be said to be abnormal.

[108] Ibid.

[109] R. SONG, *Human Genetics, op. cit.,* p. 41; E. PARENS, "Is Better Always Good?" *Hastings Cent Rep,* 1998; 28 (1): S-I-S-17.

tors tend to merge intra-normal and proper enhancements, Wachbroit stresses the need to maintain the distinction between the two: while the former involves differences in degree, the latter involves differences in kind.[110] Undoubtedly, the technology is still not scientifically feasible, but successes in several experiments with plants and animals suggest that it is attainable in humans. Eventually, scientists will collect genetic material from an individual and modify it in the laboratory to produce desired traits—hair colour, eye colour, skin colour, tallness, intelligence, musical ability, and so forth—which some authors refer to as the genetic design of a human being.[111] In theory, the technology makes it possible to improve people's physical ability or intellectual capacity at the level of the human genome, as an attempt to make them more attractive, more athletic, more artistic, or more intelligent.[112] As Flaman observes, it could lead to a situation in which it will be possible "to use DNA combinations not currently in existence to produce human beings by *recipe.*"[113]

Human genetic enhancement modification as presented above may not be as easy as it seems. In certain cases, it may eventually turn out to be a very complex procedure requiring more than the alteration of particular genes in a person to enhance a trait. This is clear in Wachbroit's assertion:

> And it may turn out that enhancing certain traits requires not only genetic modifications but also certain alterations in the individual's environment. That is to say, a particular genetic modification might not by itself bring about an enhanced trait; it might give the person a capacity to develop the enhanced trait whose realization demands a special exercise regime, diet, or other efforts. The idea of genetic enhancement technologies therefore does not rest on the assumption of genetic determinism—that a genetic alteration alone is sufficient to bring about a particular trait. While a popular

110 Ibid. For instance, Wachbroit views cosmetic surgeries more as intra-normal modifications rather than proper genetic enhancement.

111 P. FLAMAN, *Genetic Engineering…, op. cit.,* pp. 66-67.

112 A. SUTTON, "The New Genetics: Facts, Fictions and Fear," *Linacere Quarterly,* August 1995, 76–87.

113 P. FLAMAN, *Genetic Engineering…, op. cit.,* pp. 67.

> image of genetic enhancements is that of some magic-wand transformation in which the person is a passive recipient, the matter can be more complex. Realizing a genetic enhancement might involve hard work.[114]

This implies that to engineer or enhance certain traits in a person, it may not be sufficient to alter the particular genes governing those traits. Genetic modification will only give the individual the *capacity* to develop the enhanced traits, not necessarily the realization thereof, which may depend on other non-genetic factors.[115] For instance, an individual may naturally have a high IQ that can make him one of the most intelligent human beings in the world, but to actualize this potential, other factors must come into play, such as good education, discipline, exposure, hard work, opportunities, and luck.

TYPES OF HUMAN GENETIC ENHANCEMENT

As we have repeatedly noted, the two types of cells in the human being are somatic cells and germ-line cells. Depending on the purpose of the intervention, genetic enhancement modification can be applied to either type. At the level of somatic cells, the modification will affect the bodily cells but not the reproductive cells. It will affect only the individual and not his offspring, unless, perhaps, his modified cells are used to perform somatic nuclear transfer as in reproductive cloning. In contrast, genetic enhancement of the germ-line cells[116] will result in changes that can be passed on to future generations,[117] since genetic heredity is transmitted through the gametes. As Wachbroit asserts, this latter application

---

[114] R. WACHBROIT, "Human, Enhancement Uses of Biotechnology..., *op. cit.,* p. 550. In general, human enhancement can also be accomplished with drugs and blood transfusion, although not in the same way as genetic enhancement.

[115] Ibid., p. 550.

[116] D. RESNIK, "Genetic Engineering, Human," in S. POST (ed.), *Encyclopedia of Bioethics..., op. cit.,* p. 962. In 2001, a working group convened by the American Association for the Advancement of Science proposed the term inheritable genetic modification as a more appropriate term to describe germ-line genetic therapy or enhancement.

[117] E. PARENS, "Is Better Always Good..., *op. cit.,* S-1-S-17.

of the technology might require "inserting the modification in the few cells of the early embryo stage, which would likely affect the individual's germ cells."[118]

[118] R. WACHBROIT, "Human, Enhancement Uses of Biotechnology…, *op. cit.,* p. 550.

CHAPTER 7

ETHICAL ISSUES IN ARTIFICIAL REPRODUCTIVE TECHNOLOGIES

With such a wide array of ART procedures currently available, infertility can often be circumvented. However, with this diversity of techniques comes a diversity of ethical problems. This chapter examines the ethical and human rights issues associated with ART. There are numerous questions that must be confronted: Is science or technology morally neutral? Does the fact that something is technically possible make it morally permissible? Should the pragmatic value of an act be the only determinant of its moral rightness or wrongness, especially in the life sciences? Is the appeal to reproductive right sufficient reason for making every form of ART available to the public? These issues have polarized public opinion and even philosophers, bioethicists, and theologians; many stand poised between the moral acceptability and non-acceptability of the ART techniques, making it necessary to examine their arguments.

ARGUMENTS IN FAVOUR OF ART

Advocates of ART have proposed arguments in favour of the various techniques, ranging from the importance of their pragmatic value to the necessity of respecting the reproductive rights and autonomy of individuals.

PRAGMATIC USE OF ART

For utilitarians such as Jeremy Betham and John Stuart Mill, the moral rightness or wrongness of an action depends on its consequences. An action is morally right if it maximizes pleasure and happiness or minimizes pain and suffering for the majority of those affected by it.[1] On the basis of such consequentialist reasoning, proponents tend to morally justify ART by virtue of its pragmatic value. They claim that infertility is a traumatizing medical condition and that ART may be the only solution for many couples.[2] In other words, ART may be the last option to alleviate the suffering and create happiness for childless couples, especially those who desire children that are genetically related to at least one of the spouses.

Some advocates of ART do not approve of techniques involving donated eggs, sperm, and embryos and surrogate wombs. Those who do consider them morally acceptable argue that "for some couples egg donation may provide the only chance of having a child that the woman can carry to term, and which is the genetic child of her husband."[3] Similarly, surrogacy may be the only way for a couple to have a child that will be genetically related to one of the partners. Opponents argue that to resort to every available technique to realize the desire for biological

[1] R. TONG, "Reproductive Technologies: Surrogacy," in W. REICH (ed.), *Encyclopedia of Bioethics…, op. cit.*, p. 2226.

[2] L. PURDY, "Surrogacy Mothering," in KUSHE – P. SINGER (eds.), *Bioethics: An Anthology,* Blackwell Publisher Ltd., Oxford 1999, pp. 104-105.

[3] M. WARNOCK, *A Question of Life, The Warnock Report on Human Fertilisation and Embryology,* Basil Blackwell Ltd., Oxford, U.K.1985, p. 3.

children—irrespective of the ethical consequences—would be an unfair exaltation of biological parenting as the measure of one's personal worth.[4]

Some advocates of ART compare embryo donation in surrogacy to adoption; they view it as a form of prenatal adoption with advantages over normal adoption. It allows an infertile couple to have an experience of pregnancy and childbirth, and it makes possible the normal bonding between a mother and the child during pregnancy. Surrogacy arrangements in which the gamete from one of the partners is used produce a child that will be genetically related to one of the parents; Keane, a major broker on surrogacy arrangements, contends that couples want this biological connection to the child.[5] Other advocates reject adoption to prevent the possibility of adopting a child with a genetic disease, arguing that surrogacy will provide more certainty regarding the genetic health of the child.[6] Defending third party involvement in procreation, Joseph Fletcher cites the practice of Levirate marriage in the Bible (Deut. 25:5-6) as well as its pragmatic value in emancipating people from infertility and the emotional deprivation of childlessness.[7] There are others who endorse this practice provided the woman's husband gives his informed consent and there exist safeguards for the recipient and the donor.

Other commentators object to the comparison between "prenatal adoption" in surrogacy and the usual adoption, claiming that the two are not morally equivalent. Insisting that there is a significant difference between the two, Kearon asserts that while the couple is the primary focus in ART, a child in need of social parents is the primary focus in adoption.[8] In ART procedures that involve either an egg or a sperm donor, the couple does not enjoy an equal relationship with the child, who introduces an

---

[4] J. FLETCHER, "Reproductive Technologies," in J. MACQUIRE – C, CHILDRESS (eds.), *A New Dictionary of Christian Ethics,* SCM Press, London 1967, p. 538.

[5] N. KEANE – D. BREO, *The Surrogate Mother,* Everest House New York 1981, p. 15. Quoted in L. SCHEWARTZ, *Alternatives to Infertility: Is Surrogacy..., op. cit.,* p. 110.

[6] Ibid., p. 111.

[7] J. FLETCHER, "Reproductive Technologies..., *op. cit.,* p. 536.

[8] K. KEARON, *Medical Ethics: An Introduction,* The Columbia Press, Dublin 1999, p. 83. Prenatal adoption referred to here is not that undertaken by a couple to just save a viable embryo.

imbalance from the biological standpoint[9]—the parent who is genetically related to the child is more favoured. In normal adoption, however, both parents are related to the child in the same way and are equally responsible for him. Furthermore, couples who resort to ART actually create the problem, which endangers the psychological relationship between them and the child, whereas in adoption they only attempt to rescue an existing bad situation. Besides, to permit adoption does not necessarily imply a moral approval of the situation surrounding the child's birth and abandonment;[10] the fact that such crises have been managed successfully in the past does not justify a deliberate decision to create a similar situation. Consider a child who is the outcome of an incident involving rape or incest: the fact that he might adapt to his familial circumstances does not justify such immoral acts or suggest that it is ethically acceptable to plan the conception of a child in such a way.[11] Finally, they argue that surrogacy may not necessarily guarantee the genetic health of the prospective child; the possibility of genetic mutation is present in every pregnancy because spermatogenesis is an ongoing process.[12]

RESPECT FOR REPRODUCTIVE RIGHT OR AUTONOMY

Some aspects of the ART debate touch on the issue of human rights. An example is the question of reproductive right or liberty. A major argument advanced in support of ART is the need to show respect for an individual's right to reproduce. Two crucial questions often asked in this area are the following: Who should have access to ART? and, What techniques would be morally permissible?

---

[9] S. CALLAHAN, "The Ethical Challenge of the New Reproductive Technology," in S. LAMMERS – A. VERHEY (eds.), *On Moral Medicine, Second Edition,* Wm. B. Eerdmans Publishing Co., Cambridge 1998, p. 514.

[10] D. HOLLINGER, "Sexual Ethics and Reproductive Technologies," in J. KILNER – P. CUNNINGHAM – W. HAGER (eds.), *The Reproductive Revolution,* Wm. B. Eerdmans Publishing Co., Grand Rapids, Michigan 2000, p. 89.

[11] S. CALLAHAN, "The Ethical Challenge of..., *op. cit.,* pp. 510, 515.

[12] L. SCHWARTZ, *Alternatives to Infertility..., op. cit.,* p. 111.

WHO SHOULD HAVE ACCESS TO ART?

In response to this question, some commentators appeal to respect for autonomy based on the contemporary understanding of autonomy in the works of Immanuel Kant and John Stuart Mill. Kant believed in the capacity of every individual to determine between good and bad, and he advocated respect for the decision-making capacity, or self-determination, of every autonomous (competent) subject.[13] Mill rejected government paternalism in favour of freedom, claiming that the only justifiable reason to restrict a person's autonomy is the risk of harm, that is, if the exercise of his freedom causes physical harm to another person.[14] In line with this view, Beauchamp and Childress contend that to respect the autonomy of a competent agent is "at a minimum, to acknowledge that person's right to hold views, to make choices, and to take actions based on personal values and beliefs."[15] According to this understanding, to violate a person's autonomy is tantamount to treating him as a means rather than as an end, that is, according to the goals of others without regard for his own goals.[16]

Applying this robust conception of autonomy to the generation of children, proponents of ART argue that couples (or even all adults) have both a right to reproduce and the liberty to choose how to reproduce and

---

[13] IMMANUEL KANT, *Foundations of the Metaphysics of Morals,* Translated. L. WHITE BECK, Bobbs-Merrill Company, Indianapolis 1959; ID., *The Doctrine of Virtue, Part II of the Metaphysics of Morals,* Translated by M. GREGOR, University of Pennsylvania Press, Philadelphia 1964, p. 127; K. KEARON, *Medical Ethics..., op. cit.,* pp. 14-15. Kant (1724–1804) grounds respect for autonomy on the unconditional worth of every competent individual, which requires allowing him to make his own decisions.

[14] JOHN STUART MILL, (1859), *On Liberty and Other Essays,* Edited by J. GRAY (ed.), Oxford University Press, Oxford 1991; Also cited in J. MCMILLAN, "Reproductive Technologies: Sex Selection," in S. POST (ed.), *Encyclopedia of Bioethics..., op. cit.,* p. 2268. Mill, a utilitarian, believed that liberty of action and expression was necessary to maximize happiness.

[15] T. BEAUCHAMP – J. CHILDRESS, *Principles of Biomedical Ethics, Fifth Edition,* Oxford University Press, Inc., New York 2001, p. 63.

[16] Ibid.

with whom to reproduce.[17] Thus, any attempt to deny an individual's access to ART would constitute a violation of their reproductive right.[18] This implies that ART should be available to everybody, including single parents, unmarried heterosexual partners, women who do not wish to interrupt their careers, women who do not like to be pregnant, and even homosexuals.[19] Advocates contend that if a condition is not normally imposed on fertile people, it should not be imposed on those who require ART to conceive.

This appeal to reproductive autonomy raises some concerns. For Thomas Murray, it is problematic to use this as a framework for evaluating the ethics of ART. It makes it possible for adults to use any technique of their choice to fulfil their desire to have biological offspring; this restricts the moral universe of procreation to the concept of personal autonomy. It reduces everything to the interests of the prospective parents and fails to consider the interests of the child and the values at the heart of family life.[20] Pointing out this serious defect, he maintains,

---

[17] J. HARRIS, "Rights and Reproductive Choice," in J. HARRIS – S. HOLM (eds.), *The Future of Human Reproduction: Ethics, Choice and Regulation,* Oxford University Press, Oxford 1998, pp. 34-36. Harris expands reproductive autonomy or right to include the right to use whatever genes of our choice to which we can have a legitimate access or to reproduce in ways that express our reproductive choices.

[18] S. CALLAHAN, "The Ethical Challenge..., *op. cit.,* p. 511.

[19] J. ROBERTSON, *Children of Choice: Freedom and the New Reproductive Technologies,* New Jersey University Press, Princeton, NJ 1994, pp. 23, 35. Robertson considers it a primary right because it is connected to one's personal identity, dignity and the meaning of one's life. Insisting that the only justifiable ground for restricting it would be a proof of substantial harm by those calling for restriction, he maintains that being single, a homosexual, physically disabled, HIV patient and so forth is not a sufficient ground to override this liberty.

[20] T. MURRAY, "What Are Families For? Getting to an Ethics of Reproductive Technologies," in T. SHANNON (ed.), *Reproductive Technologies, op. cit.,* pp. 113, 115. Murray maintains that in reality, the excesses of control and choice in certain AR techniques can distort and destroy the important family and parental values and "the role that enduring relationships play in our flourishing as human beings."

> It permits adults to use virtually any reproductive means for virtually any end; it prohibits or condemns almost nothing. The test of an analytic moral framework cannot be limited to those cases for which it gives the answers one wants; if it provides morally dubious or outrageous answers in other cases, or feeble answers where moral judgments should be clear and ringing. Then we have reason to doubt its insightfulness and completeness.[21]

Some fear that ART has the potential to extend reproductive right into a positive right, forcing society to provide every means necessary to reproduce.[22] In fact, Kass contends that reproductive right, understood as a positive right, is now being expanded to include the right to have the child of one's choice, such as is possible with genetic screening, sex selection, and, perhaps, genetic enhancement and design.[23] Opponents argue that reproductive right is not necessarily a positive right. While it is necessary to respect the reproductive right and privacy of others, ART also has social implications that must be considered.[24] According to Sidney Callahan, we need to go beyond the narrow focus on the biological integrity of the marital sexual act and on people's desires for children; we must consider whether or not the decision to use a particular reproductive technology will promote the good of the future child, the good of the family, and the appropriate social conditions for child-rearing.[25]

---

[21] Ibid., pp. 114-115.

[22] R. BLANK – J. MERRRICK, *Human Reproduction, Emerging Technologies, and Conflicting Rights,* Congressional Quarterly Inc., Washington D.C. 1995, p. 99; See also S. CALLAHAN, "The Ethical Challenge…, *op. cit.,* pp. 509-510.

[23] L. KASS – J. WILSON, *The Ethics of Human Cloning,* The AEI Press, Washington, D.C. 1998, p. 86. Kass claims that gay-rights organizations are already clamouring for reproductive rights in the sense of being allowed to reproduce through cloning.

[24] T. SHANNON, "Ethical Issues in Genetics," in T. SHANNON – A. WOLTER, *The New Genetic Medicine,* Rowman & Littlefield Publishers Inc., Lanham, Maryland 2003, p. 26.

[25] S. CALLAHAN, "The Ethical Challenge…, *op. cit.,* p. 510.

Some argue that ART should be available to heterosexual persons in a stable relationship, while others insist that only a legally married couple should have access to ART because the family is the safest environment for the child. But a major legal and ethical debate arises here: What constitutes family?[26] Committees set up by governments to investigate ART have taken a stand on the issue. While the U.S. Ethics Advisory Committee approved IVF only for consenting married people, the Warnock Committee in Britain approved fertility treatment for stable, non-married heterosexual couples, basing its judgment on the pluralistic nature of society. Despite these restrictions, single ladies often request to be inseminated, and serious abuses cannot be ruled out. For instance, single women may resort to AID or IVF using donor sperm.[27] In other scandalous cases, Dr. Ceil Jacobson used his own sperm to inseminate unsuspecting patients in over 60 AID procedures, and Dr. Richards Asch reportedly used, without permission, the egg and embryos from some of his women patients for other couples.[28]

WHAT TECHNIQUES SHOULD BE AVAILABLE TO PROSPECTIVE PATIENTS?

Some supporters of ART argue that every adult individual has a right to reproduce and should be allowed to do so without any interference.[29] Again, they base their call for unrestricted access to the numerous techniques on respect for reproductive autonomy. In their opinion, reproduction through non-coital sexual intercourse—such as donor techniques, surrogate contracts, IVF-PGD, and sex selection—naturally falls within the scope of the reproductive right and autonomy of individuals.

---

[26] W. WADLINGTON, "Reproductive Technologies: Artificial Insemination," in W. REICH (ed.), *Encyclopedia of Bioethics..., op. cit.*, p. 2219.

[27] L. KASS – J. WILSON, *The Ethics of Human Cloning..., op. cit.*, p. 85.

[28] S. LAMMERS – A. VERHEY, "Technological Reproduction," in S. LAMMER – A.VERHEY, (eds.*), On Moral Medicine..., op. cit.*, p. 465.

[29] W. FREEDMAN, *Legal Issues in Biotechnology and Human Reproduction,* Quorum Books, New York 1991, p. 78. Freedman asserts that in the Skinner v. Oklahoma case, the highest court recognized the right to procreate as one of the "basic civil rights" a government cannot infringe upon in the absence of any compelling reason. As such reproductive freedom is understood to include the right to resort to non-coital sexual intercourse and any AR technique to have children.

ARGUMENTS AGAINST ART

The arguments against ART can be grouped into several categories. These include respect for human life, respect for human dignity, and respect for the psycho-social integrity of the child.

RESPECT FOR HUMAN LIFE IN PROCREATION

Many critics of ART argue that it is necessary to show respect for human life in procreation; those who view the embryo as a human being with a right to life find some of the reproductive techniques, such as IVF and its variants, particularly troubling.

DESTRUCTION AND MANIPULATION OF HUMAN EMBRYOS

The current practice in the standard IVF procedure is to create many embryos and select the best for transfer into the woman; this avoids repeating the ordeal of egg retrieval should the present cycle not succeed. A crucial question arises here: If these viable embryos are no longer required by the couple, can they be destroyed, allowed to die, or used for research? Similarly, to resolve the issue of multiple pregnancy, which is common in IVF, physicians often resort to foetal reduction, which terminates the lives of some of the embryos to allow one or two to survive.

Opinions diverge sharply on the morality of this practice. Opponents of IVF argue that it is morally objectionable to deliberately bring into existence embryos that will never be implanted into the woman. This paves the way for the deliberate destruction of human life, which is worthy of respect from its origin. Those who view the embryo as a person claim that foetal reduction is morally equivalent to procured abortion.

Proponents of ART justify embryo wastage by claiming that an equally large number of embryos are wasted in natural conception.[30]

---

[30] J. HARRIS, "The Ethical Use of Human Embryonic Stem Cells in Research and Therapy," in J. BURLEY – J. HARRIS (eds.), *A Companion to Genethics*, Blackwell Publishing Ltd., Malden, MA 2004, pp. 164-165, 168. Harris argues that the sacrifice of embryos is inevitable in both natural conception and ART and if this loss is justified in the former, then it is equally justified in the latter because in either case, the objective of having a healthy baby is worth this cost. For him, the differences between embryo wastage in natural conception and the deliberate choice by parents to destroy their embryos in ART procedures do not appear material.

Moreover, some claim that the outcome of the procedure—the child—justifies such wastages. They argue that foetal reduction is not an abortion because the intention is to allow pregnancy to continue, but opponents are quick to point out the moral difference between spontaneous abortion in natural conception and a couple's deliberate and foreseeable action in artificial reproduction that exposes viable human embryos to death.

EXPERIMENTATION ON HUMAN EMBRYOS

Some of the unused embryos created in ART procedures are used for investigative research. Critics find this morally reprehensible and argue that to use human embryos for experimentation is not consistent with respect for human life and dignity. Because such research embryos are never implanted, this practice amounts to deliberate destruction of human life and experimentation on a human being without consent.[31] Non-therapeutic experimentation on a viable human embryo assaults its dignity by treating it as a means to an end. The basis of this argument is the principle that in every experiment involving a human person, his or her consent must first be obtained. Since this is not possible in the case of the embryo, to proceed with experimentation is to violate this principle.

Supporters of ART justify research on embryos on the basis of its ability to yield scientific knowledge that will assure better health for individuals and families. Arguing that it is wasteful to discard embryos given their value as research objects,[32] they insist that research is not immoral because the embryo is not yet a person with a right to life—it is only a potential person. In their opinion, although there may be uncertainty as to when personhood really begins, it certainly cannot begin before the 14th day after fertilisation[33] because of the possibility of monozygotic twinning within this time frame; thus, any experimentation within 14 days of fertilisation would pose no moral problem. Supporting this claim, Peter Singer contends that at this early stage of development, the embryo

---

[31] J. MCDOWELL, "Ethical Implantations of In Vitro Fertilisation," in S. LAMMERS – A. VERHEYS (eds.), *On Moral Medicine...*, *op. cit.*, p. 507.

[32] J. HARRIS, "The Ethical Use of Human Embryonic..., *op. cit.*, p. 168. Harris maintains that "spare" embryos from IVF protocols can serve a good purpose. They can be a source of embryonic stem cells, making it a waste to discard them.

[33] K. KEARON, *Medical Ethics...*, *op. cit.*, p. 82.

does not have the anatomical features of a human being; it does not have a brain or a nervous system and thus cannot experience pain from the experimentation. He considers an experiment on a living, sentient mouse to be of greater moral significance than experimentation on an early human embryo. Experimentation on human embryos has several potential advantages: it can improve our understanding of fertilisation, increase the success rate of IVF, and produce scientific knowledge that may result in the cure of life-threatening diseases.[34]

RESPECT FOR DIGNITY IN HUMAN PROCREATION

Opponents of ART assert that human beings have an inherent dignity, and the way we bring a child into existence should conform to this dignity. As a result, some reproductive techniques have come under intense criticism as being unworthy of human dignity. To support their claim, the critics of controversial reproductive techniques, and even some proponents of ART who merely oppose third party involvement, cite the Kantian second formulation of the categorical imperative about the intrinsic worth of human beings. According to Kant, "Everything has either a price or a dignity. If it has a price, something else can be put in its place as an equivalent; if it is exalted above all price and so admits of no equivalent, then it has dignity."[35] For him, human dignity requires that every human person be treated "never merely as a means, but always also as an end."[36] Based on this assertion, many commentators argue that some of ART's methods of bringing children into existence are not consonant with our rational human nature and dignity. Their arguments are many and varied; for the sake of clarity, we will examine them under several subheadings.

ETHICAL ISSUES IN ASSISTED INSEMINATION BY HUSBAND (AIH)

For most commentators, AIH poses no moral problem: fertilisation occurs normally in the fallopian tube, and issues regarding embryo

[34] P. SINGER, "New Assisted Reproductive Technology," in H. KUHSE – P. SINGER (eds.), *Bioethics: An Anthology, op. cit.*, p. 101.

[35] IMMANUEL KANT, *Groundwork of the Metaphysics of Morals,* Translated, H. J. PATON, Harper and Row, New York 1964, p. 102.

[36] Ibid., p. 105.

destruction and experimentation do not arise. However, some find the practice of obtaining sperm outside the marital sexual act ethically objectionable, because it separates the unitive and procreative aspects of conjugal love; rather than assist the marital sexual act, the "physical act of masturbation" actually replaces it. This objection comes mainly from the Catholic Church and is defended by most of her moral theologians.

IVF: HUMAN PROCREATION OR LABORATORY MANUFACTURE?

IVF and other forms of laboratory conception do not conform to the human way of procreating; they tend to change the generation of a new child from being an act of "generation" to an act of "production." Laboratory conception can cause society to view a child as an entitlement rather than a gift, or as a product over which we must exercise quality control.[37,38] Insisting that there is a significant moral difference between procreation and laboratory production, opponents of IVF distinguish between "making" and "doing." In natural conception, couples only "do" something (that is, perform the marital act), and the human life that ensues is not made by them. In contrast, the action of "making" (as in laboratory conception) proceeds from the agent to the product that is made,[39] and this "product" (the child) is the central focus of the entire procedure. Applying the mentality of manufacturing to laboratory conception, medical scientists employ the most efficient means to achieve the highest quality at the lowest cost. In this case, any product that does not meet the set standard is seen as defective, and it is either accepted with little appreciation or completely discarded.[40] This mentality is especially apparent in IVF-PGD, in which only embryos that "pass the test" are transferred into the woman.[41] According to May, this manner

---

[37] W. MAY, *Catholic Bioethics and the Gift of Human Life,* Our Sunday Visitor Publishing Division, Our Sunday Visitor, Inc., Huntington, Indiana 2000, p. 81.

[38] G. MEILAENDER, "A Child of One's Own: At What Price?" in J. KILNER – P. CUNNINGHAM – W. HAGER (eds.), *The Reproduction Revolution, op. cit.,* pp. 43, 45; ID., G. MEILAENDER, *Bioethics, A Primer for Christians, Second Edition,* Wm. B. Eerdmans Publishing Co., Michigan 2005, p. 20.

[39] W. MAY, *Catholic Bioethics and..., op. cit.,* p. 81.

[40] Ibid.

[41] P. FLAMAN, *Genetic Engineering, op. cit.,* p. 42.

of bringing children into existence is dehumanizing, and it conforms neither to the respect due to a person nor to responsible methods of procreation: "It treats them (children) as if they were products inferior to their producers and subject to quality controls, not persons equal in dignity to their parents."[42] Reiterating this view, some assert that laboratory conception establishes an unequal relationship between the physician and the child, which contradicts the equality among persons. More precisely, it introduces a relationship of efficient causality between the one who "makes" and the one who "is made," leading to an existential and objective relationship of dependence.[43] Stressing the need for a child to be begotten, not made or produced, Meilaender writes the following:

> A child, who is thus begotten, not made, embodies the union of his father and mother. They have not simply reproduced themselves, nor are they merely a cause of which the child is an effect. Rather, the power of their mutual love has given rise to another who though different from them and equal in dignity to them, manifests in his person the love that unites them. Their love-giving has been life-giving; it is truly procreation.[44]

A child who results from the marital act of his parents is not "caused" by them, and no relationship of dominion or inequality is established between them because they merely collaborated in the creation of a new life; this is not the case with laboratory conception. Ashley contends that IVF replaces the personal relationship and communion symbolized by the marital act and reduces the generative process to something similar to a chemist making a compound. In natural conception, the partners are

---

[42] W. MAY, *Catholic Bioethics..., op. cit.,* pp. 82, 84. The point is that a child who is generated shares an equal dignity with its parents, but when a child is treated as a product, this introduces a kind of inequality.

[43] F. FABO, "Medical Intervention and Human Sexuality," Being a Lecture delivered at the Universita Pontifica Regina Apostolorum, Rome, in February 2005, On this view, "to produce" is not the same as "to procreate." To produce has the sense of "to make" and the ensuing child is the result that is produced.

[44] G. MEILAENDER, *Bioethics, A Primer for Christians, op. cit.,* p. 14. Meilaender asserts that laboratory fertilisation destroys the features that distinguish procreation from reproduction.

the principal actors, but in laboratory conception the medical scientists are equally principal actors. In fact, they become the principal cause of generation by acting on the gametes supplied by the couple as the "raw materials" to produce a child.[45]

Not everyone agrees with this position. Some authors, including some dissenting Catholic moral theologians, make an exception for a limited use of IVF under certain conditions; they state that if the procedure utilizes the woman's natural cycle, avoids ovarian hyperstimulation, avoids the creation of multiple embryos, avoids the freezing and discarding of embryos, and refrains from other moral problems raised by IVF, it cannot be said to transform the generative process into production.[46] They have no moral objection to AIH, IVF, and its variants based on the separation of sexual love and procreation, provided a third party is not involved[47] and the couple displays a mutual love and desire to procreate.[48] In their view, procreation need not arise from a specific instance of sexual intercourse;[49] if a couple conceives with AI or IVF, the resulting child is still conceived and nurtured within the context of their marriage relationship, implying that these practices actually conform to the meaning and purpose of procreation.[50] Stressing this fact, Hollinger asserts,

[45] B. ASHLEY, "The Chill Factor in Moral Theology," *Linacre Quarterly,* 57:4, 1990, 71-72. It is important to note that the physician is the principal manager of the whole process.

[46] W. MAY, *Catholic Bioethics…, op. cit.,* p. 82.

[47] This does not mean that they have no objection to other moral problems posed by the techniques, such as embryo wastage, but the emphasis here is on the separation of sex and procreation.

[48] J. MCDOWELL, "Ethical Implications of In Vitro Fertilisation," in S. LAMMER – A VERHEYS (eds.), *On Moral Medicine, op. cit.,* p. 506. We should note that this position is clearly against the teaching of the Magisterium that IVF is fundamentally immoral, regardless of the circumstances.

[49] S. RAE, *Brave New Families: Biblical Ethics and Reproductive Technologies,* Baker Books, Grand Rapids 1996, p. 28. Cited in D. HOLLINGER, "Sexual Ethics and Reproductive Technologies," in J. KILNER – P. CUNNINGHAM – W. HAGER (eds.), *The Reproduction Revolution, op. cit.,* p. 87

[50] D. HOLLINGER, "Sexual Ethics and…, *op. cit.,* p. 87.

> While the conception does not take place from intercourse itself, as long as the conception sufficiently involves husband and wife, it takes place in the context of a loving, enjoying one-flesh relationship in which attempts to procreate have been unsuccessful. The gametes are from within the marital relationship, which involves all the basic dimensions of marriage and sex possible, with the addition of technological assistance in bringing the egg and sperm together.[51]

McCormick concurs, arguing that the physician is not the "cause" of fertilisation in the IVF protocol. In reality, fertilisation occurs when the ovum and sperm are brought together in the petri dish, making the intervention by the physician only a "condition" for its occurrence, rather than the "cause."[52] Additionally, it is possible for the couple and the physician to adopt a reverential disposition during the entire procedure, as would be the case in natural conception. On a final note, he asserts that the marital act is a preferable way of generating offspring; however, when medical conditions render that impossible, recourse to AI or IVF can be regarded as an "extension" of their marital act, in which case the child that results would still be a fruit of marital love.[53]

Opponents, such as May, reject this position and contend that the moral reasoning that underpins it is proportionalism,[54] which places emphasis on the good consequences of an act and downplays the moral object of the act. In fact, proportionalists claim that one can rightly intend pre-moral or ontic evils or disvalues, such as death and sickness, in order to achieve a proportionally greater good. But for May, resorting to laboratory conception is tantamount to using a bad means to reach a

---

[51] Ibid., p. 88.

[52] R. McCORMICK, *The Critical Calling: Reflections on Moral Dilemmas Since Vatican II,* Georgetown University Press, Washington, D.C. 1989, p. 337; Also cited in W. MAY, *Catholic Bioethics…, op. cit.,* pp. 82-83.

[53] Ibid., p. 337.

[54] POPE JOHN PAUL II, *Veritatis Splendor, On the Splendour of Truth,* 6 August 1993, *nos. 2, 3*: *AAS* 85 1993, 1133-1228. Proportionalists claim that one can rightly intend a pre-moral or ontic evils or disvalues (such as, death and sickness) in order to achieve a proportionally greater good.

good end.[55] Ashley points out that the "extension of the marital act" does not correspond to empirical fact, because what couples actually extend is the desire to have a child, rather than sexual intercourse itself.[56] Still, for other critics, laboratory conception has negative implications for human sexuality and human origin. As Kass observes, by taking the early but important stage of human generation out of the human body and into the laboratory, scientists and physicians did not only create an opportunity for couples to have children, they put "the origin of the human life literally in human hands."[57] IVF technology could lead to an increase in the "technological mastery of human generation" and a "continuing erosion of respect for the mystery of sexuality and human renewal." Thus, the very existence of the technology could justify many other steps that reduce procreation to manufacture.[58] He asserts,

> My point is simple: there are more and less human ways of bringing children into this world. I am arguing that the laboratory production of human beings is no longer human procreation, that making babies in laboratories—even "perfect babies"—means a degradation of parenthood.[59]

The experience of Paul Lauritzen and his wife, which perhaps represents that of many other couples who resort to ART, lends some support to this position. Speaking for himself and his wife, he states the following:

> The process of reproduction in a clinical environment [causes] a way of thinking of ourselves and our world in terms that are incompatible with intimacy.... Once procreation is separated from sexual intercourse, it is

---

[55] W. MAY, *Catholic Bioethics..., op. cit.,* p. 84. Besides, in producing babies, some who are considered defective come to be rejected. Hence, the producers do not only choose life for some, but they also choose death for others by discarding them.

[56] B. ASHLEY, "The Chill Factor in Moral Theology..., *op. cit.,* pp. 71-72.

[57] L. KASS – J. WILSON, *The Ethics of Human Cloning..., op. cit.,* p. 80.

[58] Ibid.

[59] L. KASS, "Making Babies – The New Biology and the 'Old' Morality," *Public Interest 26 (1972): 18-56.*

> difficult not to treat the process of procreation as the production of an object to which one has the right as a producer. It is difficult under these circumstances to place the end above the means: Effectiveness in accomplishing one's goal can easily become the sole criterion by which decisions are made.[60]

Reflecting on the embryo in the petri dish, Singer confirms the negative effects of laboratory conception on our view of human generation:

> The revolution in reproductive medicine has made the embryo a product in a way that it never was before. Looking at embryos in glass dishes on laboratory benches makes it more difficult to cling to the belief that all human life is equally precious from the moment of conception. We can say: this embryo is precious for the couples from whom the egg and sperm came, because they have been trying for many years to have a child, and this could be the child they want so much. But if—as really happened in one case that also involved Wood and Trounson—the couple from whom the egg and sperm came are killed in a plane crash while their embryos remain frozen in a tank of liquid nitrogen in a laboratory, it is hard to see that the embryo is really precious in any sense.[61]

Those who endorse laboratory conception view the various ART techniques as positive human achievements that are related to the rational control of nature. For instance, justifying the morality of genetic control in human generation, Fletcher maintains that the generation of children cannot be left to accidents of romance and meiosis; he emphasizes the need to exercise rational control and human choice in this area, instead

---

[60] P. LAURITZEN, "What Price for Parenthood?" *Hasting Centre Report 20,* March/April, 1990, 38-46. Quoted in K. O'ROURKE, *The Primer for Health Care Ethics…, op. cit.,* p. 265.

[61] P. SINGER, *Rethinking Life and Death,* Oxford University Press, Oxford 1994, p. 97. In spite of the above statement, Singer is a great supporter of all forms of ART.

of relying exclusively on nature.[62] For advocates, laboratory conception makes such a rational control over procreation possible, and they reject the view that IVF and its variants are "unnatural" and, therefore, morally unacceptable. They argue that if the line between the "natural" and the "artificial" separates moral from immoral practices, "society will have to forbid intravenous feeding as also 'unnatural.'"[63] This position is well-articulated by Singer, who maintains that our human nature is dynamic, not fixed. According to him,

> If anything at all is distinctive of human beings, and characterizes our nature, surely it is our ability to use our ingenuity to overcome impediments to getting what we want. In this sense the birth of Louise Brown was entirely in accord with human nature—perhaps more so than every previous birth, because those earlier births used means that we share with nonhuman animals, not means that are possible only for a being with our distinctive abilities.[64]

DONOR-CONCEPTION OR THIRD PARTY INVOLVEMENT

In heterologous AI and IVF techniques, couples rely on donated sperm or eggs or even on donated embryos and surrogate wombs to have babies. Such procedures have come under severe attack from the opponents of ART and from those who object to third party involvement in conception. The crux of their argument is that it jeopardizes the good of marriage and parenthood, family values, and the welfare of the child and

[62] J. FLETCHER, *The Ethics of Genetic Control: Ending Reproductive Roulette,* Anchor Press/Doubleday, New York 1974. Cited in L. WALTERS, "Reproductive Technology and Genetics," in R. VEATCH (ed.), *Medical Ethics, Second Edition,* Jones and Bartlett Publishers, Inc., p. 210.

[63] R. TONG, "Reproductive Technologies: Surrogacy," in W. REICH, (ed.), *Encyclopedia of Bioethics..., op. cit.,* p. 2226. Surrogacy challenges the traditional assumptions about parenthood and family.

[64] P. SINGER, "New Assisted Reproductive..., *op. cit.,* p. 100. The argument that IVF and certain AR techniques are unnatural is better grasped by Singer. Here, that ART is "natural" or "unnatural" is to be understood in terms of our rational human nature and dignity. So, the issue of the unnaturalness of intravenous feeding or wearing of glasses does not really arise.

that it evades sexual responsibility. Some critics even object to the use of the term "donor" because what actually takes place is gamete-selling. They assert that most men and women who donate their gametes are primarily motivated by financial compensation; this conforms to the finding that donors in almost every European country are initially attracted by the monetary benefit involved.[65]

Donor-Conception and Marriage and Parenthood: Critics argue that marriage is a life-long relationship and a mutual commitment between two individuals. A couple's true fertility is a matter of the two, not of each spouse separately, meaning that they are either fertile or infertile together.[66] Resorting to gametes, embryos, or wombs from donors introduces a third party into the marriage, which is not morally acceptable. In fact, some equate such a practice with resorting to adultery to have children, although others merely claim that it could weaken the taboo against adultery, because once women are granted the right to receive donor insemination, they may begin to prefer actual extramarital sex. Other critics argue that the use of donated gametes and the transformation of procreation into a laboratory procedure—or even a commercial enterprise—will adversely affect human relationships and society's perception of parental responsibility. In this light, Ramsey finds donor-conception theologically objectionable; he insists that keeping sexuality and procreation within marriage is the only way couples can remain faithful to God, Who established the unity between love and procreation.[67] Similarly, Rahner contends that a child should be "an embodiment of the abiding unity of the marriage-partners which is expressed

---

[65] T. IGLESIAS "Using Donor Egg and Sperm," in J. KILNER – P CUNNINGHAM – W. HAGER (eds.), *The Reproduction Revolution, op. cit.,* pp. 96-97. Cited J. SCHENKER, "Assisted Reproduction Practice in Europe: Legal and Ethical Aspects," *Human Reproduction Update 3,* no. 2, 1997: 177. Iglesias refers to The 1979 European Convention and she notes that the compensation for sperm sample in the US is about $150 to $200 and that some students donate their sperm often to meet their financial needs, such as paying for their studies in the university.

[66] Ibid., p. 109.

[67] J. FLETCHER, "*Reproductive Technologies…, op. cit.*, p. 536.

in marital union,"[68] rather than result from donated sperm and ova that are technologically manipulated. Arguing from the ethical perspective, Richard McCormick maintains that the use of a third party in conception disrupts the continuity of love necessary for an optimal expression of sexuality and parenthood. According to this view, once the foundation of procreation in marriage is violated, the parental obligation to love and care for children will be undermined.[69] This rupture is visible in the refusal of the donor to fulfil his parental role under the guise of anonymity, without considering its implication for the child. On this, Rahner writes,

> For the child produced by such a method is, in this sense, the child of the mother and of the donor. The latter refuses, however, to acknowledge his fatherhood in an act of personal love: he remains anonymous or at least does not wish to be the donor in respect of this particular mother; precisely through his anonymity he robs the child of the right and the ability to fulfil the obligation of his existence, namely to accept himself as the child of these particular parents.[70]

Gamete Donation is Demeaning to Donors: Critics of donor conception argue that it not only exposes women to many risks for financial compensation, but it also demeans the donors, whose relevance is tied to their gametes. This view is well-articulated by Iglesias:

> The donor is important only because his or her body is a reproductive resource; it produces the gametes "cell," from which a child might be conceived. The donor as a person, as a human being, remains faceless, anonymous; he or she is irrelevant. The fact that a donor has a name, history, and life story about who he or she is means

[68] K. RAHNER, "The problem of Genetic Manipulation," in S. LAMMERS – A. VERHEY (eds.), *On Moral Medicine…, op. cit.,* p. 543.

[69] J. FLETCHER, "*Reproductive Technologies…, op. cit.*, p. 536.

[70] K. RAHNER, "The Problem of Genetic Manipulation…, *op. cit.,* p. 543. Although Rahner's principal focus here is genetic manipulation, his view on the implication of donor-conception for the child is relevant.

> relatively little in this mode of generation. The child's origin is taken to be from the gamete—an "anonymous" cell—not really from a parent, as the person who engenders. The genetic connection to the one who possesses the engendering powers, the actual parent, is deemed inconsequential. When the donor gives the gametes, he or she disassociates and is disassociated from them. Once the gametes are given away, they have no more connection with the donor. In the whole process, what matters are the gametes, not the donor as a person; what matters is relevant "reproductive material" from which a child might develop. The donor as a person and the "reproductive material" are severed. The human body and the human will go separate ways. Human wholeness is broken down.[71]

Because the child is the real focus of the entire procedure, donors are dispensed from the parental responsibility that arises naturally from the gametes they freely contributed towards the generation of the child. This reduces them to mere "providers and distributors of raw material," whereas in reality, donating one's gamete makes one a genetic parent of a child; if this is done 10 times, he or she is the genetic parent to 10 children and possibly 10 different families.[72] Moreover, the practice does not respect bodily integrity as it reduces body parts to marketable commodities.

Donor-Conception and Family: For many critics, donor-conception, including surrogacy arrangement, challenges the traditional notions of family and carries serious negative consequences for family structures, values, and relationships.[73] Donor-conception makes it possible for a woman to give birth to her own grandchild using the egg from her daughter, or to give birth to her own nephew using the egg from her

[71] T. IGLESIAS, "Using Donor Eggs and…, *op. cit.,* p. 101.

[72] Ibid., p. 102. There is another dimension to the problem. Each child could have half-brothers and/or half-sisters in other families, thus creating the possibility of marriage between brothers and sisters.

[73] R. ROWLAND, "Human Embryo Research: A Global Social Experiment," in H. KUHSE – P. SINGER (eds.), *Bioethics: An Anthology…, op. cit.,* p. 98.

sister, or to give birth to the biological child of a total stranger through anonymous egg donation. The use of donated sperm, ovum, and womb in some IVF-surrogacy procedures makes it possible for a child to be connected to four or five different persons at its conception;[74] as we stated earlier, seven types of motherhood are possible in surrogacy contracts. All these arrangements in ART create new forms of genetic relationships that never existed in the past.[75]

Donor-Conception and Kinship: One of the major ethical and legal concerns about donor-conception is the issue of kinship that arises when the sperm from a donor is used to achieve conception in several women. Rejecting the practice, critics argue that siblings who are related by half blood through a common sperm or egg donor might marry and have children, oblivious to their blood relationship. Since most states and religions prohibit marriage within a certain degree of consanguinity, if this is discovered at a later period, it would automatically render the marriage null and void.[76] Unfortunately, the rule prohibiting an individual from donating sperm more than 10 times to minimize this risk is arbitrary.[77]

Donor-Conception and Sexual Responsibility: Procreation is a serious matter that can have irreversible consequences for parents, the child, and society.[78] Critics of donor-conception argue that since the way we use our generative power can affect or harm others, it is necessary to assume personal responsibility for our actions in this area. They insist that there is a significant moral difference between donating a gamete or embryo

---

[74] R. ROWLAND, "Human Embryo Research..., *op. cit.,* p. 98. In this case, the child can be related to three women (genetic, gestational and social) and two men (genetic and social).

[75] ASRM ETHICS COMMITTEE REPORT, AMERICAN SOCIETY OF REPRODUCTIVE MEDICINE, "Family members as gamete donors and surrogacy," *Fertility and Sterility 80,* No. 5, November 2003. From the facts emerging from the genetic sciences, a womb donor actually contributes genetically to the child.

[76] W. WADLINTON, "Reproductive Technologies: Artificial..., *op. cit.,* p. 2218.

[77] L. MASTROIANNI, "Reproductive Technologies: Introduction," in W. REICH (ed.), *Encyclopedia of Bioethics..., op. cit.,* p. 2208.

[78] S. CALLAHAN, "The Ethical Challenge..., *op. cit.,* p. 516.

and donating an organ. Unlike the latter, the former involves the generation of a new human being with dignity. Thus, to donate or, worse still, to sell one's gamete or embryo to others (especially unknown persons) is to reject present and future parental responsibility. Such an attitude clearly erodes a basic foundation of morality, which is the need to take responsibility for our actions. Donor-conception does not measure up to the standard of morally responsible sexual behaviour.[79] Hollinger repudiates sperm donation for this very reason, adding that it debases fatherhood. To support this point, he cites the view of Daniel Blankenhorn, who asserts, "The sperm father completes his fatherhood prior to the birth of his child. His fatherhood consists entirely of the biological act of ejaculation. He spreads his seed, nothing more. He is a minimalist father, a one-act dad."[80] Iglesias remarks that no matter how much we attempt to view the bond between the genetic parent and the prospective child as non-existent, in reality it does exist "genetically, materially, in the flesh."[81] Some perceive the action of the donor or the partial surrogate who relinquishes her child as an indication that the child is not wanted, but advocates of the practice repudiate this claim, stating that we cannot fairly describe the child as unwanted. As Harris contends, the fact that the prospective mother or couple endures the complications of using donated gametes shows that the child is ardently wanted.[82] However, Harris fails to acknowledge that the child is not wanted by the anonymous gamete donor, who is the real genetic parent.

COMMODIFICATION OF HUMAN GAMETES, EMBRYOS, AND CHILDREN

The intrusion of profit motives into the human generative process occurs frequently in donor-conceptions and surrogacy contracts; this raises profound ethical problems because it touches directly on the dignity of the human person. This intrusion produces a situation in which children, gametes, and embryos are treated as commodities to

---

[79] Ibid., pp. 514-517. In donor conception, the donor has no responsibility for the life that ensues partly from his action.

[80] D. BLANKENHORN, *Fatherless America: Confronting our Most Urgent Social Problem*, Basic Books, New York 1995, p. 171. Cited in D. HOLLINGER, "Sexual Ethical and Reproductive..., *op. cit.,* p. 87.

[81] T. IGLESIAS, "Using Donor Egg and..., *op. cit.,* p. 103.

[82] J. HARRIS, "Right and Reproduction Choice..., *op. cit.,* pp. 13-14.

be bought and sold, and in which women are treated as commodities to be rented as a means of procreation.[83] As Meilaender adds, there are even custom-made embryos that allow prospective parents to choose the combination of sperm and egg donors that best meet their expectations for the future child.[84] Commenting on the increasing commercialization of ART, Chris Raymond observes, "Buffeted by the pressures of commercial interest and near-desperate patients searching for a technological miracle, the technique has become a major player in the increasingly lucrative fertility market."[85] In accord with this observation, Blank and Merricks point to the aggressive marketing techniques employed by some private centres,[86] and Shannon describes ART as "a multi-million dollar per year market," noting the serious competition for clients on the part of the fertility clinics.[87]

Some feminists contend that the commercialization of ART destroys the integrity of women. Elizabeth Anderson argues that the reproductive abilities of women, and the children that result from them, are qualitatively different from manufactured products and cannot be treated as such. A woman's relationship to her body is so intimate that the body cannot be viewed as property, and the value of money is not comparable to the value of a person's body and the intrinsic worth of children.[88] Margaret Tighe remarks that IVF has created "horrendous possibilities"

[83] OFFICE OF TECHNOLOGY ASSESSMENT, U.S. CONGRESS, *Reproductive Health Hazards in the Work Place,* Government Printing Office, Washington D.C., 1988, p. 327.

[84] G. MEILAENDER, "A Child of One's Own: At What Price..., *op. cit.,* p. 44.

[85] C. RAYMOND, "In Vitro Fertilisation Enter Stormy Adolescence as Experts Debate Odds," *Journal of American Medical Association,* 1988, 259 (4): 464-466; Cited by R. BLANK – J. MERRICKS, *Human Reproduction..., op. cit.,* p. 95.

[86] R. BLANK – J. MERRICKS, *Human Reproduction..., op. cit.,* p. 95.

[87] T. SHANNON, "Ethical Issues in Genetics," in T. SHANNON – A. WOLTER (eds.), *The New Genetic Medicine, op. cit.,* p. 25.

[88] B. MINOGUE, *Bioethics: A Committee Approach..., op. cit.,* pp. 167-168.

for the manipulation of human beings, creating a situation in which a certain category of persons can be treated as consumer products.[89]

THE RISKS OF IVF FOR THE CHILD AND DONORS

An argument against IVF and similar techniques is that they carry higher rates of ectopic pregnancy, multiple pregnancy, premature delivery, and low birth weight. Because of these risks and IVF's low success rate, some have come to view it as a failed technology.[90] Some, however, consider the risks to offspring to be minimal, and this justifies it in their opinion. In comparison to natural conception, they cite only an additional 3% risk that an IVF child will be born with abnormalities.[91]

An ethical evaluation of the acceptable level of risk to offspring reveals a wide divergence of opinion. While John Biggers accepts the 3% additional risk,[92] Paul Ramsey insists that even "a 1% chance of error in any artificial reproductive procedure involving an unborn child is not negligible" and that such a possibility creates a "conclusive argument against any attempt at IVF."[93] Kass insists on a level of risk that is equivalent to or less than that of natural conception, while Charles Curran settles for a figure that is almost the same as in the natural process.[94] Further, the deleterious effects of ART on the egg donors and surrogate mothers pose a moral problem, especially as treatment does not always succeed in one cycle. But those who approve of the techniques dismiss this, claiming that any minor harm involved in IVF and its variants is outweighed by the benefit of bringing a child into existence[95] and the happiness that will result from it.

---

89 M. TIGHE, "A Pandora's Box of Social and Moral Problems," in H. KUSHE – P. SINGER (eds.), *Bioethics: An Anthology, op. cit.,* p. 91.

90 R. ROLAND, "Human Embryo Research: A Global Social Experiment," in H. KUSHE – P. SINGER (eds.), *Bioethics: An Anthology, op. cit.,* pp. 96-97.

91 A. JONSEN – R. VEATCH – L. WALTERS (eds.), *Source Book in Bioethics: A Documentary History,* Georgetown University Press, Washington, D.C. 1998, p. 95.

92 Ibid.

93 J. FLETCHER, "Reproductive Technologies..., *op. cit.,* p. 538.

94 A. JONSEN – R. VEATCH – L. WALTERS (eds.), *Source Book in Bioethics..., op. cit.*, p. 95.

95 L. PURDY, "Assisted Reproduction..., *op. cit.,* p. 165.

OLDER WOMEN AND IVF

The news of an Italian woman who gave birth at age 62, using donated eggs, and of a British woman who had twins at age 56[96] provoked a mixed reaction in many places; the crux of the matter is whether it is appropriate to offer ART to older women. Some claim that offering IVF to women who have reached menopause will create a market in which eggs from younger women can be purchased. As Shannon observes, although some of these eggs come from successful IVF patients who no longer require them, most are harvested in donor programmes where younger women are paid to undergo the IVF egg retrieval procedure, which exposes them to short- and long-term health risks.[97]

For some commentators, the real controversy in offering ART to older women is that some of them will not live long enough to rear the children to adulthood;[98] those who defend the practice find such an assumption unreasonable, pointing out the differences in life expectancy for women in different parts of the world. They maintain that the probability of rearing a child to adulthood would be higher for women who give birth in their 50s in developed countries than for women who give birth in their late 20s in places where life expectancy is below 50 years.[99]

RESPECT FOR THE PSYCHO-SOCIAL INTEGRITY AND WELL-BEING OF THE CHILD

Although several people are intimately involved in an ART procedure, the potential child will undoubtedly be most affected; fairness demands that any ethical evaluation should accord priority to the child's future welfare, especially because he is not in a position to consent to it.[100] According to Robert Snowden and others, "In making decision

[96] R. ROLAND, "Human Embryo Research..., *op. cit.,* p. 98.

[97] T. SHANNON, "Reproductive Technologies: Ethical and Religious Issues," in T. SHANNON (ed.), *Reproductive Technologies, op. cit.,* pp. 40-41.

[98] L. PURDY, "Assisted Reproduction..., *op. cit.,* p.168.

[99] J. JACKSON, "Can Older Women Cope with Motherhood?" in H. KUSHE – P. SINGER (eds.), *Bioethics: An Anthology, op. cit.,* p. 118.

[100] K. O' ROURKE (ed.), *A Primer for Health Care Ethics..., op. cit.,* p. 266. O'Rourke maintains that as far as ART is concerned, any sound ethical evaluation must consider the overall effects (physical, psychological, social and

and undertaking procedures to fulfil the wishes of the would-be parents, it would be improper to forget that some child must live with the consequences of those decision and procedures."[101] The impact of donor-conception on the child has received a great deal of publicity. For opponents as well as some staunch supporters of homologous AI and IVF, donor-conception is harmful and morally reprehensible because it separates the various aspects of normal parenthood (genetic, gestational, and rearing) and poses potentially serious risks to the dignity and well-being of the future child.[102] Resorting to donated gametes to provide children for infertile couples, single people, and homosexuals satisfies their desire to have children, but it ignores the interest of the child. It violates the dignity of the child, who deserves to be treated as an end in itself rather than as a means to fulfil the desires of others. It also overlooks the growing need for family therapy and family system analysis in modern medicine, which may require a child to identify the biological parents.[103] On the basis of the aforementioned reasons, Callahan strongly rejects donor-conception, claiming that

> The assumption seems to be that why and how one gets a baby makes no difference in what happens afterwards. They may be true of hens or cows, but it is hardly true of complex, thinking, emoting, imaginative human beings functioning within social systems.[104]

Callahan maintains that the gradual collapse of the traditional family system will have serious negative effects on children who are the products of such collapsed families. From the psychological standpoint, to have two rearing parents is considered advantageous for the child; the father plays an important role in the holistic development of the child,

---

spiritual) on all who are principally affected by the decision to use it, especially the child who is the only one among them who is not in a position to consent to it.

[101] R SNOWDEN – G. MITCHELL – E. SNOWDEN, *Artificial Reproduction,* George Allen and Unwin, London 1983, p. 5.

[102] S. CALLAHAN, "The Ethical Challenge..., *op. cit.,* pp. 511-512.

[103] Ibid., pp. 512, 515, 517.

[104] Ibid. Cited S. HANSON – F. BONNETT, *Dimensions of the Fatherhood,* Sage Publications, Beverly Hills, California 1985.

contributing to intellectual, moral, social, and sexual-identity formation.[105] Many critics argue that the introduction of third parties into the human generative process obscures the child's origins and can endanger his sense of identity and personality development. O'Rourke asserts that the sense of identity one needs for a healthy personal development is founded on the fact that one knows one's parents: "The development of identity in each person results from gestation, nurturing, and education. These three elements are a continuum."[106] Similarly, Iglesias argues that every human being has a beginning, a middle, and an end. Each person's story forms his personal identity, but parents deliberately tell their donor-conceived children only a part of their life-story to maintain secrecy. In her words, "The story begins somewhere, but no one knows where, because everyone hides it. When it is not fully hidden, even the full story cannot be told."[107]

Oftentimes, to avoid the psychological problems associated with the practice, parents will shroud it in secrecy. In a study by Golombok and colleagues, only 8.6% of parents of AID-conceived children over age 11 have disclosed to them the nature of their conception. About 12% expressed the intention to do so in the future, while about 75% do not intend to disclose it, even though over half of them have told a friend or a family member.[108] This implies that at least 75% of those children will never know their real fathers and the manner of their conception, or they will learn the truth from someone other than a parent. Addressing this situation, some critics assert that a child has a right to know its genetic origins. The need to maintain confidentiality carries the possibility of lying or deception, in which case a child would not be told the full truth about his biological origins; this unjustly denies him the right to

[105] Ibid.

[106] K. O'ROURKE (ed.), *A Primer for Health Care Ethics..., op. cit.*, p. 266.

[107] Cf. T. IGLESIAS, Using Donor Eggs and..., *op. cit.*, p. 110.

[108] See S. GOLOMBOK – M. BREWAEYS *et al.*, "The European study of assisted reproduction families: The transition to adolescence," *Human Reproduction,* 2002. Cited in D. MORGAN – R. LEE, "Human Reproduction and Human Rights," in D. SINGER – M. HUNTER, *Assisted Human Reproduction..., op. cit.*, p. 66.

know his biological father and half-siblings.[109] These critics argue that donor-conception is harmful to the child; the deception, in addition to being objectively wrong, can hardly be sustained in many cases, and the discovery of the truth can harm the child severely and disrupt relationships within the family; such a discovery burdens the child with adverse psychological and social repercussions,[110] which may include a distressing search for the real father or parents. Discussing the ways that donor-conception can harm the child and disrupt the family, Callahan writes the following:

> When there is one or more third party donors—of sperm, eggs, or embryo—the child is cut off from either half or all of its genetic heritage. If deception is practiced concerning the child's origins, then both the child and the extended family will be wronged. Since family secrets are rarely kept completely, the delayed revelations produce disillusionment and distrust among those deceived. When the child and relatives are not lied to, the identity of the donor (or donors) becomes an issue for all concerned.[111]

For many, the discovery that they were conceived with sold gametes and embryos or through commercial surrogacy is devastating to their sense of worth and personal identity.[112] Reacting to her conception with anonymously donated sperm, Suzanne Rubin poignantly questions, "How do I reconcile my sense of integrity with knowing that my father sold what was the essence of my life for $25 to a total stranger.... What

---

[109] J. RICHARDS, "Ethical Issue – The Major Faiths: A Personal View," in D. SINGER – M. HUNTER (eds.), *Assisted Human Reproduction, op. cit.,* p. 42.

[110] Ibid., p. 51.

[111] S. CALLAHAN, "The Ethical Challenge..., *op. cit.,* p. 513.

[112] A. KIMBRELL, *The Human Body Shop: The Cloning Engineering and Marketing of Life, Second Edition,* Roguery Publishing Inc., Washington, D.C. 1997, p. 82.

kind of man sells himself and his child so cheaply and so easily?"[113] Besides the fact that donor-conception exalts deception, it is a mere instrument for satisfying some adults' desires for money or biological children, and it cannot be in the best interest of the child that results. On this basis, critics contend that it should be completely outlawed.

This issue also raises questions about the child's right to information. While some support partial secrecy, advocates of the child's right to know insist on total information, arguing that the child's right to know should override the benefits that will accrue to parents and gamete donors through secrecy and anonymity;[114] such information should include the manner of the child's conception, the medical and genetic condition of the donor, and his or her identity. Rejecting this, some advocates of donor-conception argue for total secrecy because divulging such information will harm the child and parents, violating the principle of non-malfeasance. Critics respond to this by asserting that secrecy cannot be an application of the principle of beneficence.

The need to protect the donor's anonymity must also be considered. The Council of Europe insists on the protection of the identities of all the parties involved, including the donor; under the European Convention, a single woman or even a lesbian couple is entitled to have a child, despite the possible absence of a legal father.[115] On the other hand, respect for

[113] S. RUBIN, "Reproductive Option 1: A Sperm Donor Baby Grows Up," Cited in E. BLYTH – C. POTTER, "Paying For It? Market Force..., *op. cit.,* p. 235.

[114] J. THEVOZ, "The Rights of Children to Information," in D. EVANS – N. PICKERING (eds.), *Creating the Child: The Ethics, Law and Practices of Assisted Procreation,* Martinus Nijhoff Publishers, The Hague 1996, pp. 197, 203.

[115] EUROPEAN CONVENTION, 1978, Cited in J. SCHENKER, "Assisted Reproduction Practice in Europe: Legal and Ethical Aspects," *Human Reproduction Update 3,* No. 2, 1997, p. 1175. For some, it is one of the basic human rights of a person to decide when and how to conceive and following the position of the Council of Europe, the donor's identity is never to be disclosed. In Europe, only Sweden insists on the right of the child to obtain information about the identity of the donor.

private and family life requires that each person should be able to establish details of his identity, even if he was donor-conceived.[116]

[116] D. MORGAN – R. LEE, "Human Feproduction and Human Rights," in D. SINGER – M. HUNTER (eds.), *Assisted Human Reproduction…, op. cit.* p. 66.

OTHER ARGUMENTS IN ART

The artificial reproductive technologies have received serious attention from many feminists. In this section, we intend to examine commercial surrogacy in greater detail and consider the general opinions of feminists regarding ART.

SURROGACY AND COMMERCIAL SURROGACY

One of the most widely attacked of all the ART procedures is the surrogacy contract. In this area, we can distinguish three main positions: those who disapprove of every form of surrogacy, those who oppose only commercial surrogacy, and those who approve of commercial and non-commercial surrogacy. We will discuss arguments and counter-arguments regarding the morality of these practices.

COMMERCIAL SURROGACY AND THE DIGNITY OF WOMEN

Some feminists argue that surrogacy contracts do not respect the integrity and worth of women. Such contracts offer wealthy individuals the opportunity to exploit poor women, forcing them to surrender control over their bodies. This treats the poor women as objects or as baby-machines and selfishly exploits them.[117,118] May maintains that commercial surrogacy and the sale of eggs introduce the practices and symbols of the market place into the human generative process; by treating women and children as commodities that can be traded, they distort the very meaning of bearing and parenting a child. In his view, a society demeans itself when it allows a poor person to sell a part of his or her body. This was the opinion of the New Jersey Supreme Court trial judge who reviewed the Stern/Whitehead case: he declared the payment of money to Beth Whitehead for Baby M to be illegal and potentially degrading to women.[119] Corea alleges that in commercial surrogacy, the

[117] B. MINOGUE, *Bioethics: A Committee Approach, op. cit.*, p. 157.

[118] Cf. S. HOLDER, "Surrogate Motherhood: Babies for Fun and Profit," *Law, Medicine and Health Care,* 11 June 1984, 115-117.

[119] W. MAY, "The Gestated and Sold," in S. LAMMERS – A. VERHEY (eds.), *On Moral Medicine…, op. cit.,* pp. 519-520. Cited excerpts from the New Jersey Supreme Court decision in: "The Matter of Baby M," *The New York Times,* February 4, 1988.

woman is reduced to a mere vessel for the man's seed, a fact that is clear from her being described as various inanimate objects, such as incubator, receptacle, or rented property.[120] Others compare it to prostitution, noting that the principle that underlies both practices is the degradation of one's body for monetary benefit. As Kass insists, the practice is tantamount to the buying and selling of a human body and is therefore dehumanizing; it denies the close relationship between sexuality, love, and procreation.[121] As in prostitution, in which a woman degrades her own body for money by using it to satisfy another's lust, a paid surrogate mother denies the meaning and worth of her body by treating it as a mere incubator.[122]

Commercial surrogacy does not respect human dignity. The worth of the surrogate is reduced to her ability to carry a pregnancy to term; this reduction violates her dignity even though she gave her consent. Such a reduction is evident in the rules a surrogate mother may have to observe. She may be required to refrain from acts that will promote bonding with the child, reducing pregnancy to something mechanical. Also, the commissioning couple may cut her off completely after she gives birth and hands over the baby,[123] failing to consider the adverse psychological impact this will have on her, especially if she is also the genetic mother.

RISKS AND EXPLOITATION OF SURROGATE MOTHERS

A surrogacy arrangement does not guarantee that surrogate mothers are safe from exploitation by those who contract them; for this reason, some feminists view it as a threat to feminist values.[124] Singer admits that once money is introduced into surrogacy arrangements, it will create possibilities for the exploitation of surrogate mothers.[125] Other critics

---

[120] G. COREA, *The Mother Machine*, Perennial Library, New York 1986, pp. 221-222. She maintains that the surrogates themselves have come to see themselves this way.

[121] L. KASS, *Life, Liberty…, op. cit.*, p. 101.

[122] Ibid.

[123] G. MEILAENDER, *Bioethics, A Primer for Christians, op., cit.*, p. 22.

[124] B. MINOGUE, *Bioethics: A Committee Approach…, op. cit.*, p. 157.

[125] P. SINGER – D. WELLS, *The Reproductive Revolution,* Oxford University Press, New York 1984, p. 125. This does not mean that Singer repudiates the practice.

argue that although surrogate mothers freely consent to such arrangements, they are often compelled to do so by their socio-economic situations. Following interactions with several surrogate mothers and with people who have dealt with them, Chesler describes the kind of woman who will likely accept such a project:

> She is a fertile woman of childbearing years who has already proven herself as a biological mother; a relatively uneducated and impoverished woman who is married to a low-income husband and whose own economic options are so limited that less than a dollar an hour (for doing "nothing"—that is, carrying a child) sounds good to her—given that she is also a full-time but unpaid housewife and mother.[126]

According to one school of thought, the mere fact that a surrogate mother agrees to sign a contract does not prove that she was not exploited.[127] Hence, some argue for the prohibition of commercial surrogacy on the grounds that it is harmful and exploitative of women who engage in it. According to Rosemarie Tong, "Since there is evidence that surrogacy harms contracted mothers, a ban on commercial surrogacy needs only to rely on the harm principle."[128] Some surrogate mothers are indeed exploited in certain surrogacy contracts, such as when they are paid only part of the agreed wages if they give birth to a dead or disabled child. Both advocates and opponents of the technique agree that this practice is exploitative and cannot be justified, because these problems can also occur in natural conception; besides, the physicians and the contracting lawyers often receive their full payment in such contracts even though their efforts did not yield a child. Other critics argue that

---

[126] P. CHESLER, *Sacred Bond: The Legacy of Baby M.,* Times Book, New York 1988, pp. 44-45; Cited in L. SCHWARTZ, *Alternatives to Infertility..., op. cit.,* pp. 114, 119. For Chester, the other possible motives for surrogacy are: religious (to make a sacrifice) and psychological. The surrogate's husband may consent to the contract for altruistic reasons, the need to please his wife or for the money that will accrue from it.

[127] B. MINOGUE, *Bioethics: A Committee Approach, op. cit.*, p. 167.

[128] R. TONG, "The Overdue Death of a Feminist Chameleon: Taking Stand on Surrogacy Arrangements," *Journal of Social Philosophy 21,* (1999), 47.

the amount the surrogate is paid—perhaps $10,000—is insufficient considering the physical and psychological risks and considering that the lawyer may receive the same amount.[129]

Though proponents condemn the exploitation of surrogate mothers, they argue that this is insufficient justification for prohibiting surrogacy contracts. Instead, they prefer the approach of regulating the practice in order to eliminate exploitation. They also dismiss the argument that it should be prohibited because it is risky to women who engage in it: if people are allowed to engage in far riskier activities, such as using toxic chemicals, operating dangerous machinery, and climbing mountains, it would be unreasonable to prohibit surrogacy.[130] They assert that surrogacy allows the risks of pregnancy to be transferred to healthier women, who also are likely to produce healthier children.[131] For some, infertility is a medical problem, and surrogacy is the medical solution to it;[132] the benefits it offers surpass the risks involved. They reject the argument for the prohibition of surrogacy contracts, claiming that this argument is motivated by paternalistic tendencies or by the unjustified desire to protect those who wish to avail themselves of surrogacy's potential benefits.[133]

SURROGACY AND THE DEONTOLOGICAL RULE

The deontological rule guiding experimentation with human subjects stipulates that their informed consent must first be obtained, particularly in experiments that expose them to serious risks. Some argue that surrogacy violates this principle because the child has no say in the arrangement; they assert that surrogacy poses a threat to the welfare of the prospective child—a threat that outweighs the benefits it offers to the contracting parties.[134]

---

[129] L. PURDY, "Surrogate Mothering," in H. KUHSE – P. SINGER (eds.), *Bioethics: An Anthology, op. cit.,* pp. 107-109; ID., "Assisted Conception," in H. KUHSE – P. SINGER (eds.), *A Companion to Bioethics, op. cit.,* p. 169.

[130] L. PURDY, "Surrogacy Mothering…, *op. cit.,* pp. 105, 109.

[131] Ibid.

[132] B. MINOGUE, *Bioethics: A Committee Approach, op. cit.,* pp. 154-159.

[133] Ibid, pp. 160-163.

[134] Ibid., p. 160.

SURROGACY AND THE ISSUE OF BONDING

Under normal circumstances, a woman is expected to "pour" herself (physically and emotionally) into the gestation of a child, but in surrogacy contracts, a surrogate mother is encouraged to suppress any emotional attachment to the child and avoid actions that may increase natural bonding between her and the child.[135] Objecting to this, opponents contend that pregnancy is not a neutral biological experience; rather, it is a period during which a natural, intimate relationship develops between mother and child, and this relationship may not be easy to break.[136] By eliminating this natural bonding between mother and child, surrogacy reduces pregnancy to an empty experience; it is a process of manufacturing in which the surrogate is reduced to, and actually views herself as, a mere incubator.[137] It is perhaps this reductionist and destructive tendency[138] that led Warnock to assert that a surrogacy contract "seems to degrade the phenomenon of pregnancy and childbirth."[139]

SURROGACY IS HARMFUL TO THE CHILD

Surrogacy arrangements can be harmful, not only to the parties directly involved, but also to the family[140] and society. Young children of a surrogate who see their mother pregnant and begin to look forward to the birth of a baby may be harmed psychologically when she gives the baby away; older children may grow up to view motherhood in terms of commercial transactions rather than in terms of a life-long commitment.[141] To support this point, critics often cite protracted legal battles surrounding the custody of children resulting from surrogacy arrange-

---

[135] S. RAE, "Surrogate Motherhood..., *op. cit.*, pp. 122-123.

[136] S. CALLAHAN, "The Ethical Challenge..., *op. cit.*, p. 515; See also K. O'ROURKE (ed.), *A Primer for Health Care Ethics...*, *op. cit.*, p. 266.

[137] F. BASTERRA, *Bioethics*, St Pauls, Kindare, Ireland 1994, pp. 82-83; See also S. CALLAHAN, "The Ethical Challenge..., *op. cit.*, p. 515; See also K. O'ROURKE (ed.), *A Primer for Health Care Ethics...*, *op. cit.*, p. 266.

[138] S. RAE, "Surrogate Motherhood..., *op. cit.*, pp. 122-123.

[139] M. WARNOCK, *Nature and Morality*, Continuum, London – New York 2003, p. 103.

[140] J. RICHARDS, "Ethical Issues – The Major Faiths..., *op. cit.*, p. 53.

[141] Ibid.

ments; one example is the famous Stern/Whitehead battle for Baby M in 1985 in the United States.[142] Kiss argues that donor-conception and surrogacy will further compromise "the virtues of family, lineage and heterosexuality" and weaken the taboos against adultery and incest.[143] In contrast, supporters argue that surrogacy will not be detrimental to the family if people resort to it for good reasons.

Critics who consider commercial surrogacy to be harmful to the surrogate mother[144] and the child[145] call for its prohibition based on the principle of non-maleficence: "not to inflict evil or harm." Others vehemently oppose surrogacy contracts as a form of baby-selling, arguing that handing over a child at birth in exchange for money treats him as a commodity. Thus, commercial surrogacy degrades the child, whose intrinsic dignity raises him above the vicissitudes of the markets.[146,147] The Warnock Committee recommended that commercial surrogacy be outlawed in the United Kingdom, arguing that it involves child-selling and therefore contradicts human dignity.[148]

Proponents of surrogacy do not consider it a form of baby-selling; they claim that a man whose sperm was used to inseminate a surrogate cannot be buying a child that was already genetically his, and the fact that he will be the child's social father makes the charge of baby-selling untenable.[149] Since a child is not property that another can own, the surrogate

---

142 Beth Whitehead who was contracted for $10,000 as a surrogate was artificially inseminated with Stern's sperm, but after the delivery of Baby M, she changed her mind and wanted custody of the baby.

143 A. JONSEN – R. VEATCH – L. WALTERS (eds.), *Source Book in Bioethics…, op. cit.* p. 96.

144 If the surrogate is also the genetic mother, a serious psychological burden may be imposed on her if she has to give away the child with whom she has bonded for months.

145 The prospective social parents may refuse to accept the child if he is born with a disability whereas the surrogate did not enter into the contract with an intention to rear it.

146 S. RAE, "Surrogate Motherhood…, *op. cit.,* p. 117.

147 S. CALLAHAN, "The Ethical Challenge…, *op. cit.,* p. 515.

148 M. WARNOCK, *Nature and Morality, op. cit.,* pp. 45-46.

149 S. RAE, "Surrogate Motherhood…, *op. cit.,* p. 116.

cannot sell what she does not own. On the contrary, the parents pay for the biological services of the woman and the surrogate's "parental right to have a relationship with the child," not the child itself.[150] Thus, the practice does not treat the child as a commodity.

Insisting that commercial surrogacy is baby-selling, other critics argue for its prohibition from the standpoint of the right of the child; they cite the prohibition of slavery as proof that human beings, irrespective of race or colour, are not items that can be traded for financial gains. In their opinion, such a prohibition will safeguard the interests of the potential child and prevent the exploitation of the surrogate or of the commissioning couple.[151] They repudiate the advocates' claim that a man cannot buy what is already his, insisting that it is based on the mistaken assumption that the child is only his; they compare a surrogacy contract to a quit claim deed in a piece of property because the father buys out the surrogate's interest in the child, making it "a commercial transaction for the rights to the child or baby selling."[152]

Nowadays, surrogacy contracts are carefully structured such that the payment to the surrogate is related to her gestational services rather than to the transfer of her parental right to the child. Critics view this new development as a bid to disguise the true nature of the contract, claiming that "most surrogacy contracts are structured around the product, not the process or the surrogate's gestational services."[153] As George Annas asserts,

> Surrogacy brokers need a dose of realism. They should not be permitted to hide behind the grief of infertile couples. They are not in business to help them; they are in business to make money. What the primary

[150] N. MALM, "Selling Babies and Selling Bodies: Surrogate Motherhood and the Problem of Commodification," At the Eastern Division APA Meetings, 30 December 1987; Quoted by L. PURDY "Surrogate Mothering..., *op. cit.,* p. 108.

[151] S. RAE, "Surrogate Motherhood..., *op. cit.,* p. 117.

[152] Ibid., p. 115.

[153] Ibid., p. 116.

> screening brokers do is monetary; does the couple have the $25,000 fee?[154]

Some opponents contend that surrogacy carries serious psychological risks that are absent when the mother does not have to give up her child. It may be paternalistic to restrict the reproductive choices of women, but this does not make it morally wrong to prohibit surrogacy on the grounds that it is harmful.[155] Surrogacy, as practised now, is not aimed at transferring the burden of pregnancy from a high-risk woman to a low-risk woman. Instead, the emphasis seems to be on making it possible for the contracting man to have a child that will be genetically related to him, given that such contracts are often signed by him, the surrogate, and the surrogate's husband (if she is married).[156]

SURROGACY OBSCURES AND DEGRADES MOTHERHOOD

In the past, it was generally believed that the sperm and ovum alone determined the paternity of a child, but today, genetic science indicates that genetic inheritance combines with the environment of the womb and the disposition and health of the mother to determine the constitution and personality of the child. The genetic materials from the couple determine the child's physical traits and predispositions, while the gestational environment makes substantial contribution to the child's personality. As such, it is no longer possible to claim that the gestational mother contributes only her womb. Consequently, some critics allege that surrogacy obscures motherhood and parental rights because the birth mother contributes more than just her womb;[157] she perhaps makes a greater investment in the child than does the egg donor in terms of effort, physical

---

[154] G. ANNAS, "Death Without Dignity for Commercial Surrogacy: The Case of Baby M," *Hastings Centre Report 18,* April–May 1998: 22. Cited in S. RAE, "Surrogate Motherhood…, *op. cit.,* pp. 117.

[155] S. DODDS – K. JONES, "A Response to Purdy," in H. KUSHE – P. SINGER, *Bioethics: An Anthology, op. cit.,* p. 114.

[156] Ibid., p. 115.

[157] J. RICHARDS, "Ethical Issues – The Major Faiths…, *op. cit.,* p. 52; See also K. BARTLETT, "Re-expressing Parenthood," *Yale Law Journal 98,*1988: 329-330. Cited in S. RAE, "Surrogate Motherhood…, *op. cit.,* p. 120. In gestational surrogacy, two women make biological contributions to the future child.

and psychological risks, personal sacrifice, and the time expended on carrying the pregnancy to term. In this light, her claim to motherhood would be quite understandable; if she decides to keep the child, contrary to the terms of the contract, to deny her this right would be inconsistent with her biological and relational connections to the child.[158] In addition, critics find surrogacy degrading to both womanhood and motherhood because it introduces a division into the genetic, gestational, and rearing aspects. In natural conception, all these aspects are located in the same person, but in surrogacy, they are located in at least two and sometimes three different people: the woman who supplies the egg, the woman who gestates the child, and the woman who rears it.[159]

FEMINISTS' VIEWS ON ART

The woman bears the greater part of the physical and psychological burdens of most ART procedures. This makes it reasonable to consider women's views on ART.

ART AND WOMEN'S REPRODUCTIVE CHOICE

For liberal feminists, the various reproductive technologies enhance women's capacity to choose how to procreate, but others reject this, claiming that these choices are illusory. In reality, ART places a woman's reproductive choices in the hands of others who are not primarily interested in the woman's well-being. The choices offered by ART make little sense—they are merely the alternatives endorsed by society under social conditions that women did not create and are powerless to change. Most of the techniques allow intervention on healthy wives of infertile husbands and cause women to bear all the risks; this reality, however, is often explained and justified by referring to the woman's central biological role in pregnancy.[160]

---

[158] S. RAE, "Surrogate Motherhood..., *op. cit.,* pp. 119, 122.

[159] D. AWOYOKUN, "Perils of IVF and Surrogacy Motherhood," *Vanguard,* Monday, September 29, 2003.

[160] R. KLEIN, "What's 'New' about the 'New Reproductive Technologies?" in G. COREA, (ed.), *Man-made Women: How New Reproductive Technologies Affect Women,* Indiana University Press, Bloomington 1987, p. 65.

ART REDUCES WOMEN'S CONTROL OVER REPRODUCTION

Does ART enhance or diminish a woman's control over reproduction? The opinions of women diverge on this issue. Some feminists believe that the reproductive technologies enhance a woman's control over reproduction,[161] while others argue that these technologies promote women's dependence on physicians and medical techniques. Some contend that reproduction is a continuous process that should occur within a woman's body, whereas laboratory reproduction splits it into discrete and impersonal parts subject to a male-dominated medical profession.[162] Stressing this point, Corea asserts that ART strengthens men's claim to paternity and weakens women's claim to maternity by making the female reproductive experience discontinuous. Maternity is gradually being turned into an intellectual act that requires one to make "a causal connection between the extraction of an egg and the birth of a child to another woman nine months later,"[163] as in surrogacy. More importantly, by separating the various aspects of motherhood, surrogacy dismembers motherhood into genetic, gestational, and social forms. This can destroy the integrity of motherhood and weaken women's claim to maternity by making it contestable, as paternity used to be;[164] none of the three mothers has an overriding claim on the prospective child, causing women to lose one of their few sources of power.[165]

---

[161] S. SHERWIN, "Feminist Ethics and New Reproductive Technologies," in C. OVERALL (ed), *The Future of Human Reproduction,* Women's Press Toronto 1989, pp. 259–271. Also see A. BONNICKSON, "Reproductive Technologies: In Vitro Fertilisation and Embryo Transfer," in W. REICH (ed.), *Encyclopedia of Bioethics..., op. cit.,* p. 2223.

[162] Ibid.

[163] G. COREA, "The Mother Machine," in K. ALPERN (ed.), *The Ethics of Reproductive..., op. cit.,* pp. 223-224. Cited M. O'BRIEN, *The Politics of Reproduction,* Routledge & Kegan Paul Ltd., London and Boston, 1981. Here, Gena Corea also makes reference to the work of O'Brien.

[164] G. COREA, "The Mother Machine..., *op. cit.,* pp. 225-226.

[165] R. ARDITTI, "Review Essay: Reducing Women to Matter," *Women's Studies International Forum,* 1985, 8(6): 577-588.

ART AS A FORM OF DOMINATION OF WOMEN

Some feminists attribute sexist biases to ART; they see the techniques as attempts by men to control the procreative experience of women and, eventually, to remove their capacity to bring forth children. In natural conception, women play an active role by cooperating with their bodies to generate children, but in contrast, the whole process of laboratory production is "rationalized, objectified, planned and controlled by medical experts. More than ever before the woman is objectified and made passive."[166] They feel that women are deliberately targeted by these techniques, which can be employed as powerful instruments to help male scientists and physicians dominate them socially, economically, and politically.[167] In fact, some believe that once *ectogenesis* (artificial womb) or cloning techniques are perfected and approved for use, men will seek to completely remove women from society. Although the technologies affect women more than men, they "are virtually absent from the legal, scientific, and governmental bodies that are involved in the research, development, and delivery of the techniques."[168]

ART AND OVERPOPULATION

There are those who feel that ART may be unnecessary because the world is already threatened by overpopulation. Proponents of ART argue that although the issues of population may be problematic, it would be unfair to allow fertile couples to procreate freely while leaving the infertile ones to shoulder the burden of childlessness.[169]

---

[166] M. MIES, "Sexist and Racist Implications of New Reproductive Technologies," *Alternatives,* 1987, 12: 323-342. Cited in R. BLANK – J. MERRICK, *Human Reproduction…, op. cit.,* p. 103.

[167] R. KLEIN, "What's 'New' about the 'New Reproductive …, *op. cit.,* p. 65; See also L. PURDY, "Assisted Reproduction…, *op. cit.,* p. 164.

[168] R. BLANK – J. MERRICK, *Human Reproduction, Emerging…, op. cit.,* p. 104.

[169] P. SINGER, New Assisted Reproductive Technology," in H. KUHSE – P. SINGER, Bioethics: An Anthology, *op. cit.*, p. 100.

CHAPTER 8

ETHICAL ISSUES IN PGD, SEX SELECTION, AND HUMAN GENETIC ENHANCEMENT

Preimplantation Genetic Diagnosis (PGD), sex selection, and human genetic enhancement designs have been subjects of intense debate in the field of bioethics. Some thinkers approve of all the techniques, some argue for their limited application, and some disapprove of them completely.

ETHICAL ISSUES IN PGD

PGD may have a therapeutic value in preventing genetic diseases, but it is not without ethical problems. Since it relies on IVF technology, it involves all the ethical problems of IVF and other problems of its own. There are three main positions regarding PGD. The first is that it is morally unacceptable and should not be permitted. Advocates of the second position claim it would be morally acceptable if its application were limited to medical conditions.[1] The third position finds PGD, for both medical and non-medical applications, ethically permissible.

PRAGMATIC USE OF PGD AND REPRODUCTIVE AUTONOMY

The primary justifications for PGD are its therapeutic benefits, its pragmatic utility, and the necessity of respecting reproductive right and individual autonomy. They claim that it helps bring healthy children to couples at risk of passing on serious genetic disorders. Couples who would have remained childless because of their objection to abortion resulting from prenatal diagnosis see PGD as an acceptable option for having a child of their own. But critics argue that PGD does not guarantee that a child will be born healthy. Since it cannot detect the presence of conditions such as anencephaly and spina bifida in the pre-implantation embryo, prenatal diagnosis may still be required to confirm that the embryo is healthy.[2] Also, mosaicism may cause a healthy embryo to be discarded or an unhealthy embryo to be implanted.

Some advocates claim that PGD is better than prenatal diagnosis followed by selective abortion. The veracity of this opinion depends on when human personhood actually begins. For those who attribute personhood to the human embryo at any stage after implantation, PGD may be better for psychological reasons. This is certainly not the case, however, for those who believe that personhood begins at fertilisation. They consider selective abortion and the discarding of human embryos

---

[1] Cf. L. SPEROFF – M. FRITZ, *Clinical Gynecologic…, op. cit.*, p. 1239; See also B. STEINBOCK, "Pre-implantation Genetic Diagnosis and Embryo Selection," in J. BURLEY – J. HARRIS (eds.) *A Companion to Genetics, op. cit.*, pp. 175-176; See also I. MURRAY, "'Designer baby' inquiry ordered," *The Times,* January 17, 1998, p. 36.

[2] J. BOTKIN, "Ethical issues and practical problems in pre-implantation genetic diagnosis," *Journal of Law Medicine and Ethics 26,* 1998, pp. 17-18.

as morally equivalent forms of homicide. Some even consider PGD to be worse than traditional prenatal diagnosis because numerous embryos are lost at each attempt, whereas prenatal diagnosis only leads to the abortion of one or two embryos. Also, while it is possible that information from prenatal diagnosis will be used by parents to prepare for the prenatal or postnatal care of the child, no "defective" embryos will ever be implanted in an IVF-PGD procedure.[3]

PGD PROMOTES CONSUMER CULTURE IN HUMAN GENERATION

Critics assert that PGD introduces consumer culture into the area of procreation. Although human beings are beyond monetary price, the technique treats them as commodities. It objectifies children by subjecting them to selection and quality control as with manufactured goods, which we do not purchase if they do not measure up to our standard.[4] The technique turns parents into consumers who merely accept a "product" (a child) on the "condition" that it meets a particular standard, whereas a child should be accepted unconditionally. As Song asserts,

> Such a mentality is bad enough in many other areas of life, but it is disastrous when it starts encroaching on our attitudes to children. Instead of being accepted for themselves with an unconditional love that is willing to embrace them, whatever their capacities, there is the risk that love becomes conditional on their human genetics, meeting certain performance standard.... As one writer puts it, if the baby is born and fails to meet expectations, will it be sent back to the factory? Will the parents ask for a refund or discount? Of course, PGD is not by itself single-handedly bringing about such a wholesale commodifying mentality toward children: it is part of a much broader cultural trend.[5]

---

3 See I. MURRAY, "'Designer baby' inquiry ordered," *The Times,* January 17, 1998, p. 36.

4 R. SONG, *Human Genetics, op. cit.,* p. 24.

5 Ibid., pp. 24-25. The writer to whom Song refers in this text is Ted Peters. See T. PETERS, "The Cloning Shock: A Theological Reaction," in R. COLE – TURNER, *Human Cloning: Religious Responses,* Westminster John Knox Press, Louisville KY 1997, p. 23.

PGD AND SOCIETY'S PERCEPTION OF DISABILITY

PGD[6] poses a serious problem related to society's perception of disability. For some critics, the use of these procedures to abort or discard a human embryo because of disability discriminates against disabled people in a vicious and destructive way; it signals to them in clear terms that society does not want any more of their kind.[7] The practice suggests that the life of the disabled is worthless, and it may give rise to a situation in which it will be unacceptable for parents to give birth to disabled children or for society to support them. Society may come to view them as "products" of parental choice rather than of chance, as in natural conception.[8] Such a mentality stems from the ignorant and biased perception that a disability automatically makes life worthless; in fact, many disabled persons find their lives rewarding and worthwhile and do not wish they were dead or never born. Since disability can occur at birth or afterwards, neither PGD nor prenatal diagnosis can completely rid the human generative process of disability. Insisting that disability is a social construction, disability activists consider the attitude of inclusion to be more positive and realistic than the attempt to rid society of disabled persons. In their opinion, society must change its attitude towards disability because rejection could produce the desire for "perfect babies" and promote intolerance for imperfection.[9] On the other hand, supporters of prenatal diagnosis and PGD argue that a healthy life without diminished human capacities is desirable; thus it is reasonable and justified to resort to PGD to achieve it. There is nothing wrong with the desire to avoid having a

[6] The arguments used for prenatal diagnosis can also apply to PGD. The disability activists only approve of prenatal testing if it aims at giving prospective parents information that can better prepare them to cope with the birth of a disabled child or to initiate a prenatal therapy.

[7] See B. STEINBOCK, "Preimplantation Genetic Diagnosis..., *op. cit.*, pp. 179-180.

[8] Cf. S. LAMMERS – A. VERHEY, "Genetic Control," in S. LAMMERS – A. VERHEY (eds.), *On Moral Medicine..., op. cit.*, p. 527.

[9] See B. STEINBOCK, "Preimplantation Genetic Diagnosis..., *op. cit.*, pp. 179-180.

disabled child, and it does not imply that if a disabled child is born, he or she will be rejected or not loved.[10]

CREATING A CHILD TO SAVE ANOTHER CHILD

IVF-PGD and human leukocyte antigen (HLA) matching technology make it possible to screen embryos prior to implantation to find a match that can be a stem cell donor for a sick sibling. Advocates of the procedure defend its moral acceptability on the grounds that it enables a child to save a sick sibling, but opponents disagree. First of all, those who attribute personhood at fertilisation find the procedure morally unacceptable because it involves screening and discarding viable embryos that are not compatible donors for the sick sibling. Despite the noble desire to save an existing child, they find it morally objectionable to treat the prospective child as a means or an instrument.[11] Even some who attribute personhood at a later stage of embryonic development concur with this. Drawing a line between the instrumental use of an early embryo for research purposes and the "further instrumental manufacture and use" of the child that results "for the therapeutic benefit of another child," they insist that the procedure treats the new child as a means to an end.[12] In other words, it is not conceived or desired for its own sake, but because it can be a compatible bone-marrow donor[13] to the sick sibling, who then becomes the condition for its existence. Yet others argue that the procedure is potentially harmful to the donor-child and parents. The child may be psychologically harmed if he grows up to know that he was primarily conceived to save another child. This situation may worsen if the sick sibling does not survive: the child may feel like a failure for not fulfilling

---

[10] See Ibid., p.182.

[11] See R. CLARKE – J. FLETCHER – G. PETERSEN, "Conceiving a fetus for bone marrow donation: an ethical problem in prenatal diagnosis, "*Prenat-Diagn,* 1989; 329-334. Cited in F. SHENFIED – C. SUREAU, *Ethical Dilemmas in Reproduction,* The Pantheon Publishing Group, New York 2002, p. 55.

[12] See D. MORGAN – R. LEE, "Human reproduction and human right," in D. SINGER – M. HUNTER, *Assisted Human Reproduction…, op. cit.,* p. 67.

[13] J. RICHARD, "Ethical Issue – The Major Faiths…, *op. cit.,* p. 43. In other words, the primary goal or interest of this procedure is to find compatible embryos for the existing child, not the new child itself.

the purpose of his conception. The challenge of caring for a dying child while pregnant, coupled with that of giving birth to a new baby who requires regular attention like the dying child, would be extremely stressful to the woman and to the marriage, whether or not the sick child survives.[14] Further, they point out that the technique is extremely expensive and is available only to relatively rich couples.[15]

Supporters of the technique contend that the possibility of saving the sick sibling outweighs the physical and emotional risks involved. They argue that the use of HLA technology for this purpose is easier to defend than its use for gender selection, and the fact that the child is conceived to save another does not nullify the intention to love and raise it in the same way as the first.[16] Moreover, the technique is beneficial to the donor-child, who can be screened for genetic diseases and enjoy the fulfilment of knowing that he saved his own sibling.[17]

Dr. Grodin explains that, currently, this can be achieved in two ways. The first involves performing an HLA type compatibility test and screening the embryo to see if it is affected by the same disease as the sibling, whereas the second entails only the HLA matching test. The first ensures that the donor-child will be disease-free, but the second does not. He contends that the primary motive of parents who resort to the technique should be to conceive the new child for its own sake; he recommends that it must be accorded an independent respect and not merely valued as a stem cell donor.[18] He advocates the regulation of the practice to avoid abuses and to safeguard the interest of the second child. But

---

[14] TRANSPLANT COMMUNICATION INC., "Ethics of preimplantation genetic diagnosis debated. (Brief Article)," *Transplant News (Newsletter), Vol. 12 Issue 1.* January 12, 2002, p. NA. The name of the author was not supplied, but the statement cited was credited to Jennifer Girod.

[15] J. RICHARD, "Ethical Issue – The Major Faiths..., *op. cit.,* p. 43.

[16] See G. PENNINGS – I. LIEBAERS, "Creating a child to save another: HLA matching of sibling by means of preimplantation genetic diagnosis," Cited in F. SHENFIED – C. SUREAU, *Ethical Dilemmas in Reproduction, op. cit.,* pp. 55-56.

[17] M. GRODIN, "Should preimplantation genetic diagnosis be used to produce children who are suitable stem cell donor? (Pro & Con)," *Family Practice News,* June 15, 2004.

[18] Ibid.

others like Robert Boyle and Julian Savulescu do not believe that the technique is harmful to anyone, even when it is performed solely for the purpose of saving a sick sibling. They argue that the dying child and parents benefit from the technique, and the new child would not have come to exist in the first place without it. Hence, to prohibit it would amount to a violation of the reproductive liberty of the individual or couple.[19]

IVF-PGD AND EUGENICS

ART has been associated with eugenics in various ways. The eugenic mentality in the realm of human generation dates back to ancient times, when some ancient Greek philosophers like Plato and Aristotle believed that healthy and intelligent people in society should be encouraged to procreate, while those suffering from chronic illness should be discouraged. However, the term "eugenics," which means "well-born," was coined in the nineteenth century by a British physician named Francis Galton, who is widely recognised as the father of eugenics.[20] He advocated the use of selective breeding to achieve the improvement of the human race through "hereditary transmission of intelligence." This entails using science to selectively match parents with superior traits or intelligence. Later in the twentieth century, the eugenic theory was applied in the United States, Britain, and especially Nazi Germany under Adolf Hitler in an attempt to resolve certain social problems.

Eugenics can be positive or negative. It is positive if a given technical procedure seeks to increase the desirable genetic traits within a given population, thereby leading to the cure of a disease or the enhancement of the recipient's descendants. Examples include germ-line gene therapy and human genetic design and enhancement that affect the germ-line. Eugenics is negative if it seeks to reduce genetic defects, such as in prenatal diagnosis with selective abortion and in PGD involving the discarding of "defective" embryos.[21] Some fear that IVF or particularly

[19] TRANSPLANT COMMUNICATION INC., "Ethical of preimplantation..., *op. cit.,* p. NA. The name of the author is not given, but the statement cited was credited to Drs. Boyle and Savulescu.

[20] Cf. P. LOMBARDO, "Eugenics," in J. MACQUAIRRIE – J. CHILDLESS (eds.), *A New Dictionary of..., op. cit.,* p. 209.

[21] Cf. P. FLAMAN, *Genetic Engineering..., op. cit.,* pp. 89, 92.

PGD could be a slippery slope to eugenic programmes[22] by insisting that every embryo should be examined before transfer. Already there are some commercial banks that specialize in sperm from geniuses, such as Nobel Prize winners; their intention is to make the sperm available to women with high IQ to ensure that the resulting children will be highly intelligent.[23] Many critics see this as a step towards genetic perfection and as intolerant of those with congenital disorders. In the IVF-PGD procedure, only embryos that meet the standard are implanted into the woman, and some commentators see this as negative eugenics.

[22] See L. PURDY, "Assisted Reproduction..., *op. cit.*, p. 167.

[23] See T. INGLESIAS, "Using Donor Eggs and..., *op. cit.*, p. 97. Cited "Super-kids," *Time,* 10 March 1980, p. 49. Robert Graham was the project designer of the sperm bank established in California in 1980.

ETHICAL ISSUES IN SEX SELECTION

Gender selection has attracted great interest and intense debate worldwide. Although prenatal diagnosis, PGD, and the Microsort techniques were originally designed to avoid the birth of genetically affected children, they are increasingly used for sex selection for various social reasons. Most commentators agree that the use of PGD for sex selection to avoid certain medical conditions, such as the deadly X-linked diseases, is morally justified, but by contrast, sex selection for social reasons is a highly controversial issue. The ethical issues in this area revolve around two crucial questions: Should parents be permitted to select the sex of their children? and, if so, Under which conditions? The second question is related to the morality of destroying viable human embryos to arrive at this end.[24]

ARGUMENTS FOR NON-THERAPEUTIC SEX SELECTION

Those who support sex selection for non-medical purposes base their arguments on respect for reproductive autonomy, the ability of the technique to promote a better quality of life for the child, and the need to reduce overpopulation.

REPRODUCTIVE RIGHT OR AUTONOMY

Advocates of the "total parental autonomy" model for sex selection, such as Robertson, argue for unrestricted access to the technology in the absence of any compelling reason,[25] because only this conforms to respect for reproductive liberty and personal autonomy. Some geneticists and other advocates argue that sex selection is a logical extension of parents' reproductive right to choose the number, timing, spacing, and genetic health of their children; to deny them this right would amount to medical paternalism, which violates their autonomy as competent

[24] Cf. D. WERTZ, "Reproductive Technologies: Sex Selection," in W. REICH (ed.), *Encyclopedia of Bioethics…, op. cit.,* p. 2213.

[25] See J. ROBERTSON, "Ethical and legal issues in pre-implantation genetic screening," *Fertility and Sterility,* 57: 1, 1992. Robertson views sex selection as an extension of parental procreative liberty.

subjects.[26] Similarly, some advocates view sex selection as a strictly private matter between the physician and his patient that does not require outside interference.

Opponents reject this robust conception of parental reproductive autonomy. Characterizing it as "the market or consumer product model," George Annas maintains that it tends to treat children as consumer products, leaving parents with an option to buy or not to buy.[27] Others argue that while the Kantian view on respect for autonomy seems to favour sex selection, it may equally oppose it—in choosing the sex of their children, parents reduce them to mere instruments. Because a child is not a means, but rather an end with a right to an open future, it possesses a right to have its sex determined by a process that is random rather than technological.[28] To discredit the view that sex selection is a private matter, they point to the wider social implications of the technique, arguing that it could create or widen social inequalities between the sexes.

SEX SELECTION AND QUALITY OF LIFE OF THE CHILD

Supporters of sex selection for non-medical purposes argue that it will guarantee a better quality of life for the prospective child because he or she will be truly wanted. This argument is based on the idea that sex selection will save a child of the unwanted sex from unnecessary abuse, neglect, and subtle rejection, all of which can cause psychological problems. Opponents react to this by maintaining that children are gifts to be accepted for who they are and not because they meet the expectations or preferences of parents. Sex selection undermines this sense and seems to treat the child as though it is the property of its parents. To

---

[26] Cf. D. WERTZ, "Reproductive Technologies: Sex Selection..., *op. cit.*, p. 2213.

[27] G. ANNAS, "Non-invasive prenatal diagnostic technology: medical, market, or regulatory model?" *Annals of the New York Academy of Sciences 731,* 1994, pp. 264-265; See also B. STEINBOCK, "Pre-implantation Genetic Diagnosis..., *op. cit.,* p. 185.

[28] See J. MCMILLAN, "Reproductive Technologies: Sex Selection," in S. POST (ed.), *Encyclopedia of Bioethics..., op. cit.,* p. 2269.

promote the subjective preferences of parents at the expense of the child would be unjust to the child.[29]

SEX SELECTION AND POPULATION CONTROL

The world's human population is currently over six billion, and it increases at an estimated annual rate of 1.3%. This population is expected to rise to about nine billion in 2050, raising concerns about survival on earth.[30] Some proponents of sex selection, who are probably conscious of this, claim that some couples in search of a child of a particular sex end up having more babies than they desire. On this basis, they argue that permitting sex selection will likely reduce overpopulation. Also, it will be beneficial to the couple because the woman will not have to undergo more pregnancies than the couple desires.

ARGUMENTS AGAINST SEX SELECTION

Opponents of sex selection have come up with a number of reasons to show that it is not morally acceptable. Their arguments address the interests of the child, society, and the human embryos of the undesired sex.

GENDER IS NOT A MEDICAL PROBLEM

Proponents of the "medical model" accept sex selection for therapeutic uses and reject it for non-therapeutic uses. They argue that PGD, prenatal diagnosis, and even the Microsort technique were designed as medical technologies to avoid genetic disease in offspring. Gender is neither a genetic disease nor a medical problem.[31] Rather, sex selection falls more into the category of cosmetic surgery, undermining the major moral justification for the technologies on the basis of their informative value and therapeutic use. Hence, to use them merely to sex a child for

---

[29] B. ASHLEY – K. O' ROURKE, *Ethics of Health Care, Third Edition,* Georgetown University Press, Washington, D.C. 2002, p. 149.

[30] See J. MARTIN-SCHRAMM – R. STIVERS, *Christian Environmental Ethics, A Case Method Approach,* Orbis Books, Maryknoll, New York 2003, pp. 10-11.

[31] See B. STEINBOCK, "Pre-implantation Genetic Diagnosis..., *op. cit.,* p. 186.

non-medical reasons is tantamount to an inappropriate use of a medical technology.[32] Considering the cost of the techniques, this constitutes a serious waste of resources. Moreover, 100% success is not assured if the Microsort technique is used, meaning that some couples will have to make two or more attempts.

DESTRUCTION OF EMBRYOS OR SELECTIVE ABORTION

When prenatal diagnosis is used for gender selection, the embryos of the undesired sex are aborted. If PGD is used, embryos of the unwanted sex are destroyed, allowed to die, or donated to other couples. Some opponents claim that it is ethically impermissible to terminate the lives of viable embryos because of their sex or to use IVF-PGD to deliberately create embryos that will not be implanted because of their sex.[33]

SEX SELECTION AND IMBALANCES IN SEX RATIO

Some oppose sex selection because of potentially negative long-term effects. In their view, a widespread use of sex selection in favour of a particular gender could give rise to an imbalance in the sex ratio between men and women.[34] To support this claim, they maintain that such significant imbalances already exist in some parts of the world. For instance, it is estimated that in China there are about 50 million fewer women than there should be.[35] Although sex selection alone does not account for these remarkable imbalances in sex ratio, it is likely to worsen the imbalances.

SEX SELECTION AND EQUALITY

Critics argue that sex selection threatens gender equality,[36] as it may exacerbate it where it already exists and create it in the developed societies

---

[32] Cf. J. MCMILLAN, "Reproductive Technologies: Sex Selection..., *op. cit.*, p. 2270.

[33] See B. LEROY – D. BARTELS, "Reproduction, Ethics, Sex Selection," in *Encyclopedia of Ethical..., op. cit.,* p. 973. The Microsort technique with AI poses lesser ethical problems.

[34] See P. ROBINSON, "Prenatal screening, sex selection and cloning," in H. KUSHE – P. SINGER (eds.), *A Companion to Bioethics, op. cit.,* p.183.

[35] J. MCMILLAN, "Reproductive Technologies: Sex Selection..., *op. cit.*, p. 2269.

[36] Cf. M. EVANS – A. DRUGAN *et al.*, "Attitudes on the ethics of abortion, sex selection and selective pregnancy termination amongst health care

where gender preferences are quite minimal.[37] Evans and his colleagues maintain that gender is not a disease—to resort to abortion to control gender will be a step towards eugenics. Some feminists[38] reject sex selection because the techniques can be used to discriminate against women in places where preference for male children is strong. This view is well founded: prenatal diagnosis is used primarily to select male children and abort female foetuses in China, India, and other countries.[39] However, some reject the feminist argument because it appears to emphasize abuses and overlook the fundamental motive for the technology. Sex selection must be evaluated on its own merit, that is, from an objective, impersonal perspective.

SEX SELECTION IS SEXIST AND AGAINST HUMAN RIGHTS

Some commentators reject non-medical sex selection as discriminatory or sexist, claiming that gender is not a medical condition that PGD was designed to avoid. The ethics committee of the American College of Obstetricians and Gynaecologists approved the use of sex selection for avoiding sex-linked diseases, but it strongly opposed it for non-medical uses, arguing that such a practice may reflect and encourage sex discrimination. Even in the United States, where most couples use the technique to choose girls, those who attach advantages to being a firstborn believe that there will be fewer firstborn females, which gives the males

professionals, ethicists, and clergy likely to encounter such situations," *American Journal of Obstetrics and Gynecology,* 1991, 164:1092-1099.

[37] Cf. D. WERTZ, "Reproductive Technologies: Sex Selection…, *op. cit.,* p. 2215. Cited R. PEBLEY – C. WESTHOFF – F. CHARLES, 1982, "Women's Sex Preferences in the United State: 1970 to 1975," *Demography 19,* no. 2: 177–189; See also D. BUBECK, "Sex Selection: The Feminists Response," in J. BURLEY – J. HARRIS, *A Companion to Genethics, op. cit.,* p. 225.

[38] See D. BUBECK, "Sex Selection: The Feminists Response…, *op. cit.,* pp. 221-213; See also the reference to G. COREA, *The Mother Machine: Reproductive Technologies From Artificial Insemination to Artificial Wombs,* Women's Press, London 1985, p. 195. Feminists believe that such demographic sex imbalance will favour men although the more liberal ones endorse sex selection, claiming that it enhances reproductive freedom of women.

[39] See Ibid., p. 216.

an advantage.[40] Others contend that the code of ethics of the medical profession requires physicians to treat all equally without discrimination on the basis of creed, race, or sex. Non-medical sex selection violates this principle as well as the provision of the United Nations Charter of Human Rights, which also prohibits such discrimination.[41] This practice suggests that there is something inherently valuable or superior about one of the genders. Proponents respond that not all forms of sex selection are sexist. For instance, sex selection for family balancing does not necessarily imply rejection of or discrimination against a particular sex.[42] Hence, they assert that the technique should not be used to choose the sex of the first child or when a family has an equal number of male and female children.[43] The ethics committee of the American Society for Reproductive Medicine asserted that sex selection with the Microsort technique would be ethically acceptable for the purpose of family balancing. This is because it avoids the moral problem of creating and discarding human embryos and is not inherently sexist. However, the committee recognizes the discriminatory potential in the desire to select the sex of a first child, since this borders on preference rather than gender variety. The committee rejects the use of PGD for the sole purpose of sex selection

[40] Cf. AMERICAN COLLEGE OF OBSTETRICIAN AND GYNECOLOGISTS (ACOG), *Int. J Gynecol obstet. 56,* 1997, 199-202.

[41] UNITED NATIONS ORGANIZATION, Universal Declaration of Human Rights, adopted and proclaimed by the General Assembly of the United Nations Organization Meeting in Paris on December 10, 1948, Article 2:2; ID., INTERNATIONAL COVENANT ON ECONOMIC, SOCIAL AND CULTURAL RIGHTS, Part II, Article 2:2. Adopted and opened for signature, ratification, and accession by United Nations General Assembly resolution 2200 A (XXI) on 16 December 1996. Entered into force on 3 January 1976, in accordance with article 27; See also J. MANN – S. GRUSKIN *et al.* (eds.), *Health and Human Rights,* Routledge, New York and London 1999, p. 459.

[42] Cf. B STEINBOCK, "Sex Selection. Not Obviously Wrong," in T. SHANNON (ed.), *Reproductive Technologies, op. cit.,* p. 62. Steinbock sees sex selection for family balancing as an individual reproductive choice of the couple

[43] Cf. G. PENNINNGS, "Ethics of sex selection for family balancing: family balancing as a morally acceptable application of sex selection," *Human Reproduction,* 1996, 11:2339-2343.

because it is physically more cumbersome and it involves the creation and destruction of human embryos. It is important to note that, although the committee does not necessarily attribute personal status to the early embryos, it insists that they deserve "special respect" because of their potential to implant and bring forth a new person.[44]

SEX SELECTION IS HARMFUL TO THE CHILD

Some opponents repudiate the use of PGD for non-therapeutic sex selection on the basis of the risks to the future child. While such risks are justifiable when the procedure offers therapeutic benefits to the child, it is difficult to justify them when IVF-PGD is used for non-medical reasons. Although there is currently no evidence that sperm sorting involves a medical risk to the child, the possibility of psychological risks cannot be ruled out. If the sperm sorting technique fails, the child of the undesired sex may suffer psychologically if he is neglected or if he finds out that he is not of the sex desired by his parents.[45] Others reject non-medical sex selection because it tends to view and treat children as products. This does not respect human dignity and could result in harm to both the child and society. As such, neither parents nor any other authority should have the right to choose the sex of offspring when there is no medical condition involved.[46]

SEX SELECTION AND THE SLIPPERY SLOPE

Some are deeply apprehensive about the consequences of allowing couples to choose the sex of their children for non-medical purposes. The frightening question is, What will be next on the slippery slope of reproductive technology if couples are allowed to preselect the sex of their unborn children? If this drift from the primary purpose of the medical technique is permitted, it may lead to human genetic design

---

[44] ASRM ETHICS COMMITTEE, "Sex Selection: Final Word from the ASRM Ethics Committee on the Use of PGD (American Society of Reproductive Medicine: pre-implantation genetic diagnosis)," *The Hastings Centre Report,* March 1, 2006.

[45] Cf. J. MCMILLAN, "Reproductive Technologies: Sex Selection…, *op. cit.,* p. 2270.

[46] Cf. COUNCIL ON ETHICAL AND JUDICIAL AFFAIR, AMERICAN MEDICAL ASSOCIATION, "Ethical Issue Related to Prenatal Genetic Testing," *Arch Fam. Med. 3,* 1994, 633-642.

and enhancement technology that will enable parents to select certain physical and mental traits for their children.[47] The practice "sets a dangerous eugenic precedent for attempts to discard embryos based on 'undesirable' genetic characteristics such as low IQ, short stature, or poor eyesight."[48] On this issue, Lisa Belkin writes the following:

> Along the way, I have developed a healthy fear of the "slippery slope" ... if we allow parents to choose the sex of their child today, how long will it be before they order up eye colour, hair colour, personality traits and IQ?.... I cringe at the idea of treating human beings as a commodity... pay Microsort $2,500 (per try, not per pregnancy; the average pregnancy takes three tries) and purchase the sex of your choice. And I am all too aware that to people with real problems—couples who cannot have children, couples whose children are injured or ill—this talk of sperm sorting sounds shallow and vain.[49]

In this light, Kass stresses the need to limit technology from crossing a reasonable boundary, maintaining that we all have a stake in keeping human generation human.[50] Still, some commentators contend that promoting sex selection may create a situation in which children born from the different technologies would be pressured by parents according to certain expectations they have. According to Knowles, cited by Lisa Belkin,

---

[47] D. WERTZ, "Reproductive Technologies: Sex Selection..., *op. cit.*, p. 2215.

[48] See A. KIMBRELL, *The Human Body Shop, Second Edition,* Regnery Publishing, Inc., Washington, D.C. 1997, p. 146.

[49] L. BELKIN, "Getting the Girl," *The New York Times Magazine*, July 25, 1999, in http://www.nytimes.com/library/magazine/home/19990725mag-sci-gender-choice.html, p. 2 (Downloaded 4/7/2006). Lisa Belkin, a mother of two boys, is a contributing writer for the New York Times Magazine. She specialized on subjects on technology and ethics and has written a book about medical ethics. Actually, she wanted to try out the Microsort technique to have a daughter, but later gave up the idea following her reflection on the implication.

[50] See NEWSWEEK INTERACTIVE, "The Science of Sex Selection," in *New Babies – Newsweek Health* – MSNBC, in Com http://www.msnbc.com/id/3990134.

> When you are going to this length to have a girl, chances are you have a particular girl in mind. I really want someone to go shopping with; I really want her to take ballet. All these things point to a particular role that the child is envisioned as having in the family. If you are willing to spend that kind of money, you're.... heavily invested. There are going to be some very, very pressured kids.[51]

Although children who are not born from these techniques could also be pressured by parents, it is more likely after deliberately investing in the child's gender.

[51] See L. BELKIN, "Getting the Girl..., *op. cit.,* p. 13.

GENETIC ENHANCEMENT

Ethical issues abound in genetic design and enhancement engineering of humans, but we will limit our discussion to two serious concerns relating to the autonomy of parents and the interests of the child.

RESPECT FOR REPRODUCTIVE RIGHT AND AUTONOMY

Autonomy implies that individuals should have control over their own lives and should pursue their own lifestyle without coercion. Some argue that genetic design should be allowed on the basis of reproductive autonomy. Provided it does not harm the prospective child, it would fall into the category of things that generate a legal right to moral wrongness.[52] Some proponents argue that since procreation and the upbringing of children are serious tasks, parents should be at liberty to choose the genetic traits of their children out of respect for their personal autonomy. Jonathan Glover proposes a regulated form of the "genetic supermarket model," in which parents could purchase genes to enhance their children as an exercise of their reproductive autonomy.[53] Those who see the embryo as a human being respond that although respect for personal autonomy is a value we should promote, it is not the highest value: it is superseded by the embryo's right to life and respect.[54] Rejecting the genetic supermarket model, some opponents argue that it will aggravate the existing inequality between the rich and the poor because only the rich will be

[52] See M. CLAYTON, "Individual Autonomy and Genetic Choice," in J. BURLEY – J. HARRIS (eds.), *A Companion, op. cit.*, p. 191.

[53] J. GLOVER, *What Sort of People Should There Be?* Pelican Books, Harmondsworth 1984, pp. 45-56; Cited in M. CLAYTON, "Individual Autonomy and Genetic Choice," in J. BURLEY – J. HARRIS (eds.), *A Companion to Genethics, op. cit.*, p. 198. However, he stresses the need to decentralize such powers to avoid abuse by a group and adds that the genetic supermarket should be regulated to avoid the collective consequences of unrestricted individual choices (for example, imbalance between males and females in society and the attendant social problems) and to ensure that such choices do not limit a child's capacity to develop a sense of justice and power that guarantee an autonomous life.

[54] See M. CLAYTON, "Individual Autonomy and..., *op. cit.*, p. 191.

able to afford the more desirable genes. Besides, the existence of such a supermarket will be harmful to those already living with disabilities.[55]

Some critics claim that the child also has a right to autonomy, which is violated in non-therapeutic genetic manipulation and design. In response, advocates insist that since autonomy connotes non-interference with other people's choices, it is impossible to justify or condemn any particular conduct towards children before they are born.[56] Rejecting this view, opponents argue that it would be morally wrong and against the rights of children for parents to manipulate their genes in a non-therapeutic way after birth; thus, to perform similar manipulation before implantation is also wrong. Genetic manipulation and design pre-conditions the child such that his or her future life will always be influenced by the genetic choice made by the parents. Hence, in the exercise of their reproductive autonomy, parents have a duty to respect the autonomy of their future offspring.[57]

The expressions of particular traits depend on complex interactions among different genes as well as interactions between genes and the environment. Nevertheless, genes largely, if not completely, determine individuals in the sense of "genetic determinism." From this perspective, it is clear that parental reproductive choice, understood in an absolute sense, can conflict with the future autonomy of a child. As some opponents assert, non-therapeutic determination of a child's gender or the selection of certain genes would be a manipulation of the future child's characteristics according to the subjective opinions and tastes of the parents.[58]

IMPACT OF GENETIC DESIGN ON THE CHILD

Many commentators emphasize genetic enhancement design's potential to harm the child. They assert that parental over-investment in designing children can be a source of profound psychological difficulty; they insist that every child should be free from this and able to maintain

---

[55] See Ibid., p. 199.

[56] See Ibid., p. 192.

[57] See Ibid., pp. 200-202.

[58] Ibid; See also R. PINON JR., *Biology of Human Reproduction, op. cit.*, pp. 325-347.

its own unique identity.[59] Shannon asserts that once it becomes scientifically feasible to choose a child's genetic characteristics, parents may be pressured to select the "best" genetic heritage in order to have a perfectly designed child, leading to certain underlying expectations that can create a complex and difficult childhood.[60] Further, others contend that genetic enhancement design treats a child as a product intended to satisfy the desires of parents. Pointing out the inherent danger in viewing a child as a means to an end, rather than as a gift, Shannon asserts the following:

> While I would argue that there is nothing inherently immoral with any form of assisted reproduction, there is danger that we may lose the sense of a child as a gift and come to look upon children as means to an end, an end that is as carefully designed and programmed as possible. Such social determinism closes a child's future and violates a child's dignity. How we use our power of reproduction will reveal much about us and our priorities.[61]

Similarly, Rahner rejects genetic manipulation and design, arguing that it treats the child as a product of its parents' own free action; the child "has been planned and calculated" rather than accepted with openness and love. He insists that bringing a child into existence need not become "an act of neurotic anxiety"—the child must remain one who is both made and unconditionally accepted.[62] Putnam's observation on reproductive cloning to "choose" one's children is equally applicable here. In his opinion, it brings about a situation in which we can have "designer children" in the same way we have "designer cloth." In such

---

[59] Cf. S. CALLAHAN, "The Ethical Challenge..., *op. cit.,* p. 515.

[60] T. SHANNON, "Ethical Issues in Genetics..., *op. cit.,* p. 26.

[61] Ibid., p. 26.

[62] K. RAHNER, "The Problem of Genetic Manipulation..., *op. cit.,* pp. 542-543. Rahner sees the driving force behind genetic manipulation as 'hate of one's destiny' and the inner despair of a man arising from his inability to dispose of existence. By engaging in it, such a man goes beyond what could licitly count as a precautionary (therapeutic) eugenic measure to something illicit (for example, genetic design), which stems from the fear of destiny.

cases, children come to be viewed as if they are objects or commodities, which is demeaning to their dignity.[63] Insisting on the need to accept children as gifts, Putnam writes,

> The amazing thing about one's children is that they come into one's life as different—very different—people seemingly from the moment of birth. In any other relationship, one can choose to some extent the traits of one's associates, but with one's children (and one's parents) one can only accept what God gives one to accept.[64]

In accord with other critics, Edmund Pellegrino endorses genetic manipulation that is therapeutic, as this will clearly benefit the individual. But he insists that manipulation aimed at design and enhancement—according to "some utopian, biologically conceived image of the ideal human person"—is morally bankrupt and totally reprehensible.[65]

---

[63] H. PUTNAM, "Cloning People," in J. BURLEY (ed.), *The Genetic Revolution and Human Rights,* Oxford University Press, Inc., New York 1999, pp. 7-8.

[64] Ibid., p. 10.

[65] E. PELLEGRINO, "The Human Person, the Physician, and the Physician's Ethics, *Linacre Quarterly 62,* February 1995: 80.

CHAPTER 9

THE RELIGIONS AND ARTIFICIAL REPRODUCTIVE TECHNOLOGIES

ART has given rise to many issues of great human and religious importance. Some of these reproductive techniques, especially IVF technology, challenge certain traditional religious assumptions about procreation and the beginning of human life. Our task here is to examine the views of certain religions on the subject of ART. We will focus on Christianity (from the perspective of the Catholic Church),[1] Islam, and the African Traditional Religion (ATR), since these three are widely practised in Nigeria and Africa. From the outset, we should note that there is no deliberate attempt to reduce the Christian thought on ART to the official teaching of the Catholic Church, because some Christian denominations disagree about the morality of certain techniques and tolerate a diversity of opinions among adherents within the denomination. Besides the Church's universal character, we will primarily resort to Catholic teaching because there exists a well-articulated official Catholic position and because Catholic theologians, philosophers, and ethicists have written more on ART than those of any other religion.

1 The word Church will refer to the Catholic Church when it is not qualified.

THE CATHOLIC CHURCH ON ASSISTED PROCREATION

The Catholic Church endorses medical assistance to infertile couples. Pope Pius XII taught that the process of fertilisation could be assisted[2] under certain conditions. Such technical assistance must be within marriage; it should uphold the unitive and procreative meanings of marital sexual intercourse and respect the human embryo's right to life from fertilisation.

THE ANTHROPOLOGICAL BASIS OF THE CHURCH'S VIEW

When discussing ART, the Church substitutes the term *reproduction* with *procreation* on the basis of her anthropological vision of the human person as an incarnate spirit. Maintaining that God creates the soul of each person immediately from the moment of conception,[3] she states that a human being is neither only body nor only soul, but a unity of body and soul.[4] Gifted with rationality and fundamentally different from the animals, every human being possesses an intrinsic dignity. Man is not merely reproduced as the animals are, but on the contrary, he is *procreated*, or generated through the collaboration of a couple with God.

CRITERIA FOR EVALUATING ASSISTED CONCEPTION

Conscious of the trauma associated with infertility, the Church welcomes the possibility of technical assistance to infertile couples that would enable them to fulfil their noble desire for biological parenthood. In principle, medical techniques for assisting infertile couples should not be rejected on account of being artificial, but they must be ethically permissible. To evaluate the ethical acceptability of the various ART techniques, the Church insists on respect for three fundamental goods: the intrinsic value and dignity of a human being and his or her right to life and physical integrity from conception to natural death; the unity of marriage, which implies respect for the spouses' exclusive right to become

[2] POPE PIUS XII, Address to Catholic Doctors, September 29, 1949, *AAS* 4, 1949, pp. 559-560.

[3] VATICAN II, *Gaudium et spes* 7 Dec. 1965, *Pastoral Constitution on the Church in the Modern World,* 7 December 1965 n. 51: *AAS* 58 1996, 1023-1120. Henceforth, *GS* will be used in subsequent references to this document.

[4] To reduce man to only "body" falls into the error of biological reductionism and to reduce him to only "spirit" falls into the error of spiritual reductionism.

a father or mother only with one another; and the specifically human values of sexuality, which require a responsible means of procreation.[5]

THE DIGNITY OF THE HUMAN PERSON

The Church recognizes the existence of a human being with an inherent dignity and a right to life from the moment of conception, that is, when the ovum is fertilised. According to the Sacred Congregation for the Doctrine of the Faith (CDF) in its *Declaration on Procured Abortion*, "From the time the ovum is fertilised, a new life is begun which is neither that of the father nor of the mother; it is rather the life of a new human being with his own growth."[6] Making reference to the findings of modern genetic science, it maintains that "in the zygote resulting from fertilisation the biological identity of a new human individual is already constituted." On this basis, the embryo is an individual human being, and as such, it is a person with dignity who is worthy of the respect and protection accorded to other human beings.[7] Arguing from a theological perspective, she maintains that every human life is a precious gift of God, which carries with it a corresponding responsibility to preserve and promote it.[8] In this vision, the human being is the only creature that God made for himself. Created in the image and likeness of God, with capacities for rationality, the human being has an intrinsic dignity, which society does not confer, but only recognizes. By virtue of that dignity, every human being is always a whole rather than a part, an end and never a means.

UNITY OF MARRIAGE

The dignity of human procreation is predicated on the dignity of both parents and children. A truly responsible procreation that conforms to the dignity of spouses is that which is an expression and a sign of their mutual self-giving, love, and fidelity, which can only take place within

---

[5] SACRED CONGREGATION FOR THE DOCTRINE OF THE FAITH, *Dignitas Personae, Instruction on Certain Bioethical Questions,* The Incorporated Catholic Truth Society, London 2009, n. 12.

[6] SACRED CONGREGATION FOR THE DOCTRINE OF THE FAITH, *Declaration on Procured Abortion,* n. 7: *AAS 66* 1974, 738.

[7] Ibid.

[8] SACRED CONGREGATION FOR THE DOCTRINE OF THE FAITH, *Iura et Bona, Declaration on Euthanasia,* 5 May 1980, n. 1: *AAS* 72 1980, pp. 542-552.

the context of married life.[9] This fidelity of spouses within the unity of marriage implies an exclusive, non-transferable right to become parents only through each other[10]—marriage is a partnership of love and fidelity between two people and does not admit of a third party. Hence, to be considered responsible, any act of generating a child must respect this fundamental principle.

VALUES OF HUMAN SEXUALITY: RESPONSIBLE PROCREATION

Since a human being has an intrinsic dignity from conception, the Church insists on the right of every child to be conceived and brought into existence in a way that conforms to its dignity. This encompasses the right to be conceived normally, carried in the womb, and born and brought up within the context of marriage, which is the only setting worthy of truly responsible procreation.[11] The underlying rationale is that a child comes to discover its true identity and attain its proper development through its relationship with its own parents.

THE CHURCH'S EVALUATION OF ART

The Church rejects any form of artificial insemination or fertilisation that either substitutes the marital act or resorts to donated gametes. The introduction of a third party into procreation violates both the reciprocal fidelity of couples and the dignity of procreation; it is fundamentally harmful to the child, who has a right to be conceived and brought into the world in and from marriage.[12] In *Donum Vitae,* the CDF asserts that AI, IVF, and its variants, especially surrogacy contracts, are ethically objectionable: they "objectively deprive conjugal fruitfulness of its unity

[9] Cf. *GS* 50.

[10] SACRED CONGREGATION FOR THE DOCTRINE OF THE FAITH, *Donum Vitae, Instruction on the Respect for Human Life in its Origin and on the Dignity of Procreation: Replies to Certain Questions of the Day,* 22 February 1987, *n.* II, A, 1: *AAS* 80 1988, 70-102. We shall use *DV* in subsequent references to this document.

[11] Ibid., II, A, 1.

[12] Ibid., II, A, 2.

and integrity; they bring about and manifest a rupture between genetic parenthood, gestational parenthood and responsibility for upbringing."[13]

ARTIFICIAL INSEMINATION BY HUSBAND (AIH)

AIH is morally illicit if technical means substitute the conjugal act or if the sperm is obtained in ways other than the marital. In this case, it separates the unitive and procreative meanings of the conjugal act and the goods of marriage. Speaking about these two inseparable aspects of the conjugal act, Pope Pius XII repudiated any attempt to separate them to such a degree as to positively exclude the procreative intention from the conjugal act.[14] The CDF maintains that AIH can only be morally licit if the particular technique that is used helps the marital act to attain its natural purpose.[15]

ARTIFICIAL INSEMINATION BY DONOR (AID)

The CDF asserts that donor-conception poses a threat to the unity and stability of marriage, family, and society. It is not morally justified to use donor sperm to inseminate or perform IVF-ET for a married woman, a single woman, or a widow; it is also morally illicit to resort to surrogacy, whether on an altruistic or a commercial basis.[16] In addition to diminishing the dignity of the child, surrogacy violates the obligations of conjugal fidelity, maternal love, and responsible motherhood.

IN VITRO FERTILISATION AND EMBRYO TRANSFER (IVF-ET)

IVF-ET does not conform to the demands of responsible procreation nor to the dignity of the human being that results from it. Ethically, it is thoroughly reprehensible to deliberately create embryos with a potential for human life, yet which will eventually be frozen, destroyed, or used for research. Foetal reduction, which is used to resolve cases of multiple pregnancy, is morally equivalent to induced abortion, making it ethically reprehensible on account of the embryo's right to life. As an end

---

[13] Ibid., II, A, 2.

[14] POPE PIUS XII, Address to those taking part in the Second Naples World Congress on Fertility and Human Sterility, 19 May 1956, *AAS* 48 1956, 470.

[15] *DV.* II, B, 6; See also SACRED CONGREGATION FOR THE DOCTRINE OF THE FAITH, *Dignitas Personae, Instruction on Certain Bioethical Questions,* London: The Incorporated Catholic Truth Society, 2009, Part II, *n.* 12.

[16] *DV.* II, A, 1.

in itself, the embryo is entitled to the same profound respect and protection due to all other human beings.

MEDICAL INTERVENTION ON HUMAN EMBRYOS

Based on the ontological dignity of every human being, the Church denounces all non-therapeutic medical intervention on a human embryo, but she endorses a therapeutic type that is beneficial to the embryo and which does not carry a disproportionate risk for it and the mother. Still, for such an intervention to be licit, the informed consent of the parents must be obtained, in conformity with the deontological rule in respect of children. Stressing this point, Pope John Paul II states that only a strictly therapeutic intervention that explicitly aims at healing the individual and promoting its well-being, without harming its integrity or aggravating its condition of life, can conform to the logic of Christian moral tradition.[17] Furthermore, the CDF asserts that any medical intervention on human embryos that is not clearly therapeutic or that treats them as research materials constitutes a crime against their integrity and dignity as persons.[18] Similarly, it condemns non-therapeutic sex selection and human genetic manipulation as assaults on human integrity and dignity. A human being in his totality (body and soul) has an intrinsic dignity: all the dignity recognized to the person must also be recognized to his body. As such, the human body cannot be considered or treated as "a mere complex of tissues, organs and functions," nor can it be evaluated in the same way as the body of an animal. On the contrary, the body is a constitutive part of the person who manifests himself through it.[19] Consequently, any medical intervention on the human being does not affect only the body—it affects the whole individual, body and spirit, and must correspond to his personal dignity.

PLAYING GOD? SCIENCE IS NOT MORALLY NEUTRAL

In the standard IVF protocol, the medical scientist creates multiple embryos and then identifies the embryos that should be implanted into

---

[17] POPE JOHN PAUL II, Address to the participants at the 35th General Assembly of the World Medical Association, 29 October 1983, *AAS* 76 (1984) 392.

[18] Ibid.

[19] *DV.* I, 4.

the woman's uterus. Also, in cases of multiple pregnancy, he determines which embryos will live and which will be aborted. On account of this, the Church contends that in IVF-ET and related techniques, man is trying to play God by deciding who should be brought to life and who should die. *Donum Vitae* notes that with ART we are faced with the "temptation to go beyond the limits of a reasonable dominion over nature."[20] As *Donum Vitae* asserts,

> It would on the one hand be illusory to claim that scientific research and its application are morally neutral; on the other hand we cannot derive criteria for guidance from mere technical efficiency, from research's possible usefulness to some at the expense of others or, worse still, from prevailing ideologies.[21]

Finally, the success of the IVF procedure depends largely on the technical prowess of the physician. Hence, the Church concludes that IVF-ET "entrusts the life and identity of the embryo into the power of doctors and biologists and establishes the dominion of technology over the origin and the destiny of the human person,"[22] whereas only God is the master of life from its beginning until its end.[23]

ARE GIFT AND IUI POSSIBLE EXCEPTIONS?

The Church agrees that some form of technical assistance to infertile couples can be considered, and that some of the available techniques can be morally licit under certain conditions. First, they should facilitate rather than replace the conjugal act, as a child ought to be a fruit of the marital sexual love of its parents, which is simultaneously unitive and procreative.[24] Fertility treatment involving ovarian stimulation is morally

---

[20] Ibid., I, 2.

[21] Ibid., 2.

[22] Ibid., II, B, 5.

[23] Cf. POPE JOHN PAUL II, *Evangelium Vitae, The Gospel of Life,* 25 March 1995, nos. 53, 55: *AAS* 87 1995, 401-522.

[24] Techniques that truly "assist" procreation would be acceptable. In this case, we would no longer speak of artificial reproduction, but assisted procreation, which corresponds more to human dignity.

permissible if it is controlled and mild and if adequate precautions are taken to eliminate the risks of multifoetal pregnancies.[25]

Consequently, some Catholic moral theologians, ethicists, and medical scientists claim that GIFT has the potential, under certain conditions, to satisfy the teaching of the Church.[26] In this case, it must involve a married couple who perform the normal marital sexual act using a perforated Silastic sheath or condom, which allows the man's semen to be collected and used within 72 hours. The woman's ovum is retrieved on the exact day of the conjugal act. During the transfer into the fallopian tube, an air bubble must separate the ovum from the husband's sperm to ensure that fertilisation occurs only inside the woman's body. Likewise, IUI has the potential to satisfy the Church's position when performed under these strict conditions, although it does not require the collection of eggs.[27] There has been no official objection to these two methods when performed under these conditions,[28] but there also has been no official confirmation of their ethical acceptability.

Not everyone agrees with the above assessment of GIFT and IUI; indeed, theological opinions are polarized on the issue.[29] Despite the fact that fertilisation occurs *in vivo* in GIFT and IUI, some moral theologians argue that conception does not really result from sexual intercourse, but from the medical scientist's technical manipulation of the couple's reproductive cells.[30] As Watt observes, the act of sexual intercourse should contribute directly to the eventual union of sperm and

---

[25] B. COHLEN *et al.*, "Controlled Ovarian Hyperstimulation and Intrauterine Insemination for Treating Male Subfertility: A Controlled Study," *Human Reproduction*, 13, 6 (June 1998) 1553-1558.

[26] Cf. P. CATALDO, "GIFT as Assistance," *Ethics and Medics 22,* 12 December 1997:34; ID., P. CATALDO, J. "Beginning of Life Issues..., *op. cit.*, Part III, 9/5.

[27] Ibid.

[28] Ibid.

[29] While Peter Cataldo holds that following the normal marital act GIFT actually assists or facilitates the fruitfulness of the conjugal act, Grisez, May and Doefler repudiate the claim, insisting that it substitutes the marital act.

[30] See B. ASHLEY – K. O' ROURKE, *The Ethnics of Health Care..., op. cit.,* p. 129.

ovum, allowing the technology to complete the process. The reduction of the conjugal act to a mere means of collecting sperm for subsequent technological manipulation does not show respect for the act itself.[31] In other words, to attribute conception to the marital act, the act itself must have a direct causal relationship to the conception of the child.[32] John Doerfler proposes that the marital act would be the principal cause of conception if technical assistance only removes the obstacles to its effectiveness, allowing the marital act to be the principal cause of conception. When the technique interrupts the natural causal process by removing the sperm or ovum or by causing fertilisation to take place *in vitro*, it cannot be said to assist the marital act.[33] At present, some of the techniques for assisting conception that are commonly approved by Catholic theologians and ethicists include those listed by May, who cites Grisez. In the case of retrograde ejaculation or similar problems, a couple can use a technical means like a condom or prophylactic during the marital act to ensure that the man's sperm is deposited inside his wife's vagina, thereby removing the obstacle to the effectiveness of their conjugal act. In like manner, Low Tubal Ovum Transfer (LTOT) is morally licit because it merely relocates the ovum, before the marital act, to the lower part of an affected fallopian tube or to the uterus itself. Similarly, it is morally permissible for a physician to use a technical instrument to propel the sperm that a man deposited in his wife's vagina during sexual intercourse

---

[31] H. WATT, "Parenthood and new reproductive technologies anthropological consideration," in J. CORREA – E. SGRECCIA (eds.), *The Dignity of Human Procreation and Reproductive Technologies: Anthropological and Ethical Aspects,* Proceedings of the Tenth Assembly of the Pontifical Academy for Life, Vatican City, 20-22 February 2004, pp. 34-35. The emphasis here is that the sexual act should unite both the couples themselves and their gametes or bring them closer.

[32] Cf. W. MAY, *Catholic Bioethics…, op. cit.,* p. 87; See also G. GRISEZ, *Difficult Moral Questions, Vol. 3., The Way of the Lord Jesus,* Franciscan Press, Quincy, IL 1997, pp. 244-249.

[33] J. DOERFLER, "Assisting or replacing the conjugal act: criteria for a moral evaluation of reproductive techniques," Unpublished 1999 S.T.L. Dissertation at the John Paul II Institute for Studies on Marriage and Family, Washington, D.C.; ID., J. DOERFLER, "Technology and Human Reproduction," *Ethnics & Medics 24,* 8, August 1999, pp. 3-4. Cited in W. MAY, *Catholic Bioethics…, op. cit.,* p. 88.

into the fallopian tubes or uterus to facilitate fertilisation.[34] Other licit technical assistance to infertile couples includes hormonal treatments, surgery to unblock or repair the fallopian tubes, and treatment to resolve endometriosis.[35] The techniques described here do not in any way replace the marital act; rather, they only remove the obstacles to natural fertilisation and provide the necessary conditions for success.[36]

[34] Cf. W. MAY, *Catholic Bioethics…*, *op. cit.*, p. 87.

[35] SACRED CONGREGATION FOR THE DOCTRINE OF THE FAITH, *Dignitas Personae…*, *op. cit.*, Part II, *n.* 13.

[36] Ibid.

ISLAM ON ASSISTED PROCREATION

Adherents of the Islamic faith are principally divided between the Sunnis and the Shi'ites.[37] Although their opinions diverge on some of the reproductive techniques, they agree on most issues. The *shariah*, the body of Islamic laws put together from the Quran and hadith, regulates all the daily activities of the Muslims. As Serour maintains, it classifies all human actions into five categories,[38] one of which is "marriage and procreation." Islam sees Allah as the giver of life and attaches great importance to procreation. Although the Quran and other primary sources of the *shariah* make no mention of ART, Islam encourages its adherents to avail themselves of the opportunities offered by medicine and technology to resolve infertility and preserve procreation within marriage.[39] The salient points of Islamic teaching on ART will be examined briefly.

ISLAM ON MARRIAGE AND ART

In the Islamic religious framework, marriage is the only legitimate context for procreating and rearing a child, making it unacceptable for singles and homosexuals to have access to ART. Even then, a couple can legitimately conceive with a reproductive technology only within the validity of their marriage contract,[40] a fact that also applies to the natural conception of children. While Islam admits that sexual intercourse is the

[37] Cf. M. INHORN, "Making Muslim Babies: Sunni versus Shi'a Approaches to IVF and Gamete Donation," Being an address to the Department of Human Behavior and Human Education School of Public Health, II, University of Michigan; Also presented at Session 108 on "Infertility and New Reproductive Technologies" IUSSP Annual Conference Tours, France, July 2005, 5. Shi'a is the minority religious group of Islam found in countries like Iran, Iraq, Saudi Arabia, India and so on, while the Sunni is the more dominant form in the Islamic world.

[38] Gamal Serour lists the five categories as: The obligatory: such as praying and fasting; the recommended: such as marriage and family formation; the permitted: such as breaking off fasting during illness and travelling; the disapproved but not forbidden: such as divorce; and the absolutely forbidden: such as killing and adultery

[39] G. SEROUR, "Reproductive Choice: A Muslim Perspective," in J. HARRIS – S. HOLM (eds.), *The Future of Human Reproduction, op. cit.*, p. 196.

[40] See M. INHORN, *Local Babies, Global Science..., op. cit.*, p. 279.

basic and only means of establishing a pregnancy, it maintains that when a medical condition renders this impossible, it is morally permissible to resort to reproductive technologies under certain conditions.[41] In this context, ART's tendency to separate procreation from sex does not pose a moral problem.

ISLAM ON AI AND IVF

Islam approves of ART to resolve infertility and maintains that the children that result from these techniques are the legal children of their parents. Making certain restrictions, Islam insists that the techniques must be medically indicated and that the more complex procedures, such as IVF-ET, must be performed by an expert. More importantly, it insists on genetic and hereditary purity and forbids the use of third parties as an intrusion into the "marital functions of sex and procreation of the couple." Marriage is a contract between two people—to resort to a third party (gamete, embryo, or womb donor) is tantamount to *ziza*, that is, adultery.[42] The mixing of genes as takes place in donor-conception is ethically reprehensible, meaning that the gametes should come only from the infertile couple. Surrogacy is absolutely unacceptable in Islam, though it was permissible in the past. The rationale behind the new position is that gestational motherhood cannot be separated from the genetic and social aspects. Furthermore, commercial surrogacy is absolutely objectionable because it dehumanizes the child by treating it as a commodity[43] and because it impedes a child's ability to relate to a known father and mother.[44] However, Inhorn asserts that, in 1999, the Supreme Jurisprudent of the Shi'a group, Ayatollah Ali Hussein Khamanei, issued a *fatwa* approving the use of donated gametes. In this case, the child can only inherit from the donor of the gametes, not from the infertile spouses, who are merely recognized as its "adoptive parents."[45] In contrast to this, the Sunnis (and some Shi'ites) continue to reject third party involvement

---

[41] See Ibid., p. 277.

[42] M. INHORN, "Making Muslim Babies…, *op. cit.,* p. 3.

[43] G. SEROUR, "Reproductive Choice: A Muslim…, *op. cit.,* p. 197.

[44] Ibid.

[45] See M. INHORN, "Making Muslim Babies…, *op. cit.,* p. 5.

in procreation on the grounds of adultery, possible incest, and the need to preserve the child's biological descent.[46]

ISLAM AND ABORTION

In the IVF procedure, multiple pregnancy is resolved through foetal reduction, that is, the selective abortion of some of the foetuses to allow one or two to survive. Abortion is seen in most Islamic nations as a violation of a human life, making it morally unacceptable. Within the Islamic worldview, it is permissible only in some extreme circumstances, such as if a pregnancy poses a threat to a woman's physical or mental health, if the prospect of carrying it to term is remote, or if it is necessary to prevent the birth of a severely disabled child.[47] In the case of a life-threatening pregnancy, the *shariah* considers the life of the mother (the root) to be more important than that of the developing child (the shoot). Some Muslim theologians argue that abortion to avoid congenital anomalies should be permissible up to the fourth month of gestation, while some of the more conservative theologians limit its use to the first two months.[48] Similarly, Islam approves of contraception for family planning, but rejects contraceptive devices that also act as abortifacients.[49] In the past, some jurists permitted abortion before four months of gestation, while others allowed it only before seven weeks, during which time the life of the developing foetus was thought to be imperceptible. In Islam, as pregnancy progresses, abortion becomes a more serious issue, or even

---

[46] See. M. INHORN, *Local Babies, Global Science..., op. cit.,* pp. 276-277; ID., M. INHORN, "Making Muslim Babies..., *op. cit.,* pp. 6-7. Third party donation creates "mixture of relations" and confuses the purity of linage or clarity of origins. In this context, a donor-conceived child comes to be viewed as an illegitimate child.

[47] G. SEROUR – A. OMRAN, *Ethical Guidelines for Human Reproduction Research in the Muslim World,* IICPSR, Cairo 1992; See also M. INHORN, "Making Muslim Babies..., *op. cit.,* p. 4.

[48] Ibid.

[49] See "Reproduction Issues," in http://www.themodernreligion.com/misc/sex/s_repro.htm, p. 1 (Downloaded 16/8/2005). The author of the article is unknown. Islam makes a distinction between abortion and contraception. A device that thickens the cervical mucus to make it impenetrable to sperm is categorized as a contraceptive, not abortion.

a crime.[50] Today, the advancement in technology has made it possible to establish fertilisation as the beginning of human life.

In recognition of the developing child's right to life from conception, Islam accords it the status of incomplete *zimma*, as one author indicates. Ordinarily, *zimma* is the legal recognition that accords rights and duties to an individual; in the case of the foetus it is incomplete because the foetus possesses rights without corresponding duties. For instance, the law of inheritance recognizes it as an inheritor if born alive. Also, a pregnant woman found guilty of a crime punishable by death cannot be executed until she delivers and weans the baby.[51] However, since Islam approves of IVF and the use of the "surplus" foetuses for research, it would seem that the beginning of human life refers to when the pregnancy is established.

CRYOPRESERVATION OF HUMAN EMBRYOS

Islam permits the storage of sperm and the preservation of excess embryos from IVF. However, such embryos, which are considered the property of the couple, can only be transferred to the woman within the validity of their marriage contract.[52] In the event of a divorce or the death of the husband, the preserved sperm or embryos cannot be used to make the woman pregnant. In this case, they can be used for research purposes. From this perspective, Islam would object to every form of posthumous conception, including the use of foetal tissues from aborted foetuses to achieve conception in a woman. Nonetheless, it deems research on such tissues permissible with the informed consent of the couple who owns them.[53] Islam condemns the practice of using selective semen to achieve conception, viewing it as a threat to the existence of the family and the human race.[54] In this ethical framework, non-therapeutic sex selection

---

50 See J. RICHARDS, "Ethical Issues – The Major Faiths..., *op. cit.,* p. 45. Also cited I. HEWITT, *What Does Islam Say?* The Muslim Education Trust, London 1998.

51 See "Reproduction Issues," in http://www.themodernreligion..., *op. cit.,* p. 2.

52 G. SEROUR – A. OMRAN, "Ethical Guidelines for..., *op. cit.*

53 G. SEROUR, "Reproductive Choice: A Muslim..., *op. cit.,* p. 201.

54 Cf. M. INHORN, "Making Muslim Babies..., *op. cit.,* p. 4.

and human genetic design and enhancement will be ethically objectionable as a challenge to the will of God.

RESEARCH ON HUMAN EMBRYOS

Islam permits therapeutic intervention on human embryos as well as research on spare embryos from IVF, but it disapproves of the deliberate creation of embryos solely for purposes of commercial research. With the free informed consent of the couple, preserved embryos may be used for non-therapeutic research to improve the treatment of infertility, cancer, and other medical conditions.[55] Since embryos that are used as research materials carry medical risks if they are implanted,[56] Islam insists that such treated embryos should never be transferred into any woman.[57]

[55] G. SEROUR – A. OMRAN, "Ethical Guidelines for…, *op. cit.*

[56] J. ROBERTSON, *Children of Choice: Freedom and the New Reproductive Technologies,* Princeton University Press, Princeton 1994, pp. 198-200. Cited in J. HARRIS – S. HOLM (eds.), *The Future of Human…, op. cit.*, p. 199.

[57] G. SEROUR, "Reproductive Choice: A Muslim…, *op. cit.,* p. 200.

NIGERIAN AND AFRICAN TRADITIONAL THOUGHT ON ART

There is currently a dearth of literature or reflection by African scholars on the artificial reproductive technologies. At the time of this writing, there is no book on the practice of ART in Nigeria and no reflection on the different techniques from the standpoint of Nigerian culture and experience. This is not surprising considering that the technologies in question are not widespread in this part of the world in comparison to other parts. In reality, the influx of these techniques into many parts of sub-Saharan Africa is a recent development. Even in places where they have been in existence for many years, their availability has been limited and their practise has not been widespread. Nonetheless, on the basis of African philosophical, moral, and religious thought, the African position on some of the available techniques is discernible.

HUMAN SEXUALITY IN AFRICAN TRADITIONAL THOUGHT

In the traditional African worldview, sexuality expressions are considered sacred because they are connected with life, which is sacred in itself. Various African societies prohibited and punished the abuse of sexuality. A healthy and responsible use of human sexuality is required because, within the African religious and ethical framework, sexual relations are merely a means to an end, namely, the procreation of children.[58]

HUMAN GENERATION AND THE CONJUGAL ACT

Africans view God as the Creator and ultimate Source of every human life. A child is a precious gift from God and a privilege to its parents.[59] In reference to how human beings come into existence, the term "reproduction" is foreign to African traditional thought. Africans believe in procreation, though they may not have used the exact word in the past. For Nigerians and Africans in general, the term "human reproduction" does not adequately depict what happens in human generation, because human life and the act that generates human life are not purely

---

[58] L. MAGESA, *African Religion…*, *op. cit.*, p. 84.

[59] Cf. F. OBORJI, "African Traditional Religion Between Pluralism and Ultimate Reality," *Studies in Inter-religious Dialogue, PEETERS,* February 14, 2004, pp. 131, 141; See also E. KABORE, "Identity and Status of the Human Embryo…, *op. cit.,* p. 423.

biological.[60] Thus, to reduce human life to its biological dimension is to lose sight of man's composite nature as a unity of body and spirit—*muo* or *emi* (spirit, soul) and *ahu* or *ara* (body) among the Igbo and Yoruba of Nigeria respectively.[61,62] Human sexuality and marriage are sacred, and the act of generating children itself is sacred and should take place within marriage, which is the appropriate context for the begetting and rearing of children. In African thought pattern, conception does not merely derive from the sexual act between a man and his wife; rather, it is a blessing from God and the ancestors. Deng articulates this quite clearly:

> Mother and father copulate to "beget" jointly and give birth while God interferes [?] .... Every child is the outcome of a woman, God's creation and ancestral blessing. Hence, God is sometimes referred to as "Grandfather" or "Father" of every child.[63]

In the African worldview, the child, as a gift of God, results from a "conjugal relationship" between a man and a woman. Ordinarily, he is neither a product of masturbation nor of the laboratory, though he would still be recognized as a child no matter how he was conceived. Consequently, ART procedures, which do not involve the conjugal act or in which fertilisation occurs outside the woman's body, are considered abnormal and do not conform to the traditional African understanding of the generation of a human being. This explains why most Nigerian couples use IVF as a last resort and why they do so under absolute secrecy.

Today, rapid advances in science and technology and an increased need to have biological offspring have led to a modification of this view. Some believe that ART procedures, such as AI and IVF, would be

---

60 Cf. B. BUJO, *Foundations of An African Ethic,* p. 122.

61 L. BROWN, "Understanding and Ontology in Traditional African Thought," in L. BROWN (ed.), *African Philosophy: New and Traditional Perspectives,* Oxford University Press, Inc., New York 2004, p. 159; See also P. IROEGBU, *Metaphysics: The Kpim of Philosophy,* International University Press, Owerri 1995, p. 313.

62 Cf. B. BUJO, *African Theology in its Social Context,* Paulines Publications Africa, Nairobi, Kenya 1992, p. 113.

63 F. DENG, *The Dinka of the Sudan,* Richard and Winston, New York 1972, p. 30.

acceptable within African morality if the gametes were obtained from the couple within marriage; in this case the child would still be their biological offspring and a bona fide member of their ancestral lineage. This view was clearly reflected by some respondents who commented on the ethical acceptability of ART from the perspective of African culture. To support their claim, some respondents cited the practice of certain African societies and Nigerian subcultures in which a woman carries a pregnancy for an infertile sister or relative. In like manner, the practice of arranging a relative or friend to impregnate the wife of an infertile man is tolerated in some African societies.[64] Some see homologous ART procedures as preferable to such traditional practices because they do not involve adultery and the resulting child is the natural offspring of its parents.[65] Moreover, others view it as more acceptable than pursuing a biological child by consulting witch doctors, performing fetish rituals, or pledging the life of the prospective child to a deity, a practice that is common in some parts of Nigeria and Africa.

Africans never wish to die without an heir. Beyond the natural human desire to procreate and form a family, Africans need to preserve their ancestral lineage and attain personal immortality after death. As many African authors point out, children prolong the life of their parents, grandparents, and ancestors and perpetuate the entire family lineage.[66] This African emphasis on procreation can be linked to the conception of the ultimate end of the human person that is dominant in many parts of the continent. The Christian religion (for example, Catholicism) teaches that the end of the human person is "to know and to serve God." Some contemporary philosophers, influenced by atheistic existentialists like Sartre, tend to conceive the ultimate project of the human person as consisting in self-realization through an absolute exercise of freedom. In traditional African thought, it may be rightly said that the end of man

---

[64] Cf. J. MBITI, *Introduction to African Religion…, op. cit.,* p. 112. This is not a universal practice in Africa. However, in spite of the prohibition of adultery in Nigerian cultures, some people still resort to this practice secretly to have children.

[65] See J. ESANGBEDO, "Facts, 'Fears' about Test-tube Babies…, *op. cit.,* p. 18.

[66] J. MBITI, *Introduction to African Religion…, op. cit.,* p. 114; See also I. IGWEGBE, *The Meaning of the Beginning,* Snaap Press, Enugu 2002, p. 27. E. METUH, *African Religion in Western…, op. cit.,* p. 114.

is happiness in the afterlife, but in reality this consists in the perpetuation of humankind through the transmission of the vital force, which guarantees the personal immortality of the individual after his physical death on earth.[67] As Shorter puts it, in traditional African society, "To be alive was to transmit life, to be reproductive. One who did not procreate was not alive. His or her death was final."[68] The underlying sense is that an individual who has offspring does not die completely, and his body does not entirely decay in the physical world if there are children to survive him, because his body survives in them. This understanding of the end of the human person has a serious implication for Africans: the greatest disaster or disgrace that can befall an individual is to die leaving no descendants. Even though the soul survives in the spirit world, the person is completely dead in the physical world.[69] From this perspective, an individual that dies without a child has failed to fulfil his ultimate end; this is why some approve homologous ART for married couples as a last resort, though with some restrictions on embryo wastage, commercialization of gametes, wombs, and embryos, and experimentation on embryos.

DESTRUCTION AND EXPERIMENTATION ON HUMAN EMBRYOS

One reality that will pose a serious problem for many Africans is the high embryo wastage involved in IVF and related techniques. Although the techniques themselves are meant to foster the transmission of life, they also lead to the destruction of viable human embryos, which is inconsistent with the preservation and promotion of life that is a defining feature of African ethics. In traditional African thought, it is generally accepted that human life begins when the spiritual soul is infused into the body, though there seems to be no consensus as to when exactly this takes place.[70] While some people point to a period before birth, others think it occurs at birth. However, the dominant view among most Africans is

---

[67] See L. KAGABO, "Alexis Kagame: The Trial of an African Theology," in B. BUJO - J. MUYA (eds.), *African Theology in the 21st Century, Vol. 2,* Paulines Publications Africa, Nairobi, Kenya 2006, p. 25.

[68] A. SHORTER, African Culture, An Overview, *op. cit.*, p. 94.

[69] Cf. L. KAGABO, "Alexis Kagame: The Trial of the African Theology…, *op. cit.,* p. 25.

[70] We shall comment further on this in the next chapter, which is on the moral status of the human embryo and its significance for the debate on ART.

that the soul is infused at the time of conception. As Mbiti puts it, the time the soul joins the body is believed to take place "when the husband and wife sleep together at the conception of the child-to-be."[71] Perhaps with this in mind, a medical practitioner in Nigeria, Udumaga Obiora Okafor, rejects IVF on the basis of the destruction of many embryos to achieve the birth of a child. In his exact words, "An offspring that has been sought as such; at such a price; and in such a way has been obtained at the cost of the holocaust of innumerable human lives."[72] Esangbedo, an ART practitioner, was quick to respond that there are facilities for storing excess embryos,[73] although he did not mention that only about 50% of such embryos are successfully thawed, meaning that the remaining 50% are likely to be lost.

In view of the above, destructive experimentation on living human embryos and foreseeable foetal reduction are inconsistent with the transmission and preservation of the vital force, which is basic to African ethics. One way to rescue excess embryos created during IVF is through embryo donation or adoption; however, donor-conception is not sanctioned by African ethics, meaning that the deliberate creation of several embryos with the intention to donate the surplus is still morally unacceptable.

DONOR-CONCEPTION TECHNIQUES

Despite the exaggerated emphasis on children and the transmission of life, African morality abhors the intrusion of a total stranger into marriage, even in the case of infertility. From this standpoint, commercial surrogacy and all the artificial reproductive techniques involving gametes and embryos from unknown donors are ethically objectionable.[74] Such techniques may harm the prospective child psychologically and socially by exposing him to unimaginable ridicule and humiliation among extended family, his peers, and the community. In Nigeria and most parts of Africa, a person who does not know his paternal roots is regarded as a bastard and subjected to ridicule in society. Hence, every

[71] J. MBITI, *Introduction to African Religion..., op. cit.,* p. 124.

[72] U. OKAFOR, "Caution on IVF..., *op. cit.,* p. 21.

[73] See J. ESANGBEDO, "Caution on IVF – A Rejoinder..., *op. cit.,* p. 2.

[74] Cf. O. GIWA-OSAGIE - B. KAYODE, "A Rational Approach..., *op. cit.,* p. 5.

child has the right to know its biological origins or ancestral roots just as parents ought to know their children. Bujo sheds more light on this:

> If we take the problem of insemination or of *in vitro* fertilization with anonymous donors of sperm, the decisive and convincing argument will not be an abstract one, drawn from natural law: it is only the community dimension that supplies lasting justification for the prohibition. African society, where *cognatus sum, ergo sumus* is significant, does not admit any anonymity.... Here it is essential that each child knows his father and mother by name and remains in a living contact with them after their death; and it is equally essential that parents know their children by name and remain in warmest contact with them... it is extraordinarily important to insist on this precisely in Africa, where the desire for children and yearning for community can have disastrous consequences on some persons—for modern technology and medicine could pervert a good tradition into its opposite, for example, when the mother or the married couple desire children to satisfy their own ideals or egoistic desires, to bring about the community that they picture to themselves in egoistic terms, but to the disadvantage of the child, without concern for his true identity in the community.[75]

AFRICAN TRADITIONAL RELIGION AND ABORTION

Because the African traditional religion holds human life to be sacred, it does not sanction abortion at any moment after conception. Bujo explains that the vital force is central in African traditional ethics, and it poses to the community the need to develop a moral code of conduct that safeguards it and helps it to flourish.[76] Since the living-dead (that is, ancestors) continue to extend their own life in the physical world in their descendants, they too are concerned about the transmission and preservation of life. Hence, abortion, infanticide, and the like are not

---

[75] B. BUJO, *Foundations of an African Ethic, op. cit.*, p. 36.

[76] Ibid., p. 20.

sanctioned in African ethics because they affect the flow of life, offend the ancestors, and threaten the future survival of the clan or community. On this, Mbiti writes, "Anything that deliberately goes towards the destruction or obstruction of human life is regarded as wicked and evil" and is, therefore, viewed as a major offence in the eyes of the community.[77] However, if a pregnancy threatens the survival of the mother, indirect abortion may be permitted. In this case, African ethics gives preference to the woman and does not consider a decision to save her life to be a deliberate destruction of human life, even though it carries the consequence of terminating the life of the embryo. Moreover, in African traditional thought, every child that is conceived has a guardian in one of the ancestors. Hence, to destroy or abort a baby offends the ancestor who is the guardian of the unborn child; this offense can bring negative consequences upon the community and the individual who perpetrates the crime. Thus, in a traditional African setting, parents may strongly rebuke their daughter for an "unwanted" pregnancy outside wedlock, but the child is still welcomed with joy by the family and the community. This insistence on the sacredness of human life from conception to its natural end may seem absurd when we consider that twins were killed in some African communities of the past. But it is crucial to make a distinction between the real African position and an aberration. The practice was based on the misconception that a twin birth is an abnormality—a bad omen for the community. As Webster observes, some African people, such as the Igbo and Edo of Nigeria, considered twins to be "a sign of disharmony" and attributed such births to malicious spiritual forces, evil human beings, or even unfaithfulness on the part of a woman. The Igbo saw the birth of twins as degrading to humanity, since in their opinion such births were naturally reserved for animals.[78] As a result, twins were killed in the southern part of Nigeria, but this was not a general practice in Nigeria or Africa. On the contrary, many African societies, like the Yoruba of Nigeria, welcomed twins with great joy and gratitude to God and the ancestors, and they treated them with special respect and care.[79]

[77] J. MBITI, *Introduction to African Religion…, op. cit.*, p. 104.

[78] H. WEBSTER, *Taboo: A Sociological Study*, Octagon Books, New York 1973, pp. 61, 64; Cited in L. MAGESA, *African Religion..., op. cit.*, pp. 146-147.

[79] Cf. L. MAGESA, *African Religion…, op. cit.*, pp. 146-147.

PERSONHOOD IN AFRICAN THOUGHT

A characteristic feature of the African conception of a person is the tendency to restrict personhood to members of the biological human species. That is to say, the animals cannot acquire a personal status. As such, they do not possess a right to life, though some communities prohibit the killing of certain animals for unrelated reasons. There is no consensus among African scholars on the beginning of human personhood. While some attribute it from conception, many scholars claim that it is an acquired status, which implies ethical maturity on the part of the individual.[80] In this latter view, there is a distinction between a "human being" and a "human person."[81] While a person may be a human being, there are human beings who are not yet persons. This means that human personhood is not ontologically attributed to the individual; rather, it is understood in the sense of moral agency, in which case a person is a moral being or a bearer of norms.[82] Despite these divergent views, the consensus is that a human being with a right to life and protection comes into existence at the moment of conception.

PGD AND GENETIC DESIGN AND ENHANCEMENT

In African culture, every child is welcomed with joy and loved unconditionally.[83] A child is still a child even if it is handicapped; the issue of "quality control," which characterizes techniques like IVF, IVF-PGD, and human genetic design and enhancement, is foreign to Africans. Parents would gladly welcome a therapeutic intervention on their unborn child that has clear benefits for its health and survival, but nonetheless, every child is accepted as a precious gift from God and loved as he is. This is clear in the view of Godfrey Tangwa:

---

[80] See R. BELL, *Understanding African Philosophy*, Routledge, New York 2002, p. 61.

[81] I. MENKITI, "On the normative conception of a person," in K. WIREDU (ed.), *A Companion to African Philosophy*, *op. cit.*, pp. 326-326. African traditional thought in this area can be discerned in the different African languages.

[82] P. NWAEZEAPU, *When Does a Human Person Begin? Moral Status of the Embryo and Technology*, Leberit S.R.L. Press, Rome 2007, pp. 89-98. The African view on human personhood is treated in greater detail in this book.

[83] G. TANGWA, "Some African Reflections on Biomedical..., *op. cit.*, p. 391.

> Quality-talk in the domain of human reproduction is, perhaps, a case of adapting inappropriate concepts and vocabulary from the domain of economics and marketing propaganda under the influence of a calculative moral approach, such as utilitarianism.[84]

In spite of the physical and behavioural differences that we observe in human beings, it is absurd to consider one human being to be "of better or higher quality than another,"[85] since human beings are not products that can be measured in economic terms. Every human individual is an end in itself and enjoys an equal dignity and respect with every other human being, irrespective of the observable differences in physical makeup and behavioural characteristics. In this light, using human genetic design and enhancement to produce a "customized baby" would be ethically reprehensible within the African moral framework because it brings the culture of consumerism into the sacredness of human generation. In like manner, prenatal diagnosis with selective abortion and PGD for sex selection are offensive to African ethics regarding the transmission and preservation of life. Nevertheless, some couples in a desperate search for male children to assure the continuity of their lineage will find PGD and the Microsort technique extremely attractive. In fact, the latter has the potential to satisfy the African moral code because it does not obstruct the transmission and protection of life. However, this is open to further debate among African scholars.

COMMERCIALIZATION OF HUMAN SEXUALITY AND CHILDREN

The commercialization of human gametes, wombs, viable embryos, or any other reproductive tissue treats them as mere commodities. This does not conform to the African sense of the responsible transmission of the vital force—it ridicules the process and attempts to deprive it of its sacred character, thus making such commercialization ethically unjustifiable. Commenting on this, Bujo maintains that human sexuality can never be exchanged for money or other goods.[86] While women in

---

[84] Ibid., p. 392.

[85] Ibid.

[86] B. BUJO, *Foundations of an African Ethic, op. cit.,* pp. 60-61. Bujo sees the present day prostitution as a banalization of human sexuality, which replaces its "dynamic and humane character" by the "anonymous power of money" as

southwestern Nigeria and some other African societies may carry pregnancies for their infertile sisters or relatives on a strictly altruistic basis,[87] commercial surrogacy arrangements are ethically reprehensible in Africa. In most African cultures, a child's origin is traced through the paternal lineage; as such, the extended family and the community as a whole may not fully accept a child that results from anonymously purchased semen, leading to negative psychological and social consequences for the child.

WHO SHOULD HAVE ACCESS TO ART?

The strong emphasis on procreation as the end of one's existence and the only way to achieve personal immortality makes ART extremely attractive to infertile couples in Nigeria and Africa as a whole. Nonetheless, the African moral framework would consider it morally unacceptable to make the techniques available to everyone, such as gays, lesbians, and unmarried men or women. For instance, active homosexuality and same-sex "marriage" are considered both abnormal and immoral in Africa. As Magesa rightly observes, "Active homosexuality is morally intolerable," especially as it frustrates the whole purpose of human sexuality, which is the transmission and preservation of the vital force to provide the ancestors with continued remembrance and honour among their living descendants.[88] In other words, making ART accessible to homosexuals or single parents does not conform to the African notion of family or community. This can be inferred from Bujo's statement:

> It has been rightly noted that homosexuality is rare in the traditional Black Africa, and the reason for this is precisely the communal dimension: south of the Sahara, the fundamental anthropological conception in Africa is both bipolar and tripolar. One is a human being only in the duality of man and woman, and this bipolarity generates the triad man-woman-child, which leads to full community. Against this background, a man-man or woman-woman relationship would not

---

the aftermath of the damage inflicted by western industrialization on African structure and life.

[87] Usually, such a practice would involve having a sexual intercourse with the spouse of such a relative for the child to be his biological offspring.

[88] L. MAGESA, *African Religion…, op. cit.*, p. 146.

> only be looked on as an egoistic isolation which dares not take the step to full human existence; it also leads to sexist discrimination against part of the human race and shows an unwillingness to accept the enrichment that comes from heterogeneity.[89]

In Nigeria, and perhaps in Africa as a whole, the natural setting for bringing forth and educating children is the family, which consists of mother, father, and children. Because single parenthood and homosexuality are not sanctioned in African cultures, making ART available to this category of people is morally unacceptable and can confuse or corrupt the African understanding of marriage and family.

[89] B. BUJO, *Foundations of an African Ethic, op. cit.*, p. 25.

CHAPTER 10

REFLECTING FURTHER ON THE ARTIFICIAL REPRODUCTIVE TECHNOLOGIES

So far in our discourse, we have elaborated on the moral issues involved in ART. In this section, we will attempt to critically evaluate some of the important issues raised in this book and make some recommendations.

GENERAL ASPECTS

Before we undertake an ethical appraisal of the various techniques of artificial reproduction, we must ask some important questions: What are the factors of morality? Are human actions justified only by their ends or consequences? What does it really mean to assist conception? Do human beings reproduce or procreate? Our main concerns here are to clarify some terminological issues in the debate on ART and to explain the criteria of moral judgment with which we will evaluate ART.

AN ACTION IS NOT JUSTIFIED SOLELY BY ITS CONSEQUENCES

Nowadays, a couple can conceive a child naturally or with the aid of technology. The end in the two cases—to have a child—is good in itself. Even though the circumstances differ, they do not pose a moral problem. Nevertheless, the fact that these two ways of conceiving a child lead to the same goal does not mean that the two actions are morally equivalent. For instance, to establish a pregnancy through IVF with a couple's gametes and to do the same using donated gametes attracts diverse ethical evaluations, though the goal is the same. As we noted previously, advocates defend the various reproductive technologies on the basis of their pragmatic value or good consequences. Similarly, others justify a limited use of AI and IVF on the basis of the proportionate relationship between the good and bad effects the action produces, "with a view to the 'greater good' or 'lesser evil' actually possible in a particular situation."[1] Still others approve of donor-conception and surrogacy and claim that such may be the only way for an infertile couple to have a child that is related to one of them. The moral theory that underlies this position is consequentialism. This theory tends to measure the moral rightness or wrongness of a human action solely by its consequences,[2] implying that both the motive for which an act is performed and the means that are employed are outweighed by its consequences. This account of morality raises some crucial questions: Can a morally bad means generate a morally good action? Does the good consequence of an action justify it? It is not in doubt that ART is pragmatic and offers at least some measure

1 Cf. *VS.* 75.

2 J. DRIVER, *Ethics: The Fundamentals, op. cit.*, p. 40.

of happiness to numerous couples, but the real issue is whether the rightness or wrongness of an action can be determined solely by the utility that derives from it.

Consequentialist theories of morality, such as utilitarianism, measure the rightness or wrongness of an action by the goodness or badness of the actual consequences. The first form of utilitarianism, credited to Bentham and later defended by Mill, is often known as universalistic utilitarianism, which seeks to provide the greatest happiness for the greatest number of people. While Bentham proposed "act" utilitarianism, which focuses on the goodness or badness of the consequences of every individual action, Mill favoured rule utilitarianism, which concerns itself with the consequences of adopting some general rules. Although utilitarianism as proposed by these authors has its own merits (considering that society cannot possibly satisfy the needs of everyone with its limited resources), one of its major defects is the tendency to ignore the intrinsic dignity of the individual, making him merely a means to an end. In treating him as a "part" rather than a "whole" and ignoring his interests and rights, it predicates his moral worth on the happiness of the majority. This approach is detrimental to his well-being because he can be sacrificed to satisfy the needs or wishes of the majority. Thus, utilitarianism crushes the individual, compresses his liberty, ignores his rights, and reduces him to an instrument for realizing the common good.[3] To succumb to such a theory will have disastrous social consequences. For instance, it means that it will be morally acceptable to kill an innocent rich man with the intention of distributing his wealth to the poor if this will promote the happiness of the greatest number of people in his community.

A good end cannot justify a bad means in the same way that the good consequences of an action cannot be a true measure of its moral goodness, as the utilitarian theory suggests.[4] First and foremost, an action is a human act if it is conscious and free, meaning that the actor should

---

[3] D. FURROW, *Ethics: Key Concepts in Philosophy,* Continuum, London 2005, p. 46.

[4] Cf. J. SMART, "Utilitarianism..., *op. cit.,* p. 206; Also see R. FREY, "Utilitarianism and Bioethics," in S. POST (ed.), *Encyclopedia of Bioethics, op. cit.,* p. 2531.

know what he is doing and should act without coercion.[5] To be a morally good action, the end and the means (or the *moral object*) must be good. Conscious and free actions in the medical field, such as a couple's decision to have a child with ART and the physician's decision to assist them, are not morally neutral. They cannot be evaluated exclusively on the basis of good intentions or good consequences. Rather, the moral rightness or wrongness of a human action is equally contingent upon the moral object that is used. Pointing out the danger in reducing moral judgment solely to the good intention of the agent, O'Rourke asserts that "almost any action or group of actions joined together by an ultimate intention might be evaluated as 'good' if the intention is good."[6] The consequentialist account separates the goodness of an action from the goodness and badness of the agent who performs it; this contrasts with virtue ethics, which is equally interested in the virtue of the moral agent.[7] Now, if the consequences sought in an action are viewed universally in terms of how they affect mankind, the theory is known as universalistic utilitarianism; if they are determined relative to the agent himself, even when they are detrimental to others, it is referred to as ethical egoism or egoistic utilitarianism. It is in this latter form that we see the real danger of the theory.

In view of this distinction, the decision to satisfy the present desire of a couple in a way that potentially jeopardizes the future psycho-social well-being of the child, as well as the interests of the family and society, leans more to the egoistic aspect. Thus, to provide a more balanced evaluation of the vast array of reproductive technologies currently available, we will pay attention to the end of the agent, the means, and the circumstances, including the consequences. The vital point here is that every human act has a structure. The moral agent who is capable of knowing, wanting, and willing always has an end (motive or intention) in view, which leads him to desire to complete the action. To arrive at this end, he freely chooses an object (moral means). And since he is conscious and free in completing the action, he is morally responsible for it—responsible for the end, the object he chooses to reach it, and the consequences

5 Knowledge presupposes the intellect, while freedom presupposes the will.

6 K. O'ROURKE, (ed.), *A Primer for Health Care Ethics, op. cit.*, p. 264.

7 Cf. R. POPKIN – A. STROLL, *Philosophy Made Simple, 2nd Edition,* A Made Simple Book and Doubleday, New York 1993, p. 33.

it produces. The end, the moral object he employs, and the circumstances (of which the consequences are crucial) are subject to moral scrutiny, and they should all be good for the action to be morally good. A good end does not necessarily justify the means because the agent is responsible, not only for the end, but also for the means he freely chooses and the consequences of his action. Free and conscious actions in the medical and scientific fields are not morally neutral. They are human acts because they involve a free exercise of knowledge and affect human beings. As such, they can be good or bad, and their practical utility or the good intentions of the agent cannot be the only factors considered in their ethical evaluation.

ART: ASSISTANCE OR SUBSTITUTION?

Another term used to designate ART is "medically assisted conception." Certainly, this does not pose a terminological problem, as the process of conception can actually be assisted medically. However, certain ART procedures raise serious doubts as to whether the process of conception is assisted or substituted entirely. The term "assistance" connotes "to help" or "to support," is distinct from "substitution," which implies "to take the place of something" or "to use something instead of that which is normally used."[8] Naturally, at least from the standpoint of biology, human beings procreate sexually, even though man and the process of his generation are more than biology, as we will see later. Following the marital sexual love, the gametes of the couple unite to give origin to a new diploid cell called a zygote with its own unique genetic code. On account of this, to assist conception in the true sense means "to help" or "to support" the sexual love of the couple to reach its finality, rather than "to substitute" it or "to take its place" or "to use something else instead of that which is normally used," that is, to obtain sperm outside the marital sexual intercourse for laboratory fertilisation or insemination. The critical point is that by using ART to establish a pregnancy without having recourse to a couple's "normal" sexual love, physicians do not

---

[8] See S. WEHMEIER (ed.), *Oxford Advance Learner Dictionary of Current English, Sixth Edition,* Oxford University Press, Oxford 2000, see "Assistance" and "Substitute."

really "assist" the process of conception. Instead, they merely assist the couple's desire to have a child, using a means that is circumventive.

ASSISTED REPRODUCTION OR ASSISTED PROCREATION?

Most authors designate ART as "assisted reproductive technology" or "artificial reproduction,"[9] while some others view "assisted procreation" as the more appropriate term. This raises a question: Is a human being reproduced or procreated? In response to this, it must be stressed that while the term "reproduction" is appropriate to describe the experience of animals, it is extremely demeaning to the human person.[10] First, there is a qualitative difference between animals and human beings based on the latter's rational nature, which makes him capable of knowing, evaluating, willing, and being morally responsible for his free actions. Moreover, it reduces man to his biological dimension without recognizing his spiritual reality. Man is neither only body nor only spirit, but a unity of body and spirit, although not in terms of the dualism of Plato or the *cogito ergo sum* of Rene Descartes: "I think, therefore I am." The latter refers to an anthropology in which the material body is extrinsic to the spiritual soul, whereas there is a substantial unity between the two, meaning that the body and the soul are a unity in man. What thinks or acts is not the form (the spiritual soul), but man in his unity, body and soul.[11] Given this understanding of the unity of the body and soul, it is demeaning and misleading to define him as only spiritual or only material. In fact, once these two aspects are separated in the same individual, we are no longer in the presence of a human person, but a corpse. Thus, to understand and appreciate human procreation or generation, it is absolutely necessary to incorporate both the biological dimension and the anthropological and metaphysical visions of the human person. The biological dimension looks at the physiology of human generation and speaks of fertilisation and reproduction, conveying a mechanistic

[9] Although in practice, these authors refer to the same reality, that is, techniques like AI, IVF and its variants, there is need to note the important distinction between "reproduction" and "procreation" when speaking about human beings.

[10] Objects are produced, animals are reproduced but humans are procreated.

[11] For the same reason, man's dignity touches his entire person, body and soul.

and demeaning vision of man; in the same way, the tendency to see man as only a spiritual being amounts to spiritual reductionism. In contrast to these two extremes, any true description of man must account for the unity of his physical-mental-spiritual dimensions. The spiritual principle of man, the soul, can neither be reduced to matter nor be said to originate from it since the nature of the soul is superior to the nature of matter. When we view man in his unity of body and soul, we speak of procreation rather than reproduction or production. In this light, while reproduction can be artificial, procreation cannot be artificial, though it can be assisted by technology. The conclusion that arises from this is that the term "artificial reproduction" does not capture what really takes place in the generation of a child. A more appropriate term is "assisted procreation," provided the techniques truly assist the sexual love of the couple rather than substitute it.

As *Gaudium et Spes* states, a human being is procreated through the collaboration between a couple and God, who creates every individual soul at the moment of conception.[12] But even if we leave God out of the matter, reason can still lead us to the conclusion that the profound reality that takes place in marital sexual love is not the same as what happens in animal reproduction; therefore, human procreation is not the same reality as reproduction and cannot be equated to it. Animals are governed by instinct to reproduce, whereas human beings are rational and do not procreate merely to satisfy a biological instinct. Human beings can choose when to procreate, where to procreate, and with whom to procreate; consequently, they can be held accountable for their sexual behaviour. This exercise of knowledge and freewill makes procreation a human action that attracts moral evaluation and accountability. On the other hand, animals have no intellectual capacity to evaluate the moral rightness or wrongness of their behaviour, which is why we cannot hold them morally responsible for their actions.

Without doubt, it is morally permissible to "assist" the procreative process medically, but under close scrutiny it is clear that most of the techniques do not assist procreation in the real sense. In IVF and most of its variants, the physician tries to produce babies rather than assist a couple to conceive a child in a way that allows their love and mutual

---

[12] *GS* 51.

self-giving in the marital act to contribute to the union of their gametes. In reality, what we have are two biologically separated acts of egg-retrieval and sperm collection, which make the reproductive cells available for use in the ART procedure. This practice relegates the couple to mere suppliers of gametes[13] and a womb, and it makes the physician the principal agent in the act of bringing a child into existence. Moreover, it treats the child as a "product" of the laboratory and exposes it to additional health risks and manipulations by the physician. Viewed from this perspective, one may not be wrong to allege that most of the techniques reduce human procreation even below human reproduction to human *production.* The term "reproduction" can only be applied to human beings in a restricted and derogatory sense, possibly to express displeasure at an unacceptable abuse of the generative process. Hence, it does not sufficiently respect the dignity of the child or measure up to the standard of responsible procreation. Reflecting on this, Kass writes the following:

> Consider the views of life and the world reflected in the following different expressions to describe the process of generating new life. Ancient Israel, impressed with the phenomenon of transmitting life from father to son, used a word we translate as "begetting" or "siring." The Greeks, impressed with the springing forth of new life in the cyclical processes of generation and decay, called it "genesis," from a root meaning "to come into being."... The pre-modern Christian English-speaking world, impressed with the world as given by a creator, used the term "pro-creation." We, impressed with the machine and the gross national product (our own work of creation), employ a metaphor of the factory, "re-production."[14]

This shift in the language of modern man mirrors a shift in the mentality of society and its social and ethical values. In the past, the emphasis was not only on the goodness of the action, but also on that

---

[13] In most ART methods like IVF, ICSI and others, the couple is almost reduced to passive actors, making the physician the real actor.

[14] L. KASS, *Toward a More Natural Science,* The Free Press, New York 1985, p. 48.

of the moral agent who performs the act. Nowadays, many philosophers merely focus on the good consequences of the action or the intention of the agent, as is the case with utilitarians and other consequentialists and with proportionalists, who separate the goodness of the action from that of the actor. In a world that promotes individualism and egoism, it is increasingly difficult for people to transcend the "self" or their immediate desires and ambitions to see how their choices and actions can affect the wider interests of family and society. This shortcoming, the lack of formation of a true conscience, and the growing consumerism in society also influence the behaviour of couples in the area of procreation, making it necessary to adopt a more holistic approach to the contentious moral issues raised by ART. Among other things, such an approach requires us to revisit the eroded values related to respect for human life at every stage of development. We must confront the inordinate craze for wealth and power in the scientific and medical fields, the inability of modern man to accept suffering or to transcend his desires, the growing tendency to use medicine to treat mere desires, and the trend to ignore the true or holistic good of the patient as a being with three dimensions—the physical, the mental, and the spiritual—and whose moral worth and dignity are inherent and not dependent on the ability to beget a biological child or on any other material thing.

RESPECT FOR THE DIGNITY OF HUMAN PROCREATION

Unlike human beings, who have abstractive intelligence and can morally evaluate their free actions, animals merely possess practical intelligence. They act instinctively and are controlled by their biological needs even in the area of reproduction, whereas human beings have the capacity for reason and freedom. This qualitative difference underpins the dignity of the human being, and it should be respected in the way we bring a new human being into existence. In the light of this assertion, we will now evaluate the various aspects of ART to see how they conform to the dignity of human procreation.

THE ISSUE OF MASTURBATION IN ART

In ethical evaluation, distinction is made between the physical object and the moral object that is used to arrive at an end. Ethical evaluation focuses on the moral object of an action. For instance, according to the classical moral account, if a starving man takes food from another man's farm strictly for immediate survival, the action is not condemned as evil—the moral object is not stealing, but rather the preservation of life, even though the physical object is stealing in the ordinary sense. In this case, the circumstance of the agent affects the moral meaning of the act, and what underlies this is that the right to property ceases in the face of starvation. On the other hand, if he takes the same food in order to sell it and buy a wrist watch, the action is considered morally bad because the moral object is stealing. Although AIH poses no moral problem to many theorists, the Catholic Church considers it a morally bad means to attain a good end if the procedure substitutes the conjugal love of the couple. Some questions arise on this account: What is the moral object of AIH? Why is it morally wrong? We can approach this problem from two angles. On the one hand, we can evaluate the moral object of AIH solely from the standpoint of masturbation. On the other hand, we can see it as the substitution of the marital sexual love, which destroys the profound meaning of the human generative act. Here, the distinction between masturbation and substitution may seem absurd since the former is supposed to include the latter. But in view of the definition of masturbation and the distinction between physical object and moral object, some may fail to see masturbation as the moral object of

AIH. Contrary to the impression given by some authors, the objection to AIH with sperm obtained outside the marital act does not come from the standpoint of the agent's motive, that is, "solitary sexual pleasure," but rather from the perspective of collecting gametes in a way that substitutes the marital love. The emphasis here is on the substitution of the marital love, for this substitution destroys the meaning of procreating a child. We will examine the two possibilities in greater detail.

First and foremost, is masturbation the moral means of AIH? What is masturbation? The Advanced Learner's Dictionary defines the term "masturbation" as the act of giving oneself sexual pleasure by rubbing one's sexual organs or of giving somebody sexual pleasure by rubbing the sexual organ.[15] According to the Catechism of the Catholic Church (CCC), masturbation is "the deliberate stimulation of the genital organs in order to derive sexual pleasure."[16] In light of this definition and the fact that moral evaluation focuses on the moral object of an action, one may possibly argue that masturbation is not the moral object of AIH, even though it is clearly the physical object. This is because the couple does not deliberately resort to it for sexual pleasure, as the definition requires, but only as a means to collect sperm for a medical procedure that was necessitated by the couple's inability to conceive through conjugal love. The sexual pleasure the man probably experiences may be regarded as a foreseeable but undesired effect of his action. Masturbation is clearly a distorted use of the sexual faculty, but it is problematic to take this definition, which focuses on solitary sexual pleasure, and apply it out of its context. The definition emphasizes the motive of the agent, which is solitary sexual pleasure, but in the context of AIH, the motive of the agent is not solitary sexual pleasure, but rather the need to obtain sperm for fertility treatment. Now, some circumstances enter into the meaning

---

[15] S. WEHMEIER (ed.), *Oxford Advanced Learner's Dictionary..., op. cit.,* see "Masturbate."

[16] CATECHISM OF THE CATHOLIC CHURCH, *Popular and Definitive Edition,* Burns & Oats, London 2000, no. 2352; The Church maintains that masturbation is an intrinsically gravely disordered action. In general, this solitary, essentially individualistic and disordered use of the sexual faculty is contrary to its purpose. Henceforth, any reference to the definition of masturbation will refer to the CCC. Although the two definitions are in accord, the CCC definition is more elaborate on the issue.

of an action and change its moral status. For instance, it is always wrong to kill an innocent human being. Nonetheless, if a man kills an actual, present, and unjust aggressor as a last resort to defend his life, his family, or other fundamental goods, the moral meaning of his action is not murder, but self-defence. Likewise, in resorting to masturbation for AI or IVF, the infertile man's focus is not "solitary sexual pleasure." To predicate the moral wrongness of AIH or any other technique on masturbation, understood in terms of a deliberate search for solitary sexual pleasure, may not be sufficient to show why it is a morally wrong means for satisfying the good desire to have a child. With regard to ART and in view of all we have said about moral object, this definition of masturbation is limited, although it is not the case when we consider it from the standpoint of its original context, which is solitary sexual pleasure. We will now turn to the second possibility.

If we accept that masturbation is not the moral object of AIH, since the motive of the couple who resorts to it is to collect sperm rather than to experience solitary sexual pleasure, will this way of collecting sperm be a morally acceptable means to have a child? The answer is negative. That is to say, it will still be morally objectionable on account of the dignity of the man who engages in it, the dignity of the child, and the dignity of human procreation. Sometimes, to produce the semen sample, the man is left in a room to watch a pornographic video or to have a sexual fantasy that can arouse him sufficiently to ejaculate sperm. This way of collecting sperm debases him, and the entire procedure does not correspond to his dignity and involves an approval of pornography. At a deeper level, it substitutes the marital sexual love as a means of generating a child and does not respect the profound meaning and dignity of human procreation. The action reduces the procreation of a child to something of a lesser quality in comparison to what a true "human generative act" should be. From this perspective, the official position of the Catholic Church can be better appreciated for its deep insight[17] as we attempt to show why it is wrong for AIH to substitute for marital sexual love.

[17] The underlying sense in the objection of the Catholic Church is that the unitive and procreative aspects of the conjugal act are united in the same single act, but the practice of obtaining sperm outside the conjugal act separates the two and rids the generative act of its profound meaning.

Why is the marital love absolutely necessary in the generation of a child? Man is a being with three dimensions: physical, psychological, and spiritual. The marital sexual love is an act with a profound intrinsic meaning, which ought to be respected in every act of human generation. Although it has a biological dimension, the meaning of the act goes beyond mere biology. In reality, the act touches the whole person in his three dimensions, which makes it qualitatively different from reproduction among animals. In the marital sexual act, the spouses give themselves to one another totally[18] and unreservedly; this occurs in a unique way that expresses their mutual love and at the same time remains open to procreation. This mutual self-giving is total only if it touches them in all three human dimensions. To withhold the gift of oneself at any of the three levels depersonalizes the act, making it something that is incomplete, perhaps defective, in the sense of not being what it should be: a mutual, total self-giving of one's whole person to one's spouse.

In procedures in which sperm is obtained outside the marital love, the unity of the couple in these three dimensions is ruptured.[19] The aspect we can ascertain empirically is the "physical union," since the other two can only be known by the spouses themselves. In obtaining sperm outside the marital act, this union is clearly excluded at a personal level. The sperm that will fertilise the woman's eggs may even be collected and stored before the day of the insemination. Moreover, their union at both the psychological and spiritual levels is doubtful in this circumstance. Even if we claim that it is possible to "rationally" establish a previous personal mental and spiritual union of the couple, it still remains difficult to see how we can establish the unity of the three dimensions in "a single act of bringing forth a child" when their personal union at the physical level is already excluded. Worse still, in IVF and its variants, the woman undergoes egg-retrieval, perhaps unconsciously, while at the same time the man struggles to produce sperm in another room. Because

[18] Cf. POPE PIUS XII, Discourse on Moral Problems of Married Life, October 29, 1951. He maintains that the conjugal act is an expression of the mutual, total self-giving of a couple to one another.

[19] This total mutual self-giving of couples in their three dimensions is possible in the marital act even though we cannot claim that it is so in every single case. However, it is impossible when their gametes are collected outside the marital act.

laparoscopy requires general anaesthesia, it is impossible to speak of the personal union of the couple—their total and mutual self-giving love in their physical, psychological, and spiritual dimensions—when one of them is unconscious. At best, even when both of them are conscious, the child naturally takes the centre stage[20] in the minds of the couple and the physician, whereas in natural conception the couple is the primary focus. Their mutual love and total self-giving is the primary focus of the marital act, even though it is completely open to a new human life that can result as both a sign and fruit of their love. In natural conception, parents do not merely make their gametes available, but they also contribute to their subsequent union by performing the act that is necessary to bring the unitive and procreative act to its finality. Thus, they are not the efficient cause, but only the necessary condition for the child, whom they do not make but rather accept unconditionally as a fruit of their total love and mutual self-giving. In view of the equal inherent dignity of all human beings, to claim otherwise is to unbalance the relationship of equality that exists between the child and its parents. In natural conception, parents collaborate in the procreative process through their "personal and intimate union," which is impossible when their gametes are obtained mechanically. In the latter case, the child does not truly result from the total union and mutual self-giving of its parents; rather, it results from the impersonal union of their gametes through the instrumentality of the physician. This way of bringing a new human being into existence wholly depersonalizes the generative process.[21] For instance, consider the image of a prisoner packaging his semen and sending it to his spouse, or the use of a dead man's stored sperm to conceive a child. How can we speak of a personal union between the woman and the dead spouse in their physical, psychological, and spiritual dimensions? On account of this fact, Callahan contends that "one of the foundations of a responsible

[20] Experience shows that couples who undergo egg-retrieval and sperm collection are often under tension. A man struggling to produce sperm is not likely to be preoccupied with the total donation of himself to his wife *vis-à-vis* a woman undergoing egg-retrieval who may even be unconscious. The immediate concern of each will more likely be the success of the treatment.

[21] Cf. D. BOHR, *Revised Catholic..., op. cit.,* p. 303.

ethics concerning sexuality is to see sexual acts as personal acts involving the whole person."[22]

To establish conception through the marital sexual love is more consistent with the dignity of the child that results from it. He then becomes the fruit and the sign of the total love and mutual self-giving of his parents. A child who results merely from the non-personal union of its parents' gametes cannot be described in this way. The critical point here is that a person's gamete is not equal to the person, whether in a qualitative or quantitative sense; it does not have a personal status that is independent of the subject from whom it is obtained.[23] No one can reasonably claim that to destroy a semen specimen or a woman's egg is tantamount to killing a human being, in spite of the fact that these are living human cells.

Even if we claim that a couple can give themselves to one another, both mentally and spiritually, in conceiving a child outside the marital act, their mutual self-giving will be partial at best. This is because these two dimensions would still be separated from the physical dimension. Although the child that is born still possesses an inherent dignity, such depersonalization of the human generative process does not correspond to respect for the dignity of human procreation. The situation is different, however, when normal sexual love is performed by the couple and ART truly assists procreation. But a child conceived through ART, even without recourse to the marital act, still has a personal dignity because, although physicians may fertilise an egg artificially, they do not create the spiritual soul, which is the life-giving principle of the body.

DONOR-CONCEPTION

DONOR-CONCEPTION AND SURROGACY

Ethical appraisal of ART should go beyond the pragmatic value and respect for the personal autonomy of competent subjects. The conscious and free action of an individual can have irreparable consequences for others with a legitimate interest, especially those who may not be in a

[22] S. CALLAHAN, The Ethical Challenge..., *op. cit.*, p. 515.

[23] The dignity of the human body is predicated on its unity with the spiritual soul. When the spiritual soul separates from it, it ceases to be a personal body.

position to consent to it. To critically evaluate the involvement of a third-party in the conception of a child, it is pertinent to see how this relates to the legitimate interests of the child, the donor, family, and society, aside from the moral agent himself.

DONOR-CONCEPTION AND ADULTERY OR RAPE

Adultery is an illicit sexual relationship between two persons, at least one of whom must be married, while rape involves having sex with another person against his or her will. From this perspective it is extremely difficult to justify the position that equates ART procedures involving donors with adultery or rape. This is not correct because adultery involves a personal sexual relationship at the physical level between the two people involved, but in donor-conception the recipient and donor often do not know each other. In like manner, in donor-conception, a woman is not forcefully inseminated with another man's sperm; rather, she freely consents to the procedure. As such, an ethical or philosophical appraisal should avoid such hasty conclusions that are intended, perhaps, to appeal to people's emotions.

DONOR-CONCEPTION AND KINSHIP

Donor-conception has the potential to create the problem of kinship. To minimize this risk, some guidelines prohibit an individual from donating semen more than 10 times. The discomfort in this area shows that something is wrong with the practice. Although it is possible to minimize the risk in developed countries with more sophisticated systems of storing and accessing information about prospective donors and patients,[24] the same will be extremely difficult to achieve in most developing countries like Nigeria, where there is no effective way to access information about the true identity of prospective donors. This makes it possible for a man to donate his semen a number of times at different fertility centres—for commercial motives or even out of sheer mischief—without being detected. Even in the developed countries, abuses cannot be totally prevented because most donors and physicians are primarily motivated by financial gain. If society permits or ignores the sale of gametes and embryos in ART, rather than demand personal responsibility for one's action in this area, it promotes (even if passively)

[24] Efficient documentation of patients' visits and the insistence on official documents to identify every patient or donor will minimize abuses in this area.

ethical egoism, according to which an action is right if it produces a good consequence relative to the agent himself. The implicit messages that arise from such a permissive attitude include "You may use what you have to get what you want" and "The end justifies the means." But the question is, What kind of society will result from following such morality? Even a prostitute will be able to justify her action on this basis, since she only uses her sexuality to earn the money she desires, perhaps for a good purpose.

DONOR-CONCEPTION AND DECEPTION

In some cultural zones in Nigeria and Africa, close relatives or family friends are preferred as donors. This means that both the couple and the donors will know the origin of the child and their own genetic connections to him. But the use of donated gametes can lead to biological and emotional imbalances among all parties involved.[25] Even if donor-conception is practised within family circles, there is no guarantee that the well-being of the child will be adequately safeguarded. In this case, some vital questions arise: How would the real biological parent feel if it turned out that the same child was being exposed to violence or unnecessary suffering by the social parent? How would the social parents react to a growing closeness between the donor(s) and the child? Considering the serious emphasis on children to further the family lineage in Africa, what will happen if the donors lose all their children in an accident and can no longer bear children? Is there a possibility that they will divulge the secret about the child's origin or even make claims about paternity? How does the situation safeguard the psycho-social well-being of the child? Such questions are truly serious in the context of African communalism. If the child is neglected or maltreated by the social parents, the donors will likely know about it and may feel responsible for it; they may come under serious temptation or emotional pressure to intervene in order to protect the child from further abuse. In making this observation about the possible outcome of such a technique in Nigeria and Africa, we

[25] The problem is more complex for the male. At least the woman who carries a pregnancy established with a gamete from another woman or an embryo from another couple can still feel connected to the child through bonding during pregnancy and in view of the emerging fact from genetics that the environment of the womb contributes genetically to the child's traits.

should also bear in mind that the legal system is not as developed in most African countries as it is in the developed countries.

Certain practices in donor-conception seem bizarre. For instance, why would a couple in search of a biological child accept embryo donation when they know that the prospective child will not be their biological child? If a genetic offspring is really the issue, their action is a contradiction that amounts to self-deceit since the child is not and can never be their biological child. Even though this may bring them some psychological and emotional relief, it may also give rise to a deep-seated psychological conflict, as they may have to live with this illusion for the rest of their lives. Upon closer inspection, such a decision indicates that some additional social factors may underlie the practice. The most likely explanation is that to conceive with a donated gamete or to gestate a donated embryo shields them from public ridicule, whereas adoption exposes their infertility. In the opinion of society, they have a biological child, even though they know within themselves that this is not true. This breeds deception and falsehood in an attempt to conceal the truth.

At a more profound level, such an attitude shows that the challenge posed by infertility needs more than a technological response. It calls for a careful re-evaluation of society's attitude towards involuntarily childless people, because neither ART nor technology in general can completely eradicate infertility in the world. It challenges society to re-appraise its values and behaviours, such as the growing tendency to evade responsibility for one's actions, the mentality that the end justifies the means, the erroneous notion that we have value because of our abilities (in this case, the ability to beget children), and the negative influence of materialism upon all levels of society and especially upon the medical field, where a human life or the psycho-social well-being of a prospective child may be at stake. Although there is nothing wrong with the desire to have one's own child, society needs to re-examine the exaggerated emphasis on biological parenthood. Considering that not everyone can have a child, even with technical assistance, a more respectful, inclusive, and supportive disposition towards involuntarily childless couples is necessary to diminish the desire to have a child at any cost, which is what underpins the deceptive practice of donor-conception.

In regard to the African emphasis on "personal immortality," it is vital to note that if personal immortality really arises from having strictly biological offspring, some of the marriages (levirate, ghost, and woman marriages) contracted to provide a child for a deceased childless man would be inconsistent with the desired goal, for the prospective child would still not be his biological child. From this perspective, it is easy to see the futility of some of the sociocultural factors that underpin the inordinate search for a biological child. It may be reasonable to ask if women are excluded from personal immortality since special marriages are not contracted on the behalf of deceased childless women to provide children for them. This objection is only intended to show that, in every culture, there are certain unchallenged beliefs and practices that need to be appraised rationally and objectively and be continually renewed in the light of objective moral truth and according to the overall identity and vocation of the human person.

DONOR-CONCEPTION AND RESPONSIBILITY

It is a scientific fact that the owners of the gametes used to establish a pregnancy are the real biological parents of the child that results. Once a person donates or sells a gamete, a bond of kinship is automatically established between the donor and the new child. This bond creates parental responsibility. To deny the relationship amounts to deceit on the part of the donor, who evades responsibility for his action by choosing anonymity. Rearing a child in a way that leads to his holistic development is an onerous task; as rational beings, we must approach the generation of a child with a conscious and free decision that takes into consideration his overall well-being. In other words, bringing a child into existence is a human act, a rational act, rather than an act of man on the biological level. While an act of man (for example, yawning) is a mere biological act that is beyond his control and therefore not subject to moral scrutiny, a human act is subject to moral evaluation because it arises from an interaction between the intellect and the will. Every human act implies a responsibility, and an ingredient that is essential to morality is the acceptance of responsibility for one's action and its consequences. By consciously and freely donating or selling his or her gamete to another individual for use in ART, the donor wishes to participate in the generation of a new human being with intrinsic dignity, who requires education, attention, care, and the affection and guidance of its parents to attain a full personal development.[26] This creates a responsibility, and he or she ought to accept it as well as the consequences and duties that the specific action generates, such as the duty to care for the child, not just as one desires, but as his inherent dignity demands.[27]

It does not seem responsible to make one's sperm, ovum, or embryo available to a total stranger, or even to a friend or relative. This shows neither respect nor adequate consideration for the welfare of the future child; it treats him like an object one leaves in a shop, not minding who buys it or how it is used. A child is certainly not an object and has a right to know his origins, which includes knowing the donor(s), considering that this information forms part of his personal identity and history and can affect his self-perception and overall well-being. Similarly, since a human being cannot be bought or owned, should the child come to discover his true origin, he has a right to reject the parenthood of the non-genetic parents, whose only claim on him is the contract that was signed following payment to the parties involved in the transaction.

Moreover, the fact that an individual or a couple desires a child at any cost does not imply that the child's welfare is their primary motive. Sometimes it is primarily a selfish motive, such as a couple's desire to boost their image in society or to claim an inheritance. In surrogacy contracts, prospective parents may reject the child if it is born with a disability. In such a case, what will be the fate of the disabled child? A child is not an object without emotions, and technical solutions to human problems should not disregard that. Peter Singer has a point in stating that we should not demand from infertile couples what we do not normally demand from those who are fertile, but this is not entirely correct because the circumstances surrounding an act and the consequences of the act also play a major role in ethical evaluation. It may not be possible to reach all the fertile couples and regulate their activities in this way, but we can at least reach the infertile ones that wish to resort to ART. In general, human authorities have a moral duty to guide and set standards that promote the good of a child and safeguard the interests

[26] This does not ignore the contributions from the community in the formation of a child, especially in the African context.

[27] Even society expects that much, which is why a parent may lose custody of the child in countries like the U.K. and the U.S. if he or she is found guilty of neglecting his or her duties to the child.

of family and society. In the case of donor-conception, if the donor is primarily interested in the welfare of the child, he or she will also be interested in the values and parental abilities of the prospective couple. But how is this possible when he or she does not even know who will use the gametes to have children? If the child suffers on account of this action, the gamete or embryo donors will be morally culpable.

SURROGACY AND WOMEN

The argument that commercial surrogacy should be prohibited because it is risky to women is very weak. Competent adults should be able to determine the level of risk they are willing to undertake in a given procedure. A more serious concern in this area is the quality of the consent given by a surrogate. There is need to determine the level of education a surrogate receives on the procedure, the physical and psychological risks involved, the availability of alternatives, and so forth. The compelling argument for the prohibition of the procedure should be the charge of "baby-selling," which threatens the future psycho-social well-being of the child.

THE INTEREST AND RIGHT OF THE CHILD

The individual at the centre of ART is the child that may result from the technique. As Keller observes, "The most important 'party,' the child, is the ultimate casualty in such a scenario. His legitimacy, inheritance rights, custody and perhaps his very life are left open to the caprices of the parties and of an unguided judiciary."[28] Below we will consider the fate of the child in some ART procedures.

THE INTEREST OF THE CHILD IN THIRD-PARTY CONCEPTION

The child's interest ought to be paramount in any decision to resort to ART. The tendency to consider primarily the desire of an infertile couple to have a child, rather than the psycho-social impact of the technique on the future child, is unacceptable. Since parents are expected to act in the best interest of their child, they should be concerned about how a child would react or fare in the future if he comes to discover that

[28] B. KELLER, "Surrogate motherhood contracts in Louisiana: To ban or to regulate?" *Louisiana Law Review 49,* (1988), p. 149; Cited in L. SCHWARTZ, *Alternatives to Infertility, op. cit.,* p. 135.

he was conceived with anonymous sperm obtained from a sperm bank, or that his genetic mother conceived him and exchanged him for money. As Kass points out, there have been cases of men who rejected or refused to support a child that was conceived through AID. In another case, a donor sued for visitation privileges to see a son who was conceived 10 years earlier with his sperm.[29] Again, what would be the psychological impact of this lawsuit on the innocent child, especially considering the publicity it may generate?

The feelings of pain, frustration, and anguish expressed by some donor-conceived children who wish to know their genetic origins cannot be ignored. Some claim that they do not find their sense of identity complete.[30] For instance, when it was disclosed to Christine Whipp, a 46-year-old grandmother, that her father "was a glass jar with a blob of sperm in it," she confessed feeling like "a freak, a fake… (saying) I don't feel I know who I am anymore."[31] There are donor-conceived children publicly trying to find their biological parents, and there are half-siblings trying to find each other through public outcry and DNA testing.[32]

At this juncture, one may ask how most couples who conceive with donated gametes or embryos handle this problem. Some parents choose not to disclose to their children the nature of their conception. Those who argue against the disclosure of such information to donor-conceived children point out that they might find it disturbing or alienating. In other words, they concur that the technique carries potential psychological and social harm for the child.

Deception is not only unfair to the child but also is inconsistent with the values of truth and honesty, whether or not the child discovers the truth. It is an abdication of parental duty and a mark of self-centredness to conceal such a vital aspect of a child's life merely to perpetuate a secret or protect a wrong choice for which one does not wish to take

---

[29] Cf. L. KASS, *Life, Liberty…,op. cit.,* p. 99.

[30] See F. SHEFIELD, "Issues of gamete donation and sex selection: A clinician's view," in D. SINGER – M. HUNTER (eds.), *Assisted Human Reproduction, op. cit.,* p. 29.

[31] D. SINGER – M. HUNTER (eds.), *Assisted Human Reproduction, op. cit.,* p. xxiii.

[32] Cf. Ibid.

responsibility. Even if we concede that the concealment is intended to protect the psychological welfare of the child, one wonders why this was not made the primary consideration from the beginning. One of the values we advocate in bioethics today is truth-telling, and the refusal to disclose the truth about the child's origin is a violation of this value. As Thevoz observes,

> If society expects the family to have an important role in shaping the moral values of children, then it ought to promote truthfulness in family life and encourage disclosure and communication about family ties, be they biological or not.[33]

Still, donor-conception has a wider implication for society. Today, with more and more couples resorting to donated gametes and embryos, some children who were conceived naturally may begin to doubt their own biological origins. If parents cannot tell their child the truth, what moral authority would they have to demand truth and honesty from the same child? Clearly, donor-conception is not in the best interests of the child and family; rather, it serves only the interests of the parents.

An accidental discovery of the truth is also a possibility. Regardless of whether a donor-conceived child finds out his origins himself or is told by his parents, such information can lead to an identity crisis and give rise to many questions: Who then is my real father or mother? Who are my real parents? What do they look like? Why did my mother conceive me to give me away in exchange for money? Do I have other siblings? Will I ever meet them? But why are some people so cruel? Why does society allow this? This situation puts the child under tremendous pressure and may negatively affect his psychological well-being, his perception of his personal worth, his perception of his biological parents, and his relationship with his family.

Deception has further implications for the child in Nigeria or sub-Saharan Africa, where a person may be considered a bastard if his genetic origins are not known. This could deny him certain family rights and expose him to intense ridicule, discrimination, and shame in the community. For a couple that conceived a baby with donated gametes or donated embryo, the problem of determining custody of the child

---

[33] J. THEVOZ, "The Right of the Child..., *op. cit.,* p. 200.

may arise in the event of a divorce. Should this happen when the child is old enough to comprehend the situation, the court case and negative publicity may harm him psychologically. In Nigerian society, where the culture is sensitive to such things as family background, this may have negative consequences for the child during pre-marriage investigations, especially if the child is a woman. Without doubt, we can say that the disadvantages of third-party conception clearly outweigh its ability to satisfy a couple's desire to have biological offspring.

A CHILD IS NOT AN OBJECT

Techniques that tend to turn the human generative process into mere production, such as IVF, ICSI, PGD for sex selection, and genetic enhancement design, demean the dignity of the child by treating it as a product. Similarly, HLA matching reduces the new child to a means to an end, whereas a child ought to be conceived for its own sake. Let us focus briefly on these techniques.

Pre-Selection of Genetic Traits: In placing undue emphasis on physical and mental traits, we fail to make a vital distinction between the substance and the accidents of the human person. Every child should be accepted and loved unconditionally as a new and unrepeatable gift. Although genetic traits are important, they are mere accidents of a human being and not his essence, meaning that we cannot predicate our acceptance of a child on them. They do not make a human being who he is; rather, it is his substance or essence that makes him who he really is: a person with intrinsic dignity. If we simply love a child for his physical and mental attributes or because he measures up to our desires, it is impossible to speak about love in the strict sense. This fact degrades the child whose worth is then reduced to "what he possesses" rather than "who he is." We do not show regard for a person's dignity if we claim that she has value because of her beauty, intelligence, or any other physical, mental, or spiritual capabilities. A person has intrinsic dignity irrespective of her peculiar traits. If our love or acceptance of a child is predicated on desirable attributes, it is totally impossible to speak of conceiving it for its own sake or of accepting and loving it unconditionally.[34] In reality, the

---

[34] There is a difference between accepting a person for his own sake and accepting him for the particular traits he possesses. In the first instance, what is loved, at least primarily, is the real person (not his qualities), but in

genetic enhancement design of a child, whenever it becomes feasible, will jeopardize the future child's psychological well-being, given that some of the problems faced by adolescents in today's society, like depression and suicide, are correlated with excessive parental control. The point is that when we design a child to meet certain subjective desires, we treat it as a means to satisfy the imagination of its parents.[35] Individuals have their preferences, and it is impossible for parents to know with certainty what the preferences of an unborn child would be later in life. In spite of their "good" intentions, their choice may turn out to be harmful if the child comes to know that they chose for her something she does not like. Further, when many parents choose particular physical characteristics for their children, these characteristics may become too common and thus less desirable in society. The practice will likely increase the tendency of parents to be overbearing towards their children, leading to serious negative consequences. As Callahan observes,

> The child who was wanted for all wrong reasons is pressured to live up to parental dreams of the optimal baby or perfect child. Outright rejection of imperfect or non-optimal babies contracted for by alternative reproductive technology is possible and should be a matter of grave concern.[36]

HLA Matching: It is the desire of good parents and society to have healthy children, just as every right-thinking person wishes to be healthy. Sickness is neither a human good nor does it promote human flourishing. As such, every effort to prevent genetic disorders and to promote a child's health is good, but the means that is used to arrive at this noble end must

---

the latter what is loved primarily is the quality he possesses, not the person himself.

[35] Some parents may prefer their girl to be skinny according to the present standard of selecting beauty pageants in the West whereas the girl may grow up to hate skinny people. On the other hand, where a child is conditioned to a large extent to have the predisposition for certain abilities according to the desire of its parents, we cannot claim that she is completely free. Every child should be guided and given an opportunity to develop her personality as much as she can rather than being predisposed genetically to a large extent to become what parents want her to be.

[36] S. CALLAHAN, "The Ethical Challenge..., *op. cit.*, p. 515.

also be good. In HLA matching, the worth of the new child is primarily predicated on its ability to satisfy a need. It is brought into existence, not for its own sake, but for that of another to whom it can be a donor. If it cannot be a match for the sick sibling, it is immediately rejected, that is, donated, destroyed, or allowed to die. In the opinion of its parents, its value is not intrinsic because it depends on what it is expected to be—a donor—rather than who it is: a human being with intrinsic dignity. That is to say, if it cannot fulfil the desire of the parents or the purpose for which it was brought into existence, it has no value. In opposition to this mentality, a child is a gift and not a commodity that we purchase or accept because of its utility or health status, which are mere accidents of his existence. It is necessary to make a distinction between the child as a gift that is beyond price and the child as a mere commodity. While the latter can be bought, owned, and used as we desire, a gift places some limits on how it ought to be used, making it wrong to bring a child into existence primarily for the sake of another, who then becomes the condition for the child's existence. As Campbell suggests, "Notions of welfare of the child should be based on the concept of the child as a gift rather than a commodity."[37]

Sex Selection: Some advocates of non-medical sex selection claim that it will guarantee a better quality of life for the child because he or she is completely wanted. If this is true in every case, some questions arise: Should the quality of life that parents desire for their children be dependent on their gender? What matters more, a child's status as a human being or its gender? Is the position that predicates a child's quality of life on its gender consistent with the perception of a child as a gift to be accepted and loved unconditionally? Is the generation of the child intended primarily to satisfy the desires of the parents or primarily for the child's own sake? These questions are crucial considering the fact that some of the techniques do not guarantee success, meaning that some couples will have to choose between procuring an abortion and giving birth to a child of the unwanted sex. Without doubt, this will erode an important parental value, namely, the willingness to love and care for every child as a unique gift.

---

[37] A. CAMPELL "Reproductive Medicine – The ethical issues in the twenty-first century," *Human Fertility 5,* (suppl): S33-S36.

The concern about overpopulation is not unreasonable considering an expected population of nine billion in 2050. But sex selection may not contribute significantly to population reduction. A more effective approach to achieve this goal is to embark on a worldwide campaign, especially in Asia and Africa, to educate people about the dangers of overpopulation. But any serious concern about the environment must be prepared to address the problem from its roots rather than blame it entirely on population growth. We cannot be blind to the other major contributors, such as the deplorable culture of consumerism and waste in technologically developed nations and among the rich, the use of technologies that damage ecosystems, and economic systems (such as capitalism) that seem to define human well-being from a materialistic standpoint. Man has a responsibility towards creation and must devise ways to protect it. If we wish to save the earth and mankind from self-destruction, we should not blame population growth; rather, we must revisit those things that encourage environmental degradation, such as the unrestrained production of goods, genetic engineering, and anthropocentric attitudes towards nature.[38,39]

The desire to have children of both sexes is good if it is an implicit appreciation of the value of both sexes and if the couple does not already have children of both sexes.[40] But, even if the intention is good and the circumstance poses no moral problem, the means that is used to satisfy the desire is still very important. To resort to techniques that substitute marital love and discard embryos of the unwanted sex is to employ a morally wrong means to attain a good end. In human generation, a couple is not supposed to "make" a child according to their own desires and preferences. Instead, they ought to accept and love unconditionally whatever child results as a fruit of their love.

Emerging trends in sex selection are deeply rooted in producer and consumer culture, unhealthy rivalry among individuals and nations,

---

[38] Cf. J. MARTIN-SCHRAMM – R. STIVERS, *Christian Environmental Ethics…, op. cit.,* pp. 10-18.

[39] Cf. POPE BENEDICT XVI, 'If You Want to Cultivate Peace, Protect Creation,' Message for the World Day of Peace, January 1, 2010, n. 12.

[40] Every other ulterior motive for desiring a child of a particular sex, such as to inherit a property cannot be justified.

and the desire to seek undue advantage over others. These attitudes will further erode the well-established values that have long sustained family and society. Rather than choose a child's traits to improve her competitive ability in society, a more enduring solution is to create a more humane society that values respect for persons, love, equal opportunity, and care of the poor and less-privileged. There is need to focus more attention on projects that promote the person and that can usher in a new world order characterized by love, justice, and peace[41] instead of egoism.

COMMERCIALIZATION IN ART AND HUMAN DIGNITY

Human beings have intrinsic dignity, which implies that they are always ends in themselves and never only means. In many ART procedures, human embryos and gametes are sold as products and surrogate wombs are hired. This does not respect human dignity because it treats humans—actual or "potential"—or parts of them as mere objects.

In third-party conception with sold gametes and embryos, we cannot speak of "donation" or a "donor" in the strict sense; rather, it is the commercialization of human persons and gametes.[42] More appropriate terminology would be sperm, egg, or embryo "vendors" and womb "hirers," rather than donors, because they deliver their gametes and rent their wombs in exchange for a specified sum of money. Although some ART practitioners claim that the so-called donors are only compensated for their services, in practice it is extremely difficult to draw a line between compensation and real payment, especially if we consider the serious risks that egg-donors and surrogate mothers undertake in IVF egg-retrieval procedures and surrogacy contracts. Even though there are some altruistic donors, studies indicate that the primary motive of the vast majority of so-called donors is monetary compensation. Since the embryo is biologically a human being from fertilisation with an active potential to become an adult human being, to treat it as a product constitutes a flagrant attack on its dignity. On the other hand, human gametes are connected with the transmission of human life, which has an intrinsic value. To sell a gamete from which a child will result is inconsistent with

---

[41] The technique itself is likely to eliminate justice since only the rich will be able to afford it or the more important genes, giving them and their children undue advantage over others.

[42] Cf. SHENFIELD, "Issues of gamete donations..., *op. cit.,* p. 29.

the dignity of that child. It does not seem that anyone would be proud to say, "I am the fruit of a $50 sperm, $1000 egg, and $10,000 hired womb." It seems to suggest that a child can be purchased for about $11,050, meaning that he is not beyond a price. Such a practice does not promote the common good in view of its foreseeable implications for kinship and the future child, who deserves the protection of society as one of its defenceless members. We ought to be concerned about the overall implications of our choices in the area of human generation, not just for ourselves, but also for those who are directly affected by them and for the common good of the society to which we belong.

The basic principle underlying the sale of gametes and embryos raises a serious ethical problem. As we have repeatedly stated, a person may never be used as a mere instrument. Affirming the fundamental worth of every individual, Kant asserts that we must "act so as to treat humanity, whether in one's own person or in that of another, in every case as an end and never only as a means."[43] The sale of embryos and human gametes conflicts with such a principle. Physicians tend to treat egg vendors as machines that manufacture eggs in spite of the serious health risks involved in the egg-retrieval procedure. For them, her human value consists in her ability to produce good eggs; they have little or no concern for her overall well-being and for her primary motivation, which may be abject poverty. To sell one's gamete as a means of survival may be psychologically damaging to the vendor, who may see the rich couple and the physician as "using" her for their own selfish ends. Medicine ought to look at the true good of a patient and seek to promote her overall health at the three dimensions—physical, mental, and spiritual. The risk that the egg vendor undergoes in IVF to satisfy "a couple's desire" to have a child is disproportionate.[44] By nature, the egg vendor's inherent dignity

---

[43] IMMANUEL KANT, *Grounding for the Metaphysics of Morals,* Translated by J. ELLINGTON, Hackett, Indianapolis 1981; Also see S. FROST, *Basic Teachings of the Great Philosophers,* First Anchor Books Edition, New York 1989, p. 95.

[44] Most women who undergo egg-retrieval do so primarily, if not solely, for money perhaps due to poverty or financial crisis related to basic sustenance, family welfare or the need to finance one's studies. The primary interest of the physician or the contracting couple is not to reduce their burden or to offer them meaningful financial assistance, but to obtain their eggs for their

places her beyond price, but she willingly accepts a price the same way a prostitute violates her self-worth for the purpose of making money. Finally, the couple who desperately desires a child is primarily concerned about the eggs rather than the overall well-being of the vendor as a person with dignity. Their main interest is not in the health implications of the egg-retrieval procedure or the emotional impact of giving up her genetic child. For them, she seems like a thing that can be used. Moreover, it is difficult to establish that the primary interest of the contracting couple in surrogacy arrangements is the child for its own sake, considering that they may reject the child if it is born with a disability.[45]

Such a line of reasoning suggests that a human being can be a means to an end, which again reflects the dominant social mentality that the end justifies the means. To treat others solely as a means to realize one's own end, with no consideration for their intrinsic worth and the consequences of one's action for them, is not only egoistic but also constitutes a blatant attack on the dignity of the human person. On this account, we must insist that every contact with the human embryo and other human beings (gamete vendor, surrogate mother, and similar) should reflect the profound respect, care, and protection that correspond to their intrinsic dignity.

own ends. This is very clear in the case of a surrogate mother who may not be paid fully if she has a still-birth, which may not be due to any fault of hers.

45 The point is that if the child (and not the interest of the couple) is the main concern in ART and it is wanted primarily for its own sake, then how do we explain the fact of its rejection in the event of a serious disability? This merely shows that, in some cases at least, the prospective parents are primarily after their own interest rather than the child itself. That is to say, if it is truly wanted and loved for its own sake, they will accept it no matter the disability.

RESPECT FOR HUMAN LIFE

The issue of abortion remains controversial. The Nigerian constitution, as well as those of some other countries, does not permit it. To approve any ART procedure that involves the destruction of embryos provides a tacit approval of abortion. With regard to multifoetal reduction of embryos in ART procedures, advocates of the techniques argue that it is not an abortion because the intention is to allow pregnancy to continue. Taken on its own, an indirect abortion to save the lives of some of the embryos and their mother may be covered by the principle of double effect if the couple did not freely create or foresee the situation. But their conscious and deliberate choice to resort to IVF or its variants is not covered by this principle. Since they freely consented to the laboratory creation and transfer of multiple embryos, they are morally culpable because in such a procedure the problem of multiple pregnancy and selective abortion is foreseeable. Moreover, this is explained to couples prior to initiating the treatment cycle and repeated prior to the transfer of the embryos.

MORAL STATUS OF THE HUMAN EMBRYO

The most serious objection to prenatal diagnosis with selective abortion, PGD, and IVF and its variants is the constant destruction of viable human embryos. The arguments and counter-arguments on this topic bring to the fore the issue of the moral status of the human embryo.[46] The debate in this area is very complex and has polarized the opinions of philosophers, bioethicists, and even theologians. Without repeating the positions of the different theorists, it is necessary to summarize the salient points they contain.

Different theorists define human personhood variously and locate it in various stages of the development of the human life. In general, their positions can be categorized under two main opposing trends: personalism and personism.[47] The personalist theory proposes an ontological view of a person and maintains an identity between a "human being" and a "human person" both "at the conceptual and the practical levels."[48] In this view, all human beings are persons ontologically, while animals are excluded from personal status. Moreover, a being is a person in virtue of his rational nature and not because he is capable of fulfilling certain functions. Human personhood begins at conception. Following fertilisation in which the sperm penetrates the ovum, the fusion of their pronuclei, and the mixing of the maternal and the paternal chromosomes, a zygote is formed, marking the beginning of a human being with a unique genetic code. It has an inherent dignity and possesses a morally significant life, which cannot be violated irrespective of the stage and quality of its development. For proponents of this view, fertilisation is the only substantial and qualitative change that occurs in the process of human

---

[46] See P. NWAEZEAPU, *When Does a Human Person Begin? Moral Status of the Embryo and Technology*, LEBERIT S.R.L. Press, Rome 2007, pp. 25-84.

[47] See L. PALAZZANI, "The Meanings of the Philosophical Concept of Person and Their Implications in the Current Debate on the Status of the Human Embryo," in J. CORREA - E. SGRECCIA (eds.), *Identity and Statute of the Human Embryo,* Proceedings of the Third Assembly of the Pontifical Academy for Life, Vatican City February 14-16, 1997, 74-95, p. 82.

[48] Cf. L. PALAZZANI, "The Concept of Person…, "The Concept of Person Between Bioethics and Biolaw," Being a Lecture at the Faculty of Bioethics, Pontifica Universita Regina Apostolorum, Rome, Oct. 2004, p. 3.

generation. All other changes in the later stages of embryonic development are merely quantitative. After the constitution of the zygote, the development of the new human being follows a process that is marked by biological unity, coordination, continuity, and graduality.[49]

On the other hand, the personist theories tend to assign personhood to various stages in the development of the embryo. Some theorists defend the bodily continuity theories, and others support the psychological or mental continuity theories. Their positions are discussed briefly below.

The Moment of Implantation: Some theorists propose the moment of implantation of the embryo in the mother's uterus as the significant marker of the beginning of personhood or as the minimal condition for it.[50] The basis of this argument is the philosophical theory that stresses the importance of "relationship" as a necessary component of any definition of person. Since it is at the moment of implantation that the "first primary physiological relationship" is established between the embryo and its mother, they argue that prior to this it is not a person.[51] In their view, the early embryo cannot survive or develop on its own because it requires the appropriate environment provided by the mother.[52]

14th Day Post-Fertilisation Theory: Some theorists attribute personhood after the 14th day post-fertilisation. They argue that we cannot recognize a personal status to the human embryo before it develops definitive characteristics with the appearance of the primitive streak or *gastrulation* in the third week of gestation. The main reasons that underpin this position include the *totipotency* of the embryonic cells up to the eight-cell stage and the possibility of monozygotic twinning and recombination

---

[49] Cf. D. BOHR, *Revised Catholic Moral Tradition,* Our Sunday Visitor Publishing Division, Our Sunday Visitor Inc., Huntington, Indiana 1999, p. 295.

[50] See E. SGRECCIA, *Manuale di Bioetica I, Fondamenti ed Etice Biomedica,* Vita e Pensiero, Milano 1999, p. 448.

[51] See L. PALAZZANI, The Meanings of the Philosophical..., *op. cit.,* p. 84.

[52] See M. TIGHE, "The Pandora's Box of Social and Moral Problems," in H. KUHSE - P. SINGER (eds.), *Bioethics: An Anthology,* Blackwell Publisher Ltd., Oxford 1999, p. 92; Also see L. PALAZZANI, "The Meanings of the Philosophical..., *op. cit.,* p. 84.

until the 14th day after fertilisation. Today, this appears to be the strongest objection to the attribution of personhood at fertilisation.

Viability of the Foetus: The human foetus can survive outside its mother's womb before birth. As a result, some theorists place the significant marker of personhood at the point of viability of the embryo understood as the point of gestation when the foetus is capable of surviving outside the mother's womb with the help of medicine and technology. This is what the U.S. Supreme Court in *Roe v. Wade* considered to be the most compelling indicator of the presence of a person in the mother.[53] The point of viability may be reached by 22 weeks[54] or even earlier.

Foetal Movement and Quickening Argument: Scientists can use ultrasound to detect the movement of the embryo in the womb at seven to eight weeks of pregnancy,[55] while quickening occurs at 16 to 20 weeks. Some theorists consider quickening—the first movement of the foetus *in utero*—to be a significant indicator of the presence of a human being who deserves to be accorded a full or at least a partial recognition of the personal status. The assumption that underpins this position is that the foetus acquires a personal status only when it acquires a separate existence independent of the mother, which occurs when it begins to generate its own movement. Hence, proponents argue that prior to this time it is only part of the mother with no right to life and after this time it has a right to life.[56]

Sentience—Moment of the Formation of the CNS: Some theorists claim that for a being to qualify for personhood it must possess the desire to live and capability of being harmed. Since this is impossible without sensitivity, they see sentience, understood as the capacity to feel

---

[53] See Roe v. Wade, 410 U.S. 113 (1997). Cited in R. EVANS, "The Moral Status of Embryos," in KILNER, J. - CUNNINGHAM, P. - HAGER, D. (eds.), *The Reproduction Revolution,* Wm. B. Eerdmans Publishing Co., Cambridge, UK 2000, p. 67.

[54] See P. SINGER, *Rethinking Life and Death,* Oxford University Press, Oxford 1994, pp. 101-102.

[55] Ibid., pp. 25-27.

[56] See Ibid., pp. 25-26.

pain and pleasure, as the significant marker for ascribing personhood.[57] This implies that the human embryo cannot acquire a personal status until it acquires sentience. In this view, although the embryo has a potential to become a person and experience pain and pleasure in the future, what really matters is current sentience.[58] This position is defended by utilitarian theorists who identify the beginning of the person with the moment of the formation of the CNS.[59] Even though there is no scientific certainty as to the exact time it begins, it is clear that human sentience requires a brain.[60] Still, they ascribe personal status not only on the basis of being sentient but also on being in an existential condition to maximize pleasure and minimize pain for oneself and others.

Moment of the Formation of the Cerebral Cortex: Some theorists locate the dividing line between person and non-person at the beginning of brain function, without which a being is incapable of a conscious experience.[61] This rationalistic view of the person considers reason or the capacity for its exercise indispensable to the definition of a person. Proponents attribute personal status at the moment of the formation of the cerebral cortex, which is necessary for the exercise of rationality. But they maintain that we should at least be able to verify the "presence of neuro-physiological conditions" that would guarantee its development.[62]

---

[57] See R. ROWLAND, "Human Embryo Research: A Global Social Experiment," in H. KUHSE – P. SINGER (eds.), *Bioethics: An Anthology…, op. cit.,* p. 96.

[58] See P. SINGER, *Rethinking Life and Death, op. cit.,* p. 200.

[59] See C. KACZOR, *The Edge of Life: Human Dignity and Contemporary Bioethics,* Springer Publication, Dordrecht, The Netherlands 2005, p. 29; Also see L. PALAZZANI, "The Meanings of the Philosophical…, *op. cit.,* p. 85; Also see J. SMART, "Utilitarianism," in P. EDWARDS (ed.). *The Encyclopedia of Philosophy, Vol. 7,* Macmillan Publishing Co. Inc. & The Free Press New York 1967, p. 207.

[60] See C. KACZOR, *The Edge of Life, op. cit.,* pp. 29-30. Also see J. FEINBERG – P. FEINBERG, *Ethics for a Brave New World,* Crossway Books, Wheaton, Ill. 1993, pp. 53-55. Cited in R. EVANS, "The Moral Status of Embryos…, *op. cit.,* p. 66.

[61] Cf. F. BECKWITH, "Defending Abortion Philosophically: A Review of David Boonin's A Defence of Abortion," *Journal of Medicine and Philosophy 31,* 2006, p. 185. Without consciousness a being has no desires.

[62] Ibid.

Moment of the Acquisition of Self Consciousness: Some theorists define personhood in terms of the psychological capacities a being possesses, such as rationality, self-awareness, and sociability.[63] Making a distinction between "human being" and "person," they insist that personhood comprises both human and nonhuman animals. In this view, while some human beings (such as the embryos) are not yet persons and other human beings (such as permanent comatose patients) have ceased to be persons, some animals that possess awareness are persons. David DeGrazia ascribes personhood to some linguistically trained apes and dolphins that show some evidence of moral agency in their actions and exhibit bodily self-awareness or traits of sociability. This position implies that what really counts is an empirically verifiable ability to demonstrate the use of reason.[64] Others emphasize the capacity for moral agency, which involves the ability to understand, evaluate, will, make free moral decisions, act in a morally autonomous way (that is, on the basis of moral reasoning and judgment), and take moral responsibility for one's actions.[65]

In spite of the different views on the embryo's status as a person, it is clear that the human embryo deserves profound respect. The position that reduces the human embryo to "pre-embryo," insisting it can be used for research prior to the 14th day post-fertilisation, does not foster adequate respect for it by treating it as a means to an end. Respect implies some measure of protection from harm and abuse. Considering that many of such embryos will be eventually destroyed, an important question arises: Does the destruction of a human embryo correspond to respect for it?

---

[63] See D. DEGRAZIA, "On the Question of Personhood Beyond Homo Sapiens," in P. SINGER (ed.), *In Defense of Animals, The Second Wave,* Blackwell Publishing Ltd., Oxford 2006, p. 41.

[64] See M. TUNKER-KENNY, "The Moral Status of the Embryo…, *op. cit.,* p. 69.

[65] Ibid., pp. 81-82; ID., "Viability and the Use of the Fetus," in W. BONDESON – H. ENGELHARDT *et al.* (eds.), *Abortion and the Status of the Fetus,* D. Reidel Publishing Company, Dordrecht, Holland 1983, p. 185; Also see B. STEINBOCK, *Life Before Birth,* Oxford University Press, Oxford New York 1992, p. 54.

Some claim that a developing human embryo can become a *hydatidiform mole* instead of a human being,[66] but this has been refuted. Ammer describes a hydatidiform mole as "an abnormal development of embryonic tissue (specifically the placenta) resulting in the formation of a grapelike cluster instead of a foetus. It is distinguished from a normal pregnancy in the uterus and grows far more rapidly."[67] From this definition, it is obvious that a hydatidiform mole is an abnormal product that arises from a defective fertilisation. It may look like an embryo and its growth may resemble that of an embryo, but clearly it is not an embryo. It was never one from the beginning and could never become one. This is why it ends up as that which it actually was from the outset. According to Grisez as cited by Lee,

> A hydatidiform mole does not have, and never did have, the epigenetic primordia of a human body with the capacities of a mature human (at least some intellectual act). Rather the hydatidiform mole has within itself something of which predetermines it to develop only into unorganized tissues.[68]

This point can also be inferred from the clarification made by William Hurlbut, Robert George, and Markus Grompe regarding altered nuclear transfer (ANT) in the stem cell debate. As they point out, both in natural conception and in ART, we can never have a living whole organism or human embryo if all the essential elements for self-development are not present in the organism. These include the necessary chromosomal complement and the cytoplasmic factors, which are crucial

---

[66] Cf. R. BENNETT - C. ERIN *et al.*, "Bioethics, Genethics and Medical Ethics," in N. BUNNIN – E. TSUI-JAMES (eds.), *The Blackwell Companion to Philosophy, Second Edition,* Blackwell Publishing Ltd., Malden, MA 2003, p. 506.

[67] C. AMMER, *The New A to Z of Women's Health, Fifth Edition,* Checkmark Books, New York 2003, p. 201.

[68] G. GRISEZ, "When Do People Begin?" Proceedings of the American Catholic Philosophical Association 63 (1990): 27-47. Cited in P. LEE, *Abortion and Unborn Human Life*, The Catholic University of America Press, Washington, D. C. 1996, p. 103.

for "the proper pattern and sequence of gene expression."[69] Although some "aberrant forms" arising from failures of fertilisation may have the capability to form structures that look like an embryo, they would still not be embryos because they lack the normal capacity of an embryo for "self-integration and self-directed development towards organismal maturity."[70] Stressing this point, they maintain the following:

> Even an egg without a nucleus can undergo a series of cell division when it is artificially activated, yet it is clearly not an embryo—or an organism at all. The messenger RNA for protein synthesis that drives these early cell divisions is generated during the maturation of the egg and then activated after. Like a spinning top, the cells have a certain biological momentum that propels a partial and unorganized trajectory of development, but unlike an embryo, they are not adequately constituted to establish the dynamic molecular interactions that characterize a coherent and self-regulating organism.... Biomedical science has never considered these growths to be embryonic human beings, nor have defenders of the dignity of embryonic human life in debates about abortion or embryo-destructive research. Everyone acknowledges that they are not organisms, but tumors; yet they generate cells with the functional characteristics of embryonic stem cells.[71]

The whole point here is that in this debate on the moral status of the human embryo, there is need to draw a clear line between what is truly an embryo and what merely has an appearance of an embryo and is erroneously viewed as one. Hydatidiform moles or tumours are not embryos or persons and never will be because they lack essential developmental elements. With this clarification it is evident that a real embryo cannot

---

[69] W. HURLBUT - R. GEORGE - M. GROMPE, "Seeking Consensus: A Clarification and Defense of Altered Nuclear Transfer," in *The Hasting Center Report, Vol. 36. No.5,* September – October 2006, p. 43.

[70] Ibid.

[71] Ibid.

become a tumour, a view that is supported by Hurlbut, George, and Grompe. Concurring within Hyun and Jung, they maintain,

> We do not, as Hyun and Jung suggest, develop "into members of the human species." No living being, by self-directed development, can become anything other than what it already essentially is; we do not know first come to be then become human beings. We begin as embryonic human beings and develop from the embryonic into and through the fetal, infant, child and adolescent stages, and ultimately into adulthood, without changing from one natural kind of being into another.[72]

The inability to detect the fundamental difference between "a real zygote" and "what is thought to be a zygote" at the early stage of embryonic development only shows the limitation of science and technology at this time in history. But even if the slightest possibility exists that a developing human embryo can become a hydatidiform mole, it will still be true that, following fertilisation, no one can determine with absolute certainty which embryos will end up as hydatidiform moles. Thus, if a zygote is constituted as a living organism of the human species at the end of the fertilisation process, a hydatidiform mole resulting from a mishap during fertilisation can never be a "zygote" in the first place, even though it could be mistaken for one. A more consistent position is to exercise restraint in favour of the "possibility" of the presence of a personal life. In this case, prudence would still require that we give the benefit of the doubt to life.

In actuality, the truth about the real status of the embryo cannot depend solely on science. The biological view of man is that of an organic machine, but the human person is not merely biological—he is also spiritual. Biology only tells us that the human embryo is a living organism that belongs to the human species. The evidence of biology is crucial and should in fact be the starting point in any discourse on the moral status of the embryo; nonetheless, biology alone cannot give us a satisfactory picture of man in his totality as an incarnate spirit, and it cannot tell us whether the developing organism of the human species is a person or not.

[72] Ibid., p. 47.

To complement the findings of biology, there is need for a philosophical reflection on the status of the embryo, which should be carried out within the framework of the whole identity of man. With regard to the assertion that the embryo cannot be a person until the primitive streak is formed, we emphasize that to limit our search for the truth about the embryo to biology is to make science an absolute. But is it really an absolute?

The history of the development of medical science indicates that science is never absolute. From an appraisal of that history, we come to understand that scientific medical knowledge is neither static nor absolute. In the past, there were certain scientific theories that were held to be absolutely correct and authoritative. These theories held sway over the vast majority of people and physicians in a particular period, only to be debunked in later periods. We can cite the example of Galeno (130–200), a practitioner and teacher of medicine who was regarded as the ultimate authority in anatomy and physiology until the sixteenth century. Medieval scholars believed that it was impossible to progress in knowledge beyond him, yet, during the Renaissance, Andreas Vesalius (1514–1564) developed scientific anatomy and published an authoritative book on the subject, making the startling revelation that the anatomical work of Galeno did not actually refer to man, but to animals.[73]

Another example is the history of the understanding of death. For centuries, the heart was thought to be the central organ of the human body. Because circulation and respiration were seen as the vital signs, death came to be defined according to the heart and lungs criteria, that is, the cessation of circulation and respiration.[74] These traditional criteria for determining the occurrence of death were contradicted by the invention of respirators and life-support machines that can conceal the vital signs of spontaneous breathing and heartbeat.[75] In response to this new situation, it became necessary to propose a new definition of death. Today, we know that the brain, and not the heart, is the central organ of the body; it is the "organ that integrates all other organ systems and is the basis for

[73] L. SPEROFF – R. GLASS – N. KASE, *Clinical Gynecologic Endocrinology…, op. cit.*, pp. 107-108.

[74] T. SHANNON, *An Introduction to Bioethics, op. cit.*, p. 79.

[75] Ibid., pp. 78-80.

the person's social presence in the world."[76] This constitutes a significant shift in scientific knowledge with the brain emerging as the new locus of death,[77] though it does not reject the traditional criteria of heart and lungs. These examples only serve to show that science is inexact, neither static nor absolute. As Robert Colombo maintains, "Biology is not an exact science. What we know now will be implemented and perfected by what we shall know later."[78]

This dynamic and inexact nature of science is crucial to our discourse on the moral status of the human embryo. Today, many authors who subscribe to the position of the Warnock Committee argue that the developing human embryo is not an ontological individual prior to the appearance of the primitive streak, when twinning is excluded. But this position fails to take the dynamic nature of science into adequate account. Perhaps scientific knowledge and the tools at our disposal can only determine the "physical" individuality of the embryo after the formation of the primitive streak—they cannot explain with certainty what gives rise to monozygotic twinning or determine whether it is really a division, a separation, or a duplication. Future advances in science and technology may come to establish the individuality of the human embryo before the 14th day after fertilisation—maybe the sixth, fifth, or third day, or even at syngamy.

A careful examination of the beginning of the person shows that only one significant and substantial change occurs. This takes place when the sex cells from the male and the female fuse together and give rise to a new entity known as a zygote, which is different from the life of the mother and father.[79] Apart from this single substantial change, every

---

[76] Ibid., p. 80.

[77] The brain is the new locus of death in the scientific definition, but since the human being is a unity of body and soul, it is reductive to define death solely in a biological sense.

[78] R. COLOMBO, "The Identity of the Human Embryo," in G. MIRANDA (ed.), *The Stem Cell Dilemma For the Good of all Human Beings?* Guile Foundation Press, Rome 2002, p. 79.

[79] N. FORD, *When Did I Begin? op. cit.*, p. 103. Here, Ford explains that fertilisation is not a momentary event but a process that may last for about 24 hours. It begins with the first contact of the sperm with the plasma membrane of the secondary oocyte (ovum) and ends with the mixing of the maternal

step in the course of the development of the human embryo is gradual, continuous, coordinated, and irreversible. Colombo is clear on this when he affirms the following:

> Provided that the required natural conditions are available—temperature, oxygen, nutrients, implantation opportunities—and the embryo is exempt from major genetic or somatic defects, it will develop into normal organism proceeding through the stages of fetus, new born and so on. Therefore, the embryo is naturally committed to become a fully developed organism in itself. Since an embryo generated by the fusion of two sex cells is genetically different from both parental organisms, it is a new organism.[80]

Colombo maintains further that the embryo is a living entity endowed with all the natural characteristics of a human person. At the one-cell stage, it already has its own DNA, protein, and cellular metabolism. The organization of the cells occurs early in its development, and it can respond to both physical and chemical stimuli.[81] Hence, the early human embryo cannot be said to be a cell, a cluster of cells, a tissue, or an organ, because none of these has the natural ability to give rise to a whole organism.[82] On the other hand, each of the totipotent cells of the embryo at the eight-cell stage can produce a human person if it is isolated and given appropriate conditions for development.

If the human embryo is not a person until after the 14th day following conception, how do we justify the substantial change from "nonperson" prior to this time to "person" afterwards? As Palazzani rightly remarks, such a "qualitative leap, a change of nature" from "non person" to "person" is difficult to explain or justify from simple logic or philosophy.[83] As experience testifies, a thing, a plant, or an animal cannot

---

and paternal chromosomes (syngamy) to constitute the zygote, which refers to the product of conception for a few days or even a fourth-night.

80 R. COLOMBO, "The Identity of the Human Embryo..., *op. cit.*, pp. 77-78.

81 Ibid., p. 77.

82 Ibid.

83 Cf. L. PALAZZANI, "The Meanings of the Philosophical...," *op. cit.*, p. 187.

metamorphose into a human being. Thus, if personhood begins about the 14th day post-fertilisation, what is the embryo prior to this time? Is it an object? Is it a plant? Is it an animal? If it is a human being, destroying it is tantamount to destroying a human subject.[84] If it is an object or a plant or an animal, the qualitative change after the 14th day that makes it a human subject is difficult to defend. If we say it is neither an object nor a plant nor an animal nor a person, then what exactly is it?

To avoid this dilemma, some who deny the personhood of the early human embryo have introduced the term "pre-embryo," which suggests that the developing human organism "becomes" an embryo only after the 14th day of gestation. The term "pre-embryo," suggested by McLaren[85] and others, has been criticized as unscientific dishonesty that obscures the truth about early human life. As O'Rahilly asserts,

> The term "pre-embryo" is not used here for the following reasons.... It may convey the erroneous idea that a new human organism is formed at only some considerable time after fertilisation... [and] it was introduced in 1986 largely for public policy reasons.[86]

To expose the policy reason that underlies this invention, Saunders cites Lee Silver, a professor of biology and advocate for all the new technologies. Silver states,

> I'll let you in on a secret. The term pre-embryo has been embraced whole heartedly by IVF practitioners for reasons that are political, not scientific. The new term is used to provide the illusion that there is something profoundly different between a six-day old embryo and a 16-day old embryo. The term is useful in a political arena—where decisions are made about whether to

[84] This view implies that every human being is a person ontologically.

[85] A. MCLAREN, "Prelude to Embryogenesis," in THE CIBA FOUNDATION, *Human Embryo Research: Yes or No?* London 1986, pp. 5-23. Cited in E. SGRECCIA, *Manuale di Bioetica I…, op. cit.*, p. 448.

[86] R. O'RAHILLY – F. MULLER, *Human Embryology and Teratology, 3rd Edition,* Wiley-Liss, New York 2001, p. 88; Cited in W. SAUNDERS, "The Human Embryo in Debate," in C. COLSON – N. CAMERON (eds.), *Human Dignity in Biotech Century, op. cit.*, p. 128.

> allow early embryo experimentation—as well as in the confines of a doctor's office where it can be used to allay moral concerns that might be expressed by IVF patients.[87]

Saunders argues that the term "pre-embryo" was coined and used mainly, if not exclusively, "to blur or conceal the scientific truth about human beginning, to bolster support for ART and obtain funds for research on human embryos."[88] Even Ford, an outspoken opponent of immediate animation, rejects the term. Although he does not accept that the human embryo is a person from fertilisation, he contends that it would be wrong to describe it as pre-embryo; he finds the term "pro-embryo" more appropriate.[89] In response, we need to stress that if the human embryo is not a human person ontologically from the outset, then it can never metamorphose into a human person. As Saunders states, "It will grow and develop and change its appearance, but it will never undergo a change in its basic nature. It will never grow up to be a cow or a fish. It is a human being—its nature is determined—from the first moment of its existence."[90] During the course of the development of the human being, the only substantial or qualitative change that occurs is fertilisation. On account of this, the term "pre-embryo" is confusing and extremely misleading and needs to be clarified and reappraised philosophically. Proponents of the term and all who claim that the early human embryo is not a person need to specify what it really is: a thing, a plant, or an animal?

Many renowned embryologists point to fertilisation as the crucial marker of the human beginning. Chief among these are Moore and Persuad, who assert that "human development is a continuous process that begins when an oocyte (ovum) from a female is fertilized by a sperm (spermatozoon) from a male.... A zygote is the beginning of a

---

[87] L. SILVER, *Remaking Edem: Cloning and Beyond in a Brave New World,* Avon, New York 1997, p. 39; Cited in W. SAUNDERS, "The Human Embryo in Debate..., *op. cit.,* p. 128.

[88] W. SAUNDERS, "The Human Embryo in Debate..., *op. cit.,* p. 128.

[89] N. FORD, *The Prenatal Person, op. cit.,* p. 67.

[90] W. SAUNDERS, "The Human Embryo in Debate..., *op. cit.,* p. 124.

new human being (i.e., an embryo)."[91] Elsewhere they add, "This highly specialized, totipotent cell (i.e., the zygote) marked the beginning of each of us as a unique individual."[92] Hamilton and Mossman give the following evidence in favour of fertilisation:

> Bisexual reproduction is characteristic of all vertebrates, and gametogenesis (the production of germ cells) is the first phase. The next phase, the beginning of the development of a new individual, is the fusion of two germ cells (gametes) of different nature; one, the spermatozoon from the male parent; the other, the ovum from the female parent. The result of this fusion is the formation of the first cell of the new individual, the zygote.[93]

Some theorists argue that we cannot attribute a personal status to the human embryo from fertilisation merely on the basis of its potential. As Singer asserts, the sperm or egg could also be said to have the same potential for a new human life.[94] This position ignores certain scientific facts on this issue. Biology tells us that following fertilisation a new organism with the 46 chromosomes of a human being is constituted. Given an appropriate environment, it will develop gradually into a child guided by its own genetic code. There is no other qualitative change in the entire process of human generation either before or after fertilisation, but the same cannot be said about the sperm or the ovum. Although these gametes are living human cells, they do not have an active potential to become a person. At best, they have a passive potential[95] until they

---

[91] K. MOORE – T. PERSUAD, *The Developing Human, op. cit.*, p. 2.

[92] K. MOORE – T. PERSUAD, *The Developing Human: Clinically Oriented Embryology, 6th Edition*, W. B. Saunders, Philadelphia, 1988, p. 18; Cited in W. SAUNDERS, "The Human Embryo in Debate," in C. COLSON – N. CAMERON (eds.), *Human Dignity in Biotech Century, op. cit.*, p. 127. The other references to these authors are to the seventh edition.

[93] W. HAMILTON – H. MOSSMAN, *Human Embryology, 4th Edition,* Heffer, Cambridge 1972, p. 14. Cited in N. FORD, *When Did I Begin? op. cit.*, p. 116.

[94] P. SINGER, *Rethinking Life and Death, op. cit.*, pp. 98-99.

[95] We cannot equate the potentiality of the human embryo with that of the sperm or egg because neither of them has the active potential to develop itself

fuse to constitute a zygote. In addition, neither the sperm nor the egg is the same "continuing" or "identical" being with the new zygote that is constituted following their fusion. The zygote, however, maintains its identity throughout the various stages of its development. In contrast to the sperm and egg, which need to undergo a qualitative change to "become" a new human organism, only quantitative changes (that is, increases in tissues and the development of necessary organs) take place in the embryo until the death of the new human being that results from it. To put it differently, the embryo is a human organism with an active potential to realize its determinate form as an adult human being. Perhaps the clarification made by Stephen Buckle can shed more light on this. According to him, we can understand potentiality in two distinct ways: potential to "become" or to "produce." When X has the potential to become Y, there is continuity of identity, meaning that X can equally claim the rights and privileges of Y as in the case of the embryo and the adult human being that it becomes. By contrast, if X is only a necessary component for producing Y, then no continuity of identity is maintained between it and Y as in the case of the sperm or the ovum taken individually and the zygote that results from their fusion. In this case, the rights of Y cannot be attributed to X.[96] In other words, X (the sperm or the ovum taken individually) will never be Y, but only a part of Y. On the other hand, the difference between the zygote and the adult human being that it becomes is not one of "quality" but of time.[97] Buckle's distinction leads Evans to the following conclusion:

> This conclusion helps to explain why ovum and semen do not have the same moral status as the fertilized egg. Whereas the ovum and semen have the potential of producing a human being (should a sperm penetrate

---

into a human being or a zygote nor satisfies the meta-biological criteria for individuality.

[96] S. BUCKLE, "Arguing from Potential," *Bioethics 2,* 1988: 227-253. Cited in R. EVANS, "The Moral Status of Embryos..., pp. 65-66; Also see C. STRONG, *Ethics in Reproductive and Perinatal Medicine..., op. cit.,* pp. 45-46.

[97] S. BUCKLE, "Arguing from Potential," *Bioethics 2,* 1988: 227-25; Cited in R. EVANS, "The Moral Status of Embryos..., pp. 65-66.

> and begin fertilizing the ovum), a fertilized ovum is becoming a human being. This distinction permits the destruction of ovum and sperm, but not the fertilized ovum. The fertilized ovum maintains continuity of identity with the human adult that it is becoming. Therefore, the former ought to be assigned with the same moral standing and right to life as the latter.[98]

So far our review of available scientific evidence on the moral status of the human embryo shows that there is scientific uncertainty regarding when a human person begins. Although the theories that point to diverse periods after fertilisation have their own positive elements, they equally have serious weaknesses. The possibility of monozygotic twinning and recombination until the 14th day post-fertilisation, which seems to be the strongest argument against the attribution of personal status immediately following fertilisation, is inconclusive. In view of this scientific uncertainty, the benefit of the doubt should be given to the embryo. Until the scientific uncertainty is clearly resolved, the position that presents the least moral problem is to recognize the personal status of the human embryo and its right to life and protection following fertilisation. One thing that remains incontestable in the entire debate is that at fertilisation a new organism that is indisputably biologically human is constituted. It will not become a thing, a plant, or an animal—it can only become a human. Fertilisation itself is the precondition for the acquisition of all the functions of the human person, such as self-awareness, reflection, and freedom. In spite of Ford's claim that the human embryo is not an ontological individual prior to the formation of the primitive streak, his remark below portrays the general uncertainty on this issue and actually favours maintaining a principle of doubt in regard to the embryo's personhood following fertilisation. According to him,

> I am not alone in finding the argument that the zygote is an ongoing human individual unconvincing. But I admit it is plausible both on account of its intrinsic merit and by reason of the number of eminent scientists and philosophers who support it. So long as there

[98] R. EVANS, "The Moral Status of Embryos…, *op. cit.*, pp. 64-65; Also see N. FORD, *The Prenatal Person, op. cit.*, p. 68.

> are good reasons to believe that the zygote is already a human individual and a person, prudence requires that any reasonable doubts should be ethically resolved in favour of treating the zygote as a person.[99]

Here, Ford does not seem to defend as vigorously as he previously did the view that the early embryo is not an ontological person until the possibility of twinning is excluded. By admitting the plausibility of the argument that the zygote is an ongoing ontological human individual from fertilisation, he does not seem to be sure of his earlier position anymore. Notwithstanding the scientific uncertainty in this area, we must admit that there are some rare cases in which a human being does not begin its existence from fertilisation. This may arise from an error during the process of fertilisation or in the course of early embryonic development, as in the case of monozygotic twinning when a twin initiates a new life cycle—or technology does, should human "reproductive" cloning become scientifically feasible. In the latter case, the human embryo would still be a person even though it did not result from the process of fertilisation.[100] But we are still dealing with an assumption based on animal cloning, and we cannot extrapolate the results from experiments with one species to another species without scientific verification. This point is clear from experiments with some nonhuman primates. Even though reproductive cloning has been successful with domestic species, some studies show that the same is yet to be accomplished in experiments with nonhuman primates, such as rhesus monkeys. In one experiment, experienced technicians cloned about 135 embryos with the best oocytes obtained from rhesus and cynomolgus macaque monkeys using the Hwang's "squish" technique, which is currently the best cloning technique. In spite of the high IVF success rate for nonhuman primates, all 135 cloned embryos failed to implant.[101] Perhaps this was due to the fragility of the eggs of primates.

[99] N. FORD, *The Prenatal Person, op. cit.*, p. 64.

[100] Fertilisation does not take place in cloning.

[101] C. SIMERLY *et al.*, "Embryogenesis and Blastocyst Development after Somatic Cell Nuclear transfer in Nonhuman Primates: Overcoming Defects Caused by Meiotic Spindle Extraction, *Developmental Biology 276* (2004):

Whatever may be the case, we should be willing to accept our limitedness as human beings by admitting that our present knowledge is not absolute. What is presently known with scientific certainty is that a new organism belonging to the biological human species comes into existence at fertilisation; this new organism will develop only into a baby and subsequently an adult human being, guided by its own genetic code. Even though we cannot deny the possibility of monozygotic twinning and recombination, it is critical to note that human embryos do not have a natural active potential to twin. On the contrary, they are naturally committed to developing as single individuals. Rather than hastily conclude that this possibility denies their personhood, it may be more prudent to approach this crucial issue with greater caution in view of the serious consequences it has for life. It will be presumptuous and wrong to base our judgment on a reality that may arise from mere accident or on a cause that is not clearly understood at present. This seems to be the position adopted by the Catholic Church:

> The least that can be said is that present science, in its most evolved state, does not give any substantial support to those who defend abortion.... From a moral point of view this is certain: even if a doubt existed concerning whether the fruit of conception is already a human person, it is objectively a grave sin to dare to risk murder. "The one who will be a man is already one."[102]

Some ethicists argue that the possibility for the embryo to twin and become two individuals should in no way justify a denial of its personal status and thus expose it to death. On the contrary, it calls for additional caution and respect as there is a possibility of destroying

---

237-252; Cited in I. HYUN - K. JUNG, "Human Research Cloning..., *op. cit.,* p. 37.

[102] SACRED CONGREGATION FOR THE DOCTRINE OF THE FAITH, *Declaration on Procured Abortion,* n. 13: *AAS* 66 1974, 739; Also see R. SONG, *Human Genetics, op. cit.,* p. 35. Here, the Church adopts a precautionary position and does not take a final official position on the exact moment rational ensoulment takes place. But she maintains that in view of the gravity of the issue involved (that is, the possible destruction of a human life), benefit of doubt should be given to the developing life from fertilisation.

two persons. Further, the theorists who insist on the formation of the brain and the CNS do not even agree on the exact time these are formed during embryonic life. The scientific uncertainty in this area means that personhood can be attributed to the embryo at different times during its development. In like manner, the psychological continuity theories present with serious problems. Functions do not determine the existence of a being, but only presuppose the existence of a subject who completes them. Although barking gives evidence to the presence of a dog, it does not imply that we cannot recognize a being as a dog if it has not developed enough to bark or if it has permanently lost that capacity due to an accident. In a final analysis, in the face of the scientific uncertainty witnessed in the debate on the beginning of a human person, the fertilisation theory seems the most consistent with our current knowledge of human developmental biology; the more cautious and prudent thing to do is use it as the basis for formulating national regulations on the limit of biomedical intervention. In this case, the burden of proof is on those who argue against immediate ensoulment at fertilisation rather than on those who defend it.

SOME HUMAN RIGHTS ISSUES IN ART

Is it possible to speak about human rights in ART? While some often speak of the reproductive right of the individual, there is no agreement concerning the right of the future child in ART. Below we will examine the reproductive right of the couple and the rights of the child.

RESPECT FOR PROCREATIVE AUTONOMY

Proponents of ART justify it on the basis of respect for the procreative autonomy of individuals. This tendency to make the autonomy of the individual the sole measure of the morality of an action is related to atheistic existentialist philosophy that exaggerates man's subjective freedom. Jean Paul Sartre, one of the most famous existentialists, contends that the only difference between man and the animals is that man is absolutely free. To accept the existence of God would limit man's freedom, hence he claims that there are no essences, implying that a predefined human nature does not exist. In his vision, existence precedes essence.[103] His whole philosophy seems an attempt to affirm the primacy of the world of human experience. Unlike Heidegger, who had some influence on him, Sartre was an atheist. For him, it is impossible to think of a given human nature in the absence of one (a God) who has a conception of it. And since there is no cosmic designer or creator who conceives it, there cannot be a pre-design or essence of the human nature. From our existence, we are free to make ourselves whatever we choose to be.[104] Condemned to freedom, we are the sole creators of meaning and value in a world that is without objective and transcendent values. We create our own essence; we are free to create our own interpretation of ourselves

---

[103] JEAN-PAUL SARTRE, *Being and Nothingness: An Essay on Phenomenological Ontology,* H. BARNES (trans.), Routeledge, London 1994, pp. 554-556. It was originally published in French in 1939; ID., "Existentialism is a Humanism," in R. SAMPLE – C. MILLS – J. STERBA, *Philosophy: The Big Questions,* Blackwell Publishing Ltd., Malden, MA 2004, p. 315. Also see S. FROST, *The Basic Teachings of…, op. cit.*, p. 266. Also see S. STUMPF – J. FIESER, *Philosophy: History and Problems, Sixth Edition,* McGraw-Hill Higher Education, New York 2003, p. 463.

[104] JEAN-PAUL SARTRE, "Existentialism is a Humanism…, *op. cit.*, p. 318. Also see S. FROST, *The Basic Teachings of…, op. cit.*, p. 266.

in relation to the world as an expression of our freedom.[105] According to this philosophical current, the individual is the sole protagonist of his own life, with absolute freedom as his only reference. He arrives at an ethics of responsibility predicated on freedom. We must do things because we choose to do them, and we choose freely to do them because they are good for us. Hence, we are responsible for the events that befall us and for everything we do; our actions[106] are good or bad depending on whether or not we acted freely.

In like manner, Stuart Mill, who was in favour of the reform of society to prevent certain social evils, was particularly concerned about the need to guarantee individual freedom. This led him to postulate that individuals should be left to pursue their own happiness as they see fit, without any interference from the government or other people. He claims that the only justifiable reasons for the state to interfere in or restrict individual freedom are "self-protection" and "to prevent harm to others." Without doubt, respect for autonomy in the area of human procreation is consistent with human dignity and should be promoted. But an ethical problem arises when the concept of autonomy is expanded to the point of making it an absolute—when it takes no cognizance of the close relationship between freedom and responsibility and when it is made the sole criterion for judging the morality of a human action.

In view of the gross misconception, exaggeration, and abuse of procreative autonomy in modern times, all of which conflict with some basic fundamental goods of the person and society, it is necessary to clarify the meaning, extent, and possible limit of such an important value. With regard to this, certain questions arise: What does autonomy entail? Is the subjective autonomy of the individual absolute? Is it the greatest human value? Should it be placed at the pinnacle of societal values to the detriment of life itself, which is the precondition for it? Can there be freedom without responsibility? Is autonomy auto-referential? Is it the measure of the moral goodness of an action? What is the extent of autonomy that society ought to recognize, respect, and promote in a crucial matter like

---

[105]Cf. C. GUIGNON (ed.), *The Existentialists,* Rowman and Littlefield Publishers Inc., New York 2004, p. 137.

[106]JEAN-PAUL SARTRE, *Being and Nothingness…,* p. 554; Also see J. REYNOLDS, *Understanding Existentialism,* Acumen Publishing Ltd., Chesham 2006, pp. 68-69.

procreation? More precisely, can we justify a human action on the basis of autonomy even when it injures the fundamental good of another person, such as the life of the embryo? Or when it puts the future psycho-social well-being of a child in jeopardy, such as in surrogacy or donor-conception? Or when it injures the common good of society as manifested in the distortion of family and human sexuality or in view of the kinship problems that third-party techniques are likely to create?

Today, people lack the moral strength to do what is right, or they are becoming unable to distinguish right from wrong as a result of inadequate formation of the conscience. For instance, how do we explain the practice in some European countries, permitted in the name of autonomy, of displaying human beings (prostitutes) in shops for customers as if they were commodities, or the practice of live sex performance before spectators?[107] This disordered conception of subjective autonomy underpins the constant appeal to procreative autonomy of the individual to justify every available ART technique. Subjective freedom cannot be the measure of the morality of an action. It only tells us that an act is free and that the moral agent is responsible for his action. But on the contrary, authentic freedom emphasizes a corresponding responsibility for our personal choices. In view of this, it is necessary to clarify, review, and redefine the concepts of autonomy in general and of procreative autonomy in particular. There is an urgent need to give autonomy a precise content and, at the same time, to set a reasonable limit that neither diminishes the freedom of the individual nor exaggerates it. Autonomy needs to be oriented towards a higher ideal that exalts the intrinsic value of every human life from its first beginning to its end and that promotes the fundamental goods of the human person, the family, and society. Any authentic concept of autonomy should exist within a moral theory that emphasizes personal responsibility for one's actions. In this orientation, an absolute conception of autonomy, understood as the liberty to do whatever one desires with one's body or to use any available techno-

[107]In a television interview in London in July 2006, one of such ladies stated clearly that she enjoys having sex when there are people to watch her. She did not see anything wrong with that. What mattered to her was that she has a right to do whatever she likes with her body. No doubt, this can influence the way others come to understand freedom with some consequences for society. But then, is this really freedom?

logical means to have a child, is annulled and replaced by a responsible and constructive exercise of subjective freedom. It is only this responsible exercise of freedom that truly corresponds to the rational nature of man and his moral dimension.

IS AN ACTION GOOD BECAUSE IT IS FREE?

Subjective autonomy cannot be the basis of the moral rightness or wrongness of an action. To make it the sole criterion for evaluating the moral goodness of an action is to destroy morality itself. In this case, two individuals in the same situation can make conflicting choices and still be said to have made good moral choices provided they acted freely. In the end, what is good or bad comes to depend on the individual, and more specifically, on whether or not he acted freely—a reality that reduces morality to something relative. If procreative autonomy is the ultimate criterion for determining the moral acceptability of a technique, and if an individual is free to procreate with whatever means he chooses, the following questions are bound to arise: On what ground does society prohibit incest between two competent individuals provided they act freely? How do we justify the law in some nations and religions that prohibits marriage between close relatives provided they are competent and freely consent to it? Why does society condemn adultery for the purpose of having a child if the spouses of the adulterous man and woman freely consent to it? From the above, it is easy to see that freedom is not what makes an action good or bad. To evaluate the moral goodness of an action, we need to look at the end for which the agent acts, the means that is used to attain it, and the circumstances in which he acts. Hence, in evaluating the ethics of ART, it is grossly misleading to make respect for procreative autonomy either the starting point or the ultimate criterion of judgment while ignoring the interests of the child, family, and society.[108] This is Murray's point when he asserts,

> Choice and control are to be valued, but not limitlessly, and not as decisive moral panaceas. Choice is not the universal moral solvent, dissolving all moral dilemmas.

---

[108] As far as the decision to resort to ART is concerned, the more important values include respect for life itself, respect for the personal identity and the psycho-social integrity of the child, respect for human dignity in procreation among others.

> We should turn first to what shapes our lives and gives them meaning, and especially to the enduring relationships.... When we avert our gaze from those tapestries, we blind ourselves to what ought to be our starting point for thinking insightfully, about ethical issues in creating child.[109]

ACCESSIBILITY TO ART

When we take into account the best interest of the child, it is difficult to justify the position that every adult individual, including singles and homosexuals, should have access to ART on the basis of respect for their procreative liberty. Undoubtedly, all human beings, including homosexuals and those who choose to remain single, possess an intrinsic dignity and should be respected. But there is need to stress that the position denying them access to ART is not a form of discrimination against them. Rather, the issue at stake here is the best interest of the child. Every choice we make has its own consequences, for which the moral agent is responsible. To choose to remain single, one should also accept the consequence—to remain childless—especially as procreation within marriage is meant primarily to safeguard the interest of the child. Similarly, those who do not have a homosexual status but choose to live that way should also be willing to accept responsibility for the consequence of their choice, which in this case is to not have a child, since nature has designed that humans should procreate through the sexual union of a man and a woman. The case of those with a homosexual status poses greater difficulty, considering that they did not freely choose this condition. Nonetheless, this does not justify granting them access to ART in view of the child's best interest.

We must not forget that family fulfils crucial psychological and social roles towards the integral development of a child. As Callahan asserts, "Psychologically and socially the family provides emotional connections, social purpose and meaning to life."[110] Children who grow

[109]T. MURRAY, "What Are Families For..., *op. cit.,* p. 120.

[110]S. CALLAHAN, "The Ethical Challenge..., *op. cit.,* p. 513.

up under a single parent (or parents who do not relate well)[111] may live with psychological pain and diminished self-confidence. In Nigerian society, such children are likely to be treated as objects of ridicule by their peers and others, a situation that jeopardizes their psychological and social well-being.

From the standpoint of human sexuality, the genes determine the biological sex of a child, but not necessarily its sexual orientation. The fact that a child is of a given biological sex does not necessarily imply that it will have a corresponding sexual orientation. In fact, an individual can be heteroerotic, homoerotic, or bierotic[112] depending on his subjective sexual orientation (that is, what he thinks he is—male or female) as opposed to the objective aspect, determined by his external sex organ. As Coleman maintains, about 90% of children develop core gender identity that corresponds to their biological sex by the middle or end of their third year.[113] Although studies in this area are inconclusive, it is clear that the sexual orientation of a child may be influenced by the social environment in which he is reared. On account of this, we cannot exclude the possibility that a child who is reared by homosexual parents is influenced towards homosexuality, a situation that jeopardizes his personal development. On the other hand, if the child grows up to be heterosexual or to despise homosexuality, the possibility of psychological suffering is aggravated. He may be unable to reconcile himself with this reality, and his confidence before his peers may be eroded due to shame over his background. In southern Nigeria, where homosexuality is taboo, his plight in the extended family and society may be worsened by stigmatization and social discrimination; he may even be forced to live in isolation to avoid unending ridicule. If a child ought to be conceived primarily for its own sake and with its best interest in mind, is it acceptable for society to satisfy the egoistic desires of some adult humans to the detriment of a child's future well-being?

---

[111] For instance, one of the reasons some youths take to drugs is because of the tensed situation in the family, for instance, when parents do not relate well.

[112] An individual is heteroerotic if he is sexually attracted to the opposite sex; he is homoerotic if he is sexually attracted to the same sex; and he is bierotic if he is sexually attracted to both sexes.

[113] Cf. G. COLEMAN, *Human Sexuality, op. cit.*, pp. 61-61.

IS HAVING A CHILD A RIGHT?

To interpret reproductive right as a positive right to have a child in an absolute sense means that individuals are free from any form of interference in choosing how to procreate. More importantly, it creates a claim on society to provide alternate means of having a child for those who cannot or do not wish to procreate naturally. Procreative right cannot be interpreted in a positive sense because society does not presently have the capacity to fulfil this demand.[114] This leaves us with an option to view it in the negative sense of non-interference with procreative liberty. Even then, non-interference cannot be understood in the absolute sense that the bearer can use every technological means available to have a child. As Martin Evans contends, "Rights of non-interference are meant to prevent or overcome wrongful interference."[115] This implies that there can be a "rightful interference" by society to prevent techniques that are ethically objectionable. Besides, to make the procreative right of individuals absolute, such that society cannot interfere with their choices, even when they are morally reprehensible, is to lose sight of the fact that society itself has a legitimate interest in ART. It is on the basis of this legitimate claim that it prohibits human reproductive cloning.

Childbearing cannot be a right just as it is not the sole purpose of marriage. There is a great difference between "a right to the conjugal act from which a child can result" and "the right to have a child." What a couple has is the former, not the latter. To claim that to have a child is a right does not only introduce the idea of an "enforceable claim" but also reduces a child to a piece of property that another can own. The Catholic Church maintains that in situations of involuntary childlessness, marriage as a vocation retains its character of being a communion of life and preserves its value and indissolubility. The Church insists that as a gift of God, a child is not a right, but a privilege whereby married

---

[114]Cf. R BLANK – J. MERRICK, *Human Reproduction…, op. cit.,* p. 99. As some commentators assert, to transform procreative autonomy into a positive right would imply a claim on society to guarantee, through whatever means possible, the capacity to procreate.

[115]See M. EVANS, "A Right to Procreate?" in D. EVANS – N. PICKERING (eds.), *Creating the Child,* Martinus Nijhof Publishers, The Hague 1996, p. 130.

couples collaborate with the Creator to bring a new life into existence.[116] This is a position that is generally held by the various religions and by most individuals.[117] Perhaps this is also the mind-set that underlies the expression "custody of the child," which is used in legal battles instead of "ownership" of a child. The tendency to think that a couple has a right to have a child rather than view a child as a gift partly explains why some people are now expanding procreative right to include the right to use technology to have a designer child that meets their own imagination. This does not conform to the child's dignity; we can only have a right "to" or "to have" an *object*, not "to" or "to have" a *person*.[118] For this reason, it is more consistent with human dignity to understand and interpret procreative right, not as a right to have a child, but as a right to the marital sexual act, from which a child can result. This latter sense makes it easier to see and appreciate a child as a gift.

The tendency to measure a person's worth by the ability to bear[119] a biological child is highly demeaning to the person. With particular reference to the African situation, this implies that the function of a woman determines her worth. To identify the worth of women with their procreative ability is to treat them as machines for making babies. Certainly, this is not correct and it should be rejected. The dignity and worth of a person does not depend on the functions he or she is able to exercise; rather, it is intrinsic to his or her nature as a rational being, a person created in the image and likeness of God. Commenting on the distortion of the woman's authentic identity that arises from such a tendency, the CDF asserts the following:

---

[116] *GS* 50.

[117] Cf. S. CALLAHAN, The Ethical Challenge..., *op. cit.*, p. 515.

[118] The fact that a human being who is already born is recognized as a bearer of right in the UN Charter of Human Rights and in the constitutions of most countries suggests that a child is not a property that can be owned. Parents are simply custodians or guardians, which is why children are granted autonomy by the law once they attain the age of maturity usually placed at 18.

[119] "To have" a child, as used here, is not in the legal sense. It is in the ordinary sense of bearing a child as distinguished from the other sense of seeing a child as a positive right.

> Although motherhood is a key element of women's identity, this does not mean that women should be considered from the sole perspective of physical procreation. In this area, there can be serious distortions, which extol biological fecundity in purely quantitative terms and are often accompanied by dangerous disrespect for women.... This means that motherhood can find forms of full realization also where there is no physical procreation.[120]

We can infer from this statement that a woman does not cease to have value and her life does not become worthless if she is unable to bear children. This worthlessness is the dominant mentality in some societies, and it is unfortunate that some women and men think this way. Every culture has its own positive and negative elements. This calls for an ongoing cultural reflection in the light of objective moral truth and values with the aim to recognize and promote those positive elements that are consistent with respect for life and human dignity. Such a reflection should also intend to purify culture and traditions of certain negative elements that demean people and women in particular. The state, the religions, and secular bodies should collaborate in this exercise as part of a united effort to build a community where everyone is valued, respected, and protected.

WHAT ARE THE MOTIVES FOR DESIRING A CHILD?

The problem of infertility should stir in everyone an important reflection: Why do people want children? Do they desire children primarily for personal reasons or for the child's own sake? Although the personal desire to procreate and preserve one's own genes has a strong genetic basis, it ought to be subjected to rational scrutiny. This is true for both natural procreation and ART. To have a child to satisfy a natural biological desire or for other selfish reasons[121] is unacceptable. Also, the

---

[120] SACRED CONGREGATION FOR THE DOCTRINE OF THE FAITH, *Letter to the Bishops of the Catholic Church on the Collaboration of Men and Women in the Church and in the World,* Pauline Books and Media, Boston 2004, n. 13.

[121] Sometimes, people beget children to satisfy personal needs and desires, which may include: to secure an inheritance, to prove one's sexual prowess, to have

means that a couple employs to achieve their noble desire to have a child is important. To conceive a child primarily for its own sake necessarily includes conceiving it in a way that is consistent with its dignity and excludes the use of technology that threatens its health or well-being. As Callahan points out, the motives for conceiving a child to a large extent influence how the child will be reared.[122] The desire to have a child should automatically include the willingness to love and rear it well. To give priority to the best interest of the future child will make parents more conscious of their responsibility towards it. Parental responsibility is not limited to providing a child with the basic human needs, formal education, and material comfort. It also includes adequate formation in enduring moral values, such as respect for human life, honesty, charity, justice, and peace, without which society will degenerate. Such formation is necessary for children and society to flourish.

THE RIGHT OF THE CHILD

Some proponents claim that we cannot talk about the violation of the rights of a child in ART since decisions are made when it does not exist. At first, this view may seem plausible in virtue of the U.N.'s definition of a bearer of human rights as a child who is already born. Despite this debatable stance, it is possible to speak about the rights of the child in ART.[123] Fundamental human rights cannot be conferred by society because they inhere in an individual—society can only recognize them. Thus, to claim that society can determine who is a bearer of fundamental human rights will endanger the right of some humans, for society may decide to move the present boundary to a time after birth, meaning that newborns would no longer qualify as bearers of rights. This is not impossible if we consider the increasing trend in philosophy and bioethics to define a person in terms of certain psychological capacities. We are

---

one to perpetuate the family name, to commit a person to marriage, to secure one's marriage, for social prestige, to be like others to secure one's old age and so forth.

[122]S. CALLAHAN, "The Ethical Challenge..., *op. cit.,* p. 515. As Callahan observes, there is a wide difference between being wanted and being well reared.

[123]Cf. SACRED CONGREGATION FOR THE DOCTRINE OF THE FAITH, *Declaration on Procured Abortion,* n. 12.

currently experiencing a gradual shift in the understanding of family. In contrast to the traditional notion of family as comprising father, mother, and children, nowadays family can also comprise two men or two women and their child. If society has the power to confer the right to life, it can equally take it away, in which case it would no longer be fundamental to the bearer. Besides, history does not favour conceding such an enormous power to society considering that in the past some human beings—namely slaves—were thought to have no rights. For instance, in surrogacy contracts the child is given away in exchange for money after it is born, that is, when he is already a bearer of human rights according to the U.N. criterion. The Warnock Committee alluded to this fact when it stated that commercial surrogacy is baby-selling. Moreover, to speak of the rights of the child when first resorting to ART does not necessarily imply that the child has rights before it begins to exist; rather, we are concerned about its future rights. Since a decision to use ART jeopardizes the future well-being and rights of a child, the choice ought to take into account these future rights. Some of the pertinent questions they should ask are the following: At any time in the future, will the child have a right to know his biological origins? In the case of embryo donation, will he have a right to reject the parenthood of his social parents in favour of his genetic parents? If the answer to the latter is negative, are we saying that parenthood can be bought? In this case, would the child not be right in thinking of himself as a thing that has been used to satisfy the desires of others? Moreover, if we cannot speak about the future rights of a child because he does not yet exist, why then do we insist that parents ought to consider the best interest of the child when it does not yet exist? Is it not in view of the fact that it will eventually come to possess interests when it begins to exist and because its future interests can potentially be compromised before conception through the selfish choices or actions of the parents?

CHAPTER 11

WHAT CAN BE DONE? SOME RECOMMENDATIONS

In the preceding chapter, we made an effort to evaluate ART in light of the intrinsic value of every human life from conception, keeping in mind the moral principle that the end does not justify the means. In this section we will make some recommendations regarding the problem of infertility.

NEED FOR A CURATIVE TECHNIQUE FOR INFERTILITY

The artificial reproductive technologies are circumventive techniques that bypass the natural procreative mechanisms of the human being. Physicians use them to provide infertile couples with children without treating the real causes of their infertility and without eliminating the profound feelings of inadequacy that many experience both before and after fertility treatment. Thus, they can have children, though medically they are still infertile. This situation makes their childbearing totally dependent on the physician. ART puts infertile couples at the mercy of the physician, who now invades their privacy in every act involved in procreation. Every attempt to have another child reminds them about their inadequacies and renews the feelings of loss of control. This is especially the case with the woman, who has to submit herself to the medical team and be exposed to fertility drugs and the risks of the procedure.

Since health necessarily extends to the physical, mental, and spiritual well-being of the individual, there is a need to address the problem of infertility more holistically. A patient needs to be cured at all three levels for healing to be holistic. As the CDF states, every medical intervention on the human body does not touch only the physical dimension of the person but also the whole person, who is a unity of body and soul.[1] As Shannon writes,[2]

> My point here is not to argue against the use of Artificial Reproduction, but to remind us that we constantly need to think of the totality of the person, not just the biological functioning or the technical elements of a solution. If the main focus is on the techniques, if the biology becomes the centre of attention, then IVF becomes much more production than reproduction.[3]

He maintains that it is not enough to assist an infertile patient to have a child with ART; there is need also to consider the overall welfare of a patient—his or her hopes, fears, and expectations—otherwise the

---

1 *DV.* 3.

2 T. SHANNON (ed.), *Reproductive Technologies, op. cit.*, p. 44.

3 Ibid., p. 45.

person may end up being harmed even when the treatment has been successful. Successful ART procedures may resolve childlessness, but they do not resolve infertility, which continues to carry risks of identity crisis, feelings of inadequacy, and psychological trauma. As Shanner remarks, in the case in which a person's "profound concept of self, gender identity, maturity and control are called into question, to provide a child through ART is not really a cure for infertility" because shame and distress over one's inadequacy are not easily relieved, even though treatment has been successful.[4] We cannot discount the important contributions of technology to human development and flourishing, but it is crucial to note that it truly serves the good of man only when it resolves a problem without endangering or destroying our human dignity and authentic values.

Considering the totality of the childless couple and their overall welfare, there is a need to recover virtue in the practice of medicine and to pursue the traditional goal of medicine to cure and care for the person in every contact with him. Since medical intervention deals with the whole patient, not merely his body, there is need to humanize medicine and see it as an instrument of service that focuses on his true good. This implies knowing what the specific medical condition and the proposed intervention represent in his or her psychic economy. According to medical practitioner Marcia Angell, "The quality of mercy is essential to the practice of medicine."[5] Also, the view of John Paul II regarding organ transplant is valuable here. He maintains that the fundamental criterion for evaluating every medical intervention is the promotion of the integral good of the person according to his peculiar dignity.[6] To truly promote the welfare of infertile couples, the state should commission intensive research into the causes of infertility for the purpose of developing curative techniques.

---

[4] L. SHANNER, "Bioethics through the back doors…, *op. cit.,* pp. 44, 131. Shanner is not necessarily arguing for the elimination of ART. Rather, her position is that the invasive and largely unsuccessful artificial techniques should be used sparingly as a last resort and not as the first suggestion.

[5] A. MARCIA, "The Quality of Mercy," *The New England Journal of Medicine 306, 2,* January 14, 1982: 98-99. Exposing people whose only motivation to undergo the risky IVF procedure is poverty cannot be an act of mercy.

[6] POPE JOHN PAUL II, Discourse for the 18th International Congress of Society of Transplantations, Tuesday August 29, 2000.

Such techniques, which should be morally acceptable, will enable a couple to have children at their own time and eliminate the negative feelings connected with infertility, dependence on the physician, and the inconvenience and stress associated with ART protocols. In this light, there is a need to popularize the Natural Procreative Technology, also known as NaPro Technology, and to train some medical personnel to deliver it at various health centres.

The NaPro Technology is a curative approach to the treatment of infertility that devotes its medical, surgical, and allied health energies to cooperate with the natural procreative methods and functions.[7] As a curative therapy, it addresses the problem of infertility by identifying the causes in every particular case and treating them. It employs surgery and drug therapy and at the same time seeks to create fertility awareness as a way of reducing the high incidence of infertility. To its credit, this curative approach to infertility neither substitutes the conjugal act nor makes the couple's procreation perpetually dependent on the physician. On the contrary, it seeks to treat the root of the couple's infertility to enable them to conceive on their own. Since it conforms to the natural process of procreation and does not involve selective abortion or the death of human embryos, it is clearly a morally acceptable method.

---

[7] T. HILGERS, *Medical Applications of Natural Family Planning,* Pope Paul VI Institute Press, Omaha 1991, p. xi.

HEALTH EDUCATION TOWARDS THE PREVENTION OF INFERTILITY

Our analysis of the causes of infertility shows that certain diseases, particularly the sexually transmitted diseases, contribute seriously to the high incidence of infertility in males and females. As a response to the plight of infertile couples, the state should embark on short- and long-term programmes that are designed to prevent and reduce the incidence of infertility and the use of ART. There is need for broad-based education in procreative and general health to create awareness throughout the country. This should incorporate both preventive and curative approaches and highlight the need for natural family planning in view of the serious problems posed by overpopulation.[8]

The preventive approach should focus on measures that can change the public carelessness with regard to the defence of one's procreative and general health. Most of the principal causes of infertility (tubal factor, STDs, smoking, alcohol, and drugs) are largely preventable. Moreover, prevention will save costs—understood in terms of financial resources, time, physical stress, and psychological trauma—for the individual, the couple, family, and society.[9] Education should create public health awareness and spell out positive measures that people can adopt to avoid health and fertility risks. It should emphasize the need to avoid shame and seek prompt medical treatment for infections or other medical problems that can compromise fertility. To assure greater success, government health departments, religious bodies, and non-governmental health organizations should collaborate in this exercise. With the help of the media,[10]

---

[8] Such methods should respect the profound meaning and the integral unity of the sexual love in all its three dimensions. It should emphasize self-discipline as a meaningful way of family planning.

[9] A. SPAGNOLO – G. GAMBINO (eds.), *Women's Health Issues,* Societa Editrice Universo, Rome 2003, pp. 271-272; Cf. GIWA-OSAGIE, "ART in Developing Countries…, *op. cit.,* p. 22. Giwa-Osagie affirms that the cost of treating infertility is by far more than the strategies and actions required to prevent infertility.

[10] Education geared towards the prevention of the preventable causes of infertility should be a shared task in society, but the media have a crucial role to play.

especially the electronic media, such education could reach all facets of society. It should begin early in the child's formation within the family and the school because some teenagers compromise their procreative ability early in life. It should highlight the causes of infertility, especially the principal causes in every locality, and it should explain the treatments that are available for the different cases. Above all, it should emphasize the need to form procreative health–oriented behaviour through personal hygiene and a healthy use of one's sexuality.

PRIMARY AND FUNDAMENTAL HEALTH CARE POLICY AND DELIVERY

Life and health are fundamental goods of the human person, though they are not his absolute good or his final condition for meaning and the attainment of ultimate happiness. The two are interrelated: life is a condition for health and health is critical to human flourishing, that is, to the enjoyment of life to the full.[11] They are basic and superior to most of the other goods of man, including procreation and the education of children; the state has an obligation to provide the basic health needs of its subjects, and the individuals themselves should pursue actions that will promote their health. Sickness in any form impedes the good of life and the other goods of man; it is an ethical duty to protect one's health with every necessary means, but only if the means is ethically acceptable. For instance, it is morally wrong to clone a sick child and then destroy the embryo that results for the purpose of curing the child from whom it was cloned, as we see in therapeutic cloning. This procedure treats the clone as a means to an end and does not respect its right to life or human dignity.

Poverty and poor health have been identified as causes of infertility, especially in developing countries.[12] Infertility is a medical problem, and infertile couples have a right to health care. But this implies a right to promote and defend one's health rather than a right to be healthy. Given our fragile nature and the limits of medicine and technology, no state can provide all the resources needed to guarantee the health of all its citizens. Even in developed countries, health needs are unlimited but the economic resources to satisfy them are not. Nevertheless, a citizen's right to health, which is founded on the ethical duty to protect one's health, creates a duty for the state to provide accessible primary health care service. According to Basterra, this defence of health is an essential aspect of the process of humanization.[13]

---

[11] Cf. F. BASTERRA, *Bioethics,* St. Pauls, Kildare Ireland, p. 276.

[12] Cf. L. PURDY, "Reproduction," in H. KUSHE – P. SINGER (eds.), *Companions to Bioethics, op. cit.,* p. 163.

[13] F. BASTERRA, *Bioethics, op. cit.*, p. 276.

Unfortunately, health care in Nigeria and most African countries is sorely inadequate: most of our public hospitals lack the medical facilities needed to respond to the growing health problems, including infertility. Describing the situation in sub-Saharan Africa (excluding South Africa) with regard to STDs, which are the major causes of infertility in the region, Giwa-Osagie maintains that "delayed diagnoses of STIs, lack of diagnosis, incomplete therapy, no therapy, or inappropriate therapy compound the problems of STIs in Africa."[14] In recognition of the value of health and the fact that basic health care delivery is a right, it is incumbent on civil authorities to respond adequately to the problem of infertility among their citizens. Conscious of its duty, the government should not only commission an official study on the causes of infertility but also formulate national policies on workable health and infertility care. This should not merely focus on curing diseases; it should incorporate preventive services, such as education and counselling. In general, people should be educated to be responsible for their health. Instead of waiting to embark on high-tech, risky, expensive fertility treatments, people should focus on prevention of infertility. Success in this area will reduce the cases of infertility, the need for ART, and the need for repeated medical diagnosis and treatment of infections that can compromise both fertility and overall health. With regard to Nigeria, collaboration with other countries in this area is necessary. Nevertheless, such workable health policies and practices need not be an importation of every reality in the developed countries with regard to ART, nor should they be morally neutral or insensitive to established social and cultural values. They should adequately take cognizance of socio-cultural realities and values[15] that promote respect for the person and the dignity of procreation. In addition, the state should embark on low-cost and workable primary health care delivery at all levels of government to ensure assistance for infertile couples who cannot afford expensive fertility treatments.[16]

[14] O. GIWA-OSAGIE, "ART in Developing Countries..., *op. cit.,* p. 22. Note that STIs means sexually transmitted infections, which is not different from STDs.

[15] Cf. S. DYER *et al.*, "Men leave me as I cannot have children: Women's experiences with involuntary childlessness," in *Human Reproduction*, Vol. 17, No. 6, June 2002: 1663-1665.

[16] Cf. Ibid.

This emphasis on low-cost and workable primary health care delivery is crucial because many of the causes of infertility can be prevented with early diagnosis and treatment. For instance, to prevent azoospermia, there should be a national medical policy to examine newborns and infants for undescended testes, which can be corrected with surgery. Oligoospermia and tubal factor infertility can be greatly reduced through public health education, the control of diseases, affordable public health care, and policies that ensure that childbirth takes place in health centres and under hygienic conditions. Further, the state should ensure that the health sector is properly financed and managed and that public hospitals and health care centres are well-equipped to meet the health needs of the citizens, including fertility care. Health professionals and workers should be well-motivated and there should be opportunities for them to update themselves from time to time. Since poverty can affect procreative and general health, there is need for civil authorities in developing countries to embark on well-articulated and goal-oriented projects centred on poverty alleviation, food production, and control of diseases. These will have a positive impact on public health, and they will reduce the rate of infertility in society and thus diminish the need for ART.

THE NEED FOR SEXUALITY EDUCATION

Unlike the animals, we are not motivated solely by emotion, instinct, or other non-rational forces.[17] In the realm of human sexuality, we emphatically state that human beings are not slaves to the powerful sexual instinct. Although we cannot claim to have an absolute control over it, our capacity for reason and reflection means that we are not slaves to it. We have the capacity to subject it to rational control, for which reason we can be held accountable for our conscious and free choices in the use of our sexual faculty.

Human sexuality is a precious gift, but like every other gift, it can be misused. Some of the causes of infertility, such as STDs, may result from indiscriminate sex or a procured abortion. The overall situation in the world today indicates that human sexuality is grossly misunderstood and degraded in the name of autonomy and sexual privacy. Until recently, sexuality education was an important aspect of traditional moral education in African families and communities. Parents, grandparents, members of the extended family, and even the community contributed to the education of young girls and boys in moral values and the right use of their sexuality. But as a result of sociocultural change arising from exposure to other cultures, sexuality education is increasingly undermined and sometimes ignored completely. Consequently, many young people, as Shorter observes, are "morally disoriented and sexually promiscuous,"[18] making it easier for some of them to compromise their fertility prior to marriage.

As part of the campaign to reduce the high incidence of infertility in Nigeria, and perhaps in other places, there is a need to resist the present depersonalization of sexual activity by unmarried people. There should be a conscious and well-calculated effort to promote a model of sex that is based on personal responsibility and the understanding of sex as a "total mutual self-giving" that arises from the permanent commitment between a man and a woman that is only possible within marriage. Sexuality

[17] Cf. IMMANUEL KANT, *Critique of Practical Reason,* Translated. L. BECK, *op. cit.,* pp. 63, 67.

[18] A. SHORTER, *African Culture: An Overview, op. cit.,* p. 95. It is important to note that this does not mean that every case of infertility is related to this problem.

education should be an integral part of the early and the ongoing formation of young people at home, in schools, and in society. Parents should see sexuality education as a vital responsibility. They should monitor the development of their children closely and spend time to educate them on matters of sexuality and relationships. The present craze for economic progress should not force them to undermine or overlook this critical aspect of child formation, for such negligence may have negative and irreversible consequences for their children. To collaborate with parents in this task, the state and the religions should incorporate sexuality education into the curriculum of their schools and make it an integral part of their ongoing moral and religious instructions. The capacity to offer such a vital service should form an essential part of the training of prospective teachers. Overall, it is necessary to enlighten the youth on the right use of human sexuality and to highlight the dangers associated with abusing it. Although education on the right use of sexuality should be a shared task in society, the state must realize that it is primarily the right and duty of parents and should be carried out under their attentive guidance.[19] In Nigeria and countries where the literacy rate is so low that some parents may be unable to fulfil this role, the state and the religions need to devise methods of educating parents. In general, education should train individuals to make a moral and responsible use of their sexuality. As taught by John Paul II, sexuality education must be oriented towards chastity and respect for moral norms as the necessary and highly valuable guarantee for responsible personal growth in human sexuality.[20] Public health education centred on a behavioural approach remains the best and most cost-effective way to prevent life-threatening STDs, prevent infertility, and curb the desperate demand for ART. With proper sexuality and moral education, coupled with the formation of a true conscience, human beings are capable of exerting a strong rational control over the sexual instinct. The prevalent public approach, which focuses on prevention of STDs through condom use, seems to

[19] POPE JOHN PAUL II, *Familiaris Consortio, On the Role of the Christian Family in the Modern World,* 22 November 1981, n. 37: *AAS* 74 1982, 81-191. Subsequently, *FC* will be used for any reference to this document.

[20] *FC.* 37; See also H. KLAUS, "Sterility & Infertility…, *op. cit.,* p. 272. It must also be affirmed that our contact with the West has equally brought many positive things.

assume that a rational control over our natural sexual inclinations is not achievable. Recently, however, there has been more attention on abstinence—when society placed high premium on the behavioural approach and emphasized "the need to marry as a virgin" as a social value, most women were able to achieve it. If the present situation is the opposite, it is because the will to pursue such an ideal as a value has been weakened by the erosion of sexual values, which is the aftermath of our contact with the more liberal West.[21]

[21] The formation of a child in the right use of sexuality and morality as a whole used to be one of the most significant aspects of African communalism. Today, this has been eroded by individualism, materialism, sexual liberty and similar.

THE NEED TO PROTECT AND STRENGTHEN THE FAMILY

The family is the natural and fundamental nucleus of every society; it is the natural forum for the regulation of values and human conduct. John Paul II sees it as the first and fundamental school of social living,[22] and Richards describes it as "the key building block of civic society, which helps to determine the shape of a particular society."[23] Values are first learnt in the family, and the quality of each family has crucial implications for society as a whole. A morally healthy family will most likely contribute to a healthy society, whereas a morally bankrupt family will negatively affect every facet of society, such as respect for persons, obedience to laws, attitude towards work, procreation, patriotism, development, peace, unity, stability, and morality in general. An essential aspect of the parental obligation is to inculcate in them positive values like integrity, respect for life, tolerance, and respect for others. To a large extent, the ugly situation in the world today is simply a reflection of the deep-seated crisis and moral decay in many families. As we noted earlier, Nigerian and African families used to be committed to the moral formation of their children and the establishment and preservation of virtue in society. Nowadays, some parents do not seem to view child formation as a crucial duty, and the day-to-day care of their wards is increasingly being sacrificed for economic pursuits and entrusted to nannies and others who may lack the necessary abilities or interest for forming a child. Stressing the importance of the family to society, the CDF observes,

> Since it is here above all that the features of a people take shape, it is here that its members acquire basic teachings. They learn to love inasmuch as they are unconditionally loved; they learn respect for others inasmuch as they are respected.... Whenever these fundamental experiences are lacking, society as a whole suffers violence and becomes in turn the progenitor of more violence.[24]

---

[22] *FC.* 37.

[23] J. RICHARDS, "Ethical Issues – The Major Faiths..., *op. cit.,* p. 41.

[24] SACRED CONGREGATION FOR THE DOCTRINE OF THE FAITH, *Letter to the Bishops...,* n. 13.

The family has a legitimate interest in evaluating ART, especially as some of the techniques (for example, donor-conception) can threaten its very foundations. Taking cognizance of the central role that family plays in the flourishing of society, no wise government would allow the erosion of family values or ignore the current trends that are destroying the family. In view of this, the state should consider it a basic duty to safeguard the family by promoting values that can strengthen and foster its growth. Religion is also concerned about a better society in which all humans can flourish. As this cannot be achieved without a vibrant and healthy family, the various religions should carry out a study on the present crisis in the family and draw up effective programmes that can help reform the family. They should devise well-articulated strategies for educating, guiding,[25] and equipping parents and prospective parents for the tasks of forming children and resisting social decay. The religions should revitalize moral education, targeting the youths, those preparing for marriage, and young couples. To realize this objective, they should engage in constant dialogue with policy makers and activists to pursue laws and policies that promote the family and the reestablishment of values in society. This is particularly important in Nigeria and other countries where religion plays a crucial role in the daily life of the people.

[25] Cf. *FC.* 70.

THE NEED FOR GUIDELINES AND LAWS TO REGULATE ART

There are laws and bodies governing ART in most countries, but no such laws and legal bodies exist in Nigeria. This gives practitioners wide powers and liberty to make decisions on a number of important issues. Such a situation is unfortunate and paves the way for abuses and malpractices, some of which may be irreversible. As Waddington observes, "To designate ART practitioners as gate keepers without clear guidelines or standards will lead to legal and proactive problems."[26] Although there are positive elements in the local culture that will make many of the artificial techniques morally unacceptable, the high rate of unemployment and poverty in Nigeria may make surrogacy contracts and the commercialization of human gametes attractive to poor people. Besides treating them as instruments in the hands of rich couples and IVF practitioners, such practices create catastrophic moral and social consequences in view of the kinship problems that will arise in the future. To forestall abuses, there is need for a national policy on ART. The federal government should establish an independent National Ethics Committee to evaluate the techniques and make recommendations to guide the lawmakers. Similarly, there is need to enact laws and set up legal bodies to regulate the practice of ART in Nigeria—to protect prospective users and donors from flagrant abuses, clandestine practices, and exploitation and to resolve legal conflicts that may arise from the practice. This will prevent or minimize irreparable damage to the child and protect the practitioners themselves. Although some of the existing centres have their own ethics committees and follow the guidelines provided by the foreign bodies with which they are affiliated, this still does not guarantee that the users of the services would be adequately protected[27] or that public interest would not be sacrificed in the desire for profit.

The laws that regulate ART should emphasize the indispensability of informed consent. As we saw earlier, over-stimulation of the ovaries carries some serious risks, and the IVF egg-retrieval procedure carries morbidity and mortality risks if laparoscopy is used. Also, multiple pregnancy can negatively impact the overall health of the woman or the

[26] W. WADDINGTON, "Reproductive Technologies..., *op. cit.*, 2217.

[27] Sometimes, people who are desperate for children may not reason clearly as their judgment is often beclouded by the desire for results.

surrogate. On account of these risks, the proposed regulatory body to oversee fertility practice in Nigeria should pay strict attention to the issue of informed consent in medical procedures. It should critically evaluate the extent to which prospective fertility patients, especially the egg donors and surrogate mothers, are informed about the procedures' potentially life-threatening risks and psychological damage.

In simple terms, consent means an agreement between two people in conscience or an agreement of wills. Within the context of medicine, it means that the physician and the patient must agree on the procedure to be followed before the former can initiate any intervention. Informed consent hinges on respect for the patient and his autonomy. As a competent subject, the patient is the protagonist of his own health. He has a right to determine what should be done to him and ought to be given the freedom to accept or reject a particular treatment. This right creates a duty for the physician to inform the patient adequately for the purpose of obtaining his consent to proceed with a medical therapy. To prevent abuse, such information must be clear, adequate, and objective, and it should be understood by the patient. Among other things, it should clearly state the medical procedure being proposed and highlight the side effects, risks, and alternative treatments available. There should be no deliberate attempt to misinform him or to hold back vital information in order to obtain his consent. The duty of the physician to inform him adequately should be marked by truthfulness and a sincere respect for his autonomy. Given the serious risks in the IVF procedure, it is recommended that consent be given in writing. For instance, an egg-donor should be made to state in writing her comprehension of the medical procedure and the attendant risks. If she is not literate, a lawyer, a public official, or a representative should be involved to ensure that she understands the information prior to giving her consent. This is necessary to protect patients who are primarily motivated by monetary benefits and patients who are not well-informed about the intricacies involved. Prior to initiating an ART procedure, proper counselling should be offered, not only to the couple that wishes to use it but also to the donors who wish to participate in this intention. This should be done in a manner that is objective and non-directive. And since most medical professionals are not specifically trained to fulfil this role, the services of professional counsellors should be sought.

THE USE OF COMMUNICATION MEDIA FOR EDUCATION

Our study shows that many people repudiate the majority of the ART techniques while others approve of them. Opponents should see it as a challenge to educate the public on the real moral issues involved in the debate on ART and on ART's adverse implications for human life, human dignity, family, and society. The information most people get today comes from the proponents of these controversial techniques, who focus on their utilitarian merit to convince the public and attract potential customers. To counteract the negative ideology fostered by them, opponents should provide balanced information on ART that will adequately highlight the grave dangers involved. In view of the critical nature of the issues at stake in ART, information and education must not be limited to the pages of books, newspapers, and journals. Instead there is need to take full advantage of the mass communications media[28]—electronic media, the Internet, and other effective tools in each locality. For instance, the Home Video Industry is a fast-growing industry in Nigeria, and it could be a powerful medium for educating the public. There should be an attempt to collaborate with the key players in the industry to produce educative films that promote desirable ethical values and the need to resist the exaggerated emphasis on respect for the reproductive autonomy of individuals. Moreover, such films could help to form people's consciences, thereby reducing the number of those who resort to ART because they cannot make a clear distinction between good and bad. Likewise, opponents should seriously consider the use of tracts, stickers, and billboards[29] to reach and educate the public. Such tracts should be worded in the national language and all the major local languages in Nigeria. They should highlight the causes of infertility (especially the preventable ones), the health risks involved in ART, and the ethical and social consequences of each of the techniques for child, family, and society. The messages contained in such tracts should be direct and easy to understand. Billboards with carefully worded messages that challenge people's consciences should be mounted at strategic points in the areas of national and local government.

---

[28] Cf. POPE JOHN PAUL II, *Catechesi Tradendae, On Catechesis in our Time*, 16 October 1979, n. 46: *AAS* 74 1979, 1277-1340.

[29] The messages on the tracts, stickers and billboards should be revised from time to time.

SEMINARS AND WORKSHOPS

To keep the public informed about the current issues in ART and other serious issues in bioethics, opponents of the controversial techniques of donor-conception, sex selection, and human genetic design and enhancement should organize seminars, workshops, conferences, and public lectures. Bioethicists, philosophers, theologians, medical scientists, lawyers, and experts in the various subjects should be invited to deliver papers and to participate in discussions and debates. In view of their special ministry to guide their faithful, religious leaders and marriage counsellors need to be informed about the current issues in ART and bioethics. To that end, workshops may be organized for them at regular intervals. Institutions for training future religious communicators and leaders should introduce or expand education in bioethics. Similarly, religious leaders should consider the establishment of centres for bioethics in their different localities that offer information and practical advice regarding ART and other important biomedical issues. Such centres should have thriving libraries and research facilities that are open to researchers and the public.

REDUCTION OF EVIL IN PRACTICE OF ART

The reality of our time is that the number of those who resort to ART to have children is growing in spite of the controversies that have engulfed many of the techniques. As such, we should at least seek to reduce moral evil in the practice of ART if we cannot yet completely change the situation. We can begin by insisting on the prohibition of certain techniques.

OUTLAW THIRD-PARTY CONCEPTION AND COMMERCIALIZATION

Third-party conception should be completely prohibited by law to safeguard the best interest of the child, to promote the integrity of marriage and family, and to eliminate the fears about kinship. In places where donor-conception cannot be prohibited, the state should promulgate a law that guarantees the right of donor-conceived children to know their biological origins; this knowledge is crucial for personal identity.[30] Since the child does not consent to the procedure in the first place, he should have a right to know his history. As such, the law should prohibit anonymity and secrecy and require adults who consciously and freely consent to the technique to accept responsibility for their actions. Secrecy in this case, whatever the fears may be, is not only deceitful, but it is a tacit admittance of the wrongness of the procedure. If the concern is that such a disclosure will harm the child, it would appear that the safest approach is to avoid donor-conception in the first place. A story by Meilaender will enable us to appreciate one of the numerous problems that can arise in this area.

> A husband and wife who thought they wanted a child "of their own" contracted for the conception of a child who would be conceived from sperm and ovum that came from anonymous donors and who would then be gestated in the womb of a hired surrogate. Shortly before the child was born, the husband and wife who had wanted this child divorced. A judge felt compelled

[30] The argument that disclosure will harm the child is self-destructive because it is a clear admittance that donor-conception is potentially harmful to the child born from it.

> to rule that the baby girl actually had no legal parents at all.[31]

The experience described here is likely to make an indelible impression on the child if she comes to learn about it. Hence, it is more prudent to prevent such a situation by banning donor-conception rather than by mitigating the potential effects through secrecy and deceit.[32] An unavoidable implication of outlawing donor-conception is the prohibition of altruistic donation and the vending of embryos, gametes, and wombs. This will ensure that a child will have a clear origin and that parenthood is not distorted and degraded by the numerous types of fathers and mothers that occur in donor-conception and surrogacy arrangements. If such prohibition is not immediately possible, outlawing payment for gametes would be a good starting point, even though it would be extremely difficult to ensure that the so-called compensation is not really payment.

LIMIT THE NUMBER OF EMBRYOS THAT ARE CREATED

The main arguments against IVF and its variants include the substitution of conjugal love, the reduction of human procreation to laboratory production, and disrespect for human life in view of the destruction of embryos. It is consistent with human dignity to prohibit such ethically unacceptable techniques; as a first step, however, we can minimize the moral evil by influencing the civil authorities to outlaw the creation and transfer of more than one or two embryos in a given cycle. This will prevent the problem of foetal reduction, the freezing of "surplus" embryos, and embryo research and destruction. But we must continue to insist on the moral wrongness of procedures that substitute the marital love of couples and lead to the creation of embryos outside the womb.

RESTRICT ACCESS TO ART

Parenting is a lifelong responsibility with serious consequences for the child and society. To accept parenthood, one must be prepared for the

---

[31] G. MEILAENDER, "A Child of One's Own…, *op. cit.,* p. 37. Even where the child is related to one of the couple, it is still not 'their' but 'his' or 'her' biological child. In marriage, however, a child should be 'their' and not 'his' or 'her' child.

[32] That is to say, complete prohibition is the best way to protect the best interest of the innocent child who did not consent to the technique.

onerous task of parenting. A woman who chooses to have a child should be prepared to conceive the child and to rear it. The practice of some career women, and others who do not like to be pregnant, to resort to surrogacy contracts should be prohibited. To ignore the natural bonding that takes place between a mother and the child in the womb is inconsistent with parental values and the best interest of the child. Parenting involves giving one's best—physically, mentally, and spiritually—to the child from its conception. Moreover, to safeguard the best interest of the child and family, the bond of marriage, which binds the couple in a lifelong relationship, provides a more stable environment for rearing a child. Thus, in spite of the pluralistic nature of society, ART should be restricted to only married people. As one expert in Jewish medical ethics, Rabbi David Feldman, observes, "Both procreation and family are two important issues and the first should be pursued without destroying the second."[33] This recommendation excludes same-sex "marriage," donor-conception, and surrogacy.

PROHIBIT NON-MEDICAL SEX SELECTION AND GENETIC DESIGN

Ordinarily, there is nothing wrong with the desire to have children of both sexes. But to resort to the strenuous, expensive, and invasive procedure of IVF-PGD to fulfil this desire calls into question a couple's notion of a child. If one truly values each sex, one must be open to accept any child with unconditional love. Rather than accept the child for its own sake, parents and physicians mete out a death sentence to viable embryos on account of their sex, as we see in prenatal diagnosis with selective abortion and in IVF-PGD. In such a case, the accident is placed above the substance and the latter is sacrificed for the former. Thus, the child that results from such a procedure is not accepted unconditionally as a gift but because his or her sex satisfies the desires of its parents.[34] If it happens to be of the "wrong sex," it is doomed to be rejected, destroyed, or accepted grudgingly and with disappointment. Its worth and its right

---

[33] D. FELDMAN, "The Jewish Response to Surrogate Motherhood," *Women's League Outlook,* (1987) 57 (4), 9-10.

[34] The real problem with this technique lies, not in the desire for a child of a particular sex, but in the 'will' to accept the child only if it is of the wanted sex. This makes the desire of parents the central interest in the procedure and the child as a means to attain it.

to life and protection depend on its sex, which violates the principle that the worth of a human being is intrinsic. This practice corrupts the love of parents for a child, making it conditional. This observation also applies to genetic design of a child, whereby the child is accepted only because it meets the expectations of its parents. As we stated earlier, what underpins both techniques are the consumer attitude in society and the inability to transcend oneself and one's desires. This should not be allowed in the area of human generation because a child is not a commodity whose worth is dependent on the subjective assessment of the consumer. Moreover, such practices are not consistent with the notion of parents as custodians or of a child as a gift to be accepted unconditionally. To safeguard the interest of the child and restrict procreative consumerism, non-therapeutic sex selection and genetic design and enhancement should be completely prohibited.

POSTHUMOUS CONCEPTION

In 1988, Mrs. Blood became the first woman to give birth to a child using her deceased husband's stored sperm; she has since had two children.[35] The rationale behind such a conception is difficult to explain, especially from the perspective of conceiving a child for its own sake and pursuing its best interest, because it deliberately renders the child fatherless. Whether the purpose is to inherit a property, to keep the late husband's memory, or to ensure that his lineage continues, the fact remains that the child itself is not the primary focus in the procedure. Furthermore, the generation of a child should result from the mutual consent of a couple, making such a procedure ethically wrong if the husband did not consent to it prior to his death. Even if he gave such consent it would still be ethically reprehensible because a dead father cannot fulfil his parental responsibility. To fully protect the interests of the child and family, it is necessary to insist on conception being the outcome of marital love.

[35] Cf. "Health: Fertility Milestones," in *BBC News World Edition,* http://www.newint.org/issue303/infertility.html (23/02/05).

PRENATAL ADOPTION TO SAVE AN EMBRYO

What should be the fate of stored human embryos that are no longer required by a couple? Can they be destroyed or used for research? Is it morally acceptable to adopt them in order to save them? Can they be sold to couples who wish to adopt them? The issue is more complex than it appears; even those with the best of intentions, who perceive the grave injustice done to these beings and wish to see it resolved, may fail to grasp the ethical nature of the problem and thus be misled in their conclusions.

There are several different ways to look at this problem. First and foremost, life is a fundamental good that we ought to protect. On this basis, some conclude that since human embryos are human beings with inherent dignity and a right to life, to adopt surplus IVF embryos is ethically permissible and justified if the primary intention is to save them. Without endorsing their creation in the laboratory, we can at least say that adoption will prevent the destruction of human life. In the case of a couple that already has children, it could even be a noble sacrifice. However, it is ethically unacceptable for the couple to cooperate formally or materially in creating them in order to adopt them later.

Regarding frozen embryos already in existence, a second question arises: Can a woman or a couple buy a frozen embryo with the sole intention to adopt it and save its life in view of its dignity as a human being, especially if another could buy it and use it for research that will eventually lead to its death? By virtue of his intrinsic dignity, a human being is beyond price, and offering him for sale violates his dignity by treating him like an object that has a price. For this reason, there are some who feel that, under such a precarious circumstance, buying an embryo in order to adopt and save it is morally permissible according to the principle of the lesser evil. This principle states that in the face of two moral evils that cannot be avoided it is morally acceptable to choose the lesser evil, especially if another person will carry out the greater evil if the lesser one is left undone. This does not make the moral evil a morally good choice, though the agent will not be culpable. If their sole or primary intention is to save the embryo, it can be said that their motive is good; they will be rescuing a moral situation that they did not create, provided they accept the child unconditionally rather than insist on particular characteristics.[36] But the same justification cannot be provided for the seller because this commodification of a human embryo would still be morally objectionable for violating the dignity of the prospective child.

These positions each have their own merit, but they are not conclusive. Perhaps, if such ethical solutions are proffered in a circumstance in which there is a total ban on further creation of laboratory embryos, meaning that we are dealing with only the existing ones, they may appear plausible. But to use this principle to justify such positions under the present situation in which embryos are continually created in the laboratory amounts to a dangerous application of a good moral principle. This is because, by so doing, we provide tacit support for the ethically reprehensible procedures of laboratory fertilisation and artificial heterologous procreation, whereas we should insist on their total prohibition. Also, such an application may obscure the sound reasoning showing that this way of bringing new human beings into existence does not conform to our inherent dignity. This is why the position taken by the CDF remains the most logical in this case. In view of the wider implications of prenatal adoption, it states that "the thousands of abandoned embryos represent a situation of injustice which in fact cannot be resolved."[37]

[36] Ordinarily, advocates may argue that, to buy an embryo in order to adopt it and save its life is a lesser evil in comparison to allowing it to be bought by another who will use it for research and destroy it. In this case, the couple is solely or primarily saving life even though this fulfils a secondary desire to have a child. Since no one can determine another's motive with certainty, benefit of doubt should be given to the couple and the life that is to be rescued.

[37] SACRED CONGREGATION FOR THE DOCTRINE OF THE FAITH, *Dignitas Personae...*, n.19.

COMBATING SOCIAL MISCONCEPTIONS OR NEGATIVE ATTITUDES

Infertility is a traumatizing experience for most couples. As we stated before, research shows that women undergoing fertility treatment have higher levels of stress than those struggling with life-threatening illnesses like cancer and heart disease.[38] If involuntary childlessness is not inherently life-threatening, what makes it so traumatizing? Why are most infertile couples desperate to use ART? Why are some willing to do "anything" to have a child? A truth that emerges from our study is that the factors that underlie their desperation are not limited to the natural biological desire to procreate. Some deep psychological imperatives with a social basis can be identified in this area. Here, we will summarize some of them.

[38] See C. TURKINGTON – M. ALPER, *Understanding Fertility and Infertility, op. cit.*, pp. 203-204.

COMBATING THE NOTION OF INFERTILITY AS A SHAME

Infertile couples all over the world face some social discomfort. In the African worldview, the inability to have a child is seen as a sign of a curse. In the more technologically advanced nations, there is a tendency to see infertile couples as hedonists. In general, there is a broad social climate that is hostile to childless couples. Due to grave misconceptions about childlessness arising from sociocultural relativism, the inability to have a genetic child connotes shame in the minds of many people. It represents negative things in the consciousness of individuals and societies, such as a curse, failure in marriage and life, the absence of meaning in life, the end of one's lineage, and exclusion from personal immortality in the case of Africans. As a result, childless couples are scorned and stigmatized in society, which is why many of them are desperate to have a child. Sometimes, infertile individuals are perceived as wicked people who are being punished for their numerous sins.

To counteract the desperation to resort to every form of ART or even adultery to have a child, there is a need to correct the relativism in this area and create a social framework that respects infertile couples. To view infertility as a shame or a curse and then stigmatize and ostracize childless individuals is akin to blaming a victim for his problems. There is nothing that makes the inability to have a child a curse or a shame. As Inhorn remarks, "Infertility is not inherently shameful, as it is a non-volitional status over which the infertile individual has little control."[39] The real shame is the hostile and inhumane attitude of individuals, families, and society towards infertile people. It worsens their plight and compels them to use everything that is technically possible as a last resort to have a child. There is a need to correct the gross misconception that connects every case of infertility to a past abortion[40] or to punishment for past sins. If a particular case of infertility is the outcome of a procured abortion, to stigmatize and reject the infertile individual is still inhumane.

---

[39] M. INHORN, *Local Babies, Global Science…, op. cit.*, p. 247.

[40] Although an unsafe abortion may cause infertility, most cases of infertility have no connection with it or with the moral standing of the infertile couple or individual. On the contrary, it cannot be rationally defended that all fertile couples or individuals are sinless or more righteous than the infertile ones.

People are greatly influenced by the dominant ideas in the culture and society in which they live. Their early learning process and personal experience in society can condition them to a great extent to see things in particular ways and without challenging the assumptions that underlie them. Knowing that even ART cannot resolve every case of infertility, there is need to safeguard the dignity and interests of involuntarily childless couples. Because what partly makes infertility so traumatic for couples is the negative social attitude, today's society must critically analyse these assumptions and ideas. This will liberate involuntarily childless couples from the negative attitude of society, from fear, stigma, and trauma, from the desperation to use every form of ART. Even if one's infertility is not resolved, the notion that one is not a failure or an accursed person will be extremely reassuring.[41]

[41] That is to say, if society replaces shame, stigma and other negative attitudes toward childless people with positive ones, infertility will be less traumatic.

COMBATING THE CONSUMER CULTURE IN SOCIETY

The present tendency to accept everything that is technically possible in ART in search of a child or a "perfect" baby arises from consumer culture and the growing tendency to define human well-being from a purely materialistic standpoint. The present reality in the world, in which many die of hunger and disease daily amidst extreme waste in pursuit of inordinate desires, is a failure on the part of society. To address this situation, we must distinguish between needs and desires and between justifiable and non-justifiable desires. Civil authorities have a leading role in this quest. They should search for effective ways to deal with the consumer mentality in society, which has the potential to erode the notion of a child as a precious gift. They should seek to limit the pursuit of self-interest and profit in scientific research and ART in favour of the collective interest of humanity. Similarly, rather than allow the forces of supply and demand to determine what should and what should not be done in the area of human procreation, they should strive to curb the growing technological mentality that sees whatever is technically possible to be ethically acceptable.

BETWEEN INDIVIDUALISM AND COMMUNALISM

In ethical deliberations, there is need to seek a midpoint between the extremes of individualism and communalism. According to John Bewaji, "The well spring of morality and ethics in African societies is the pursuit of a balance of individual with communal well-being."[42] From the African perspective, morality is first and foremost a personal thing, but it is not exclusively so because the individual himself lives with others in society. Since the structure of African society is communal, in pursuit of his personal goal the individual is expected to consider, not only his self-interest, but also how his choices can affect the community.[43] His choices should seek to maintain a healthy balance between his own interests and the interests of the community. Within this ethical framework, a human choice that endangers the goods of the community is considered a bad moral choice.[44] Wiredu contends that "humanism," or the promotion of "human welfare," is what characterizes African morality:

> But anyone who reflects on our traditional ways of speaking about morality is bound to be struck by the preoccupation with human welfare: what is morally good is what benefits a human being; it is what is decent for a man—what brings dignity, respect, contentment, prosperity, joy, to a man and his community. And what is morally bad is what brings misery, misfortune, and disgrace.[45]

[42] J. BEWAJI, "Ethics and Morality in Yoruba Culture," in K. WIREDU (ed.), *A Companion to African Philosophy…, op. cit.,* p. 396.

[43] Cf. S. GBADEGESIN, "Yoruba Philosophy: Individuality, Community and the Moral Order," in E. EZE (ed.), *African Philosophy: An Anthology,* Blackwell Publishing Ltd., Oxford 1998, pp. 131-132; See also R. BELL, *Understanding African Philosophy,* Routledge, New York 2002, pp. 60-61. Contrary to claims that individual identity or uniqueness was not recognized in African moral worldview, individuals are valued in themselves and as members of the social whole.

[44] Cf. J. BEWAJI, "Ethics and Morality in Yoruba Culture…, *op. cit.,* pp. 396-397.

[45] K. WIREDU, *Philosophy and African Culture,* Cambridge University Press, Cambridge 1980, p. 6; See J. BEWAJI, "Ethics and Morality in Yoruba

Without doubt, there is value in promoting individuality and personal autonomy. Nevertheless, we need to draw a clear line between extreme individualism, which exaggerates the autonomy of the individual, and extreme communalism, which swallows up the individual.[46] This is a good example of a case in which virtue lies in the middle. The solution is to not reject either of the two theories, but to reject their negative elements and harness the positive elements that promote the dignity and fundamental goods of the individual without jeopardizing the interests of the child, family, and society.

Culture…, *op. cit.,* p. 397.

[46] The personal choices we make as individuals can have negative or positive, short-term and long-term consequences for others and society. Neither individualism nor communalism is without some demerits. The fact that we live together in society means that it is important to maintain a balance between the two.

REDISCOVERY OF THE POSITIVE CULTURE OF SOLIDARITY

Human beings are social by nature and are constantly in need of the support of others. As Ashley and O'Rourke observe, a human cannot develop adequately or realize himself fully in the absence of relationships with others. As human beings, we need a community for material needs and because our personalities can be fulfilled only by relating with others in society.[47] Happiness is the goal of human life. A simple truth that our social nature thrusts upon us is that we can hardly be happy in isolation from others. Recognizing this, Ashley and O'Rourke assert,

> We cannot be happy in isolation because we are created as social beings. We can be truly happy only by sharing in a community of happy people, and that means that each must, not only respect the rights of others in a negative sense, but must be actively concerned to promote each other's welfare.[48]

Solidarity, an important characteristic of the primitive society, has been eroded by the individualistic tendencies of our modern world. This erosion is largely responsible for the growing demand for assisted suicide and euthanasia and also for the various ART techniques. As we noted earlier, the erroneous belief that a childless marriage is a failed marriage and society's negative attitudes towards childlessness often compel infertile couples to use every available means to resolve their problems. Against this background, there is need for family and society to rediscover the virtue of solidarity and be more supportive of those who suffer. Insensitivity and lack of solidarity means that childless couples are "alone" in such a decisive moment in their life. To allow the childless to suffer alone—or even worse, to contribute to their suffering through negative comments and attitudes—is not in consonance with the virtue of mercy or compassion. Instead, it evinces the moral rot in society and constitutes a major failure in our responsibility to love and care. This attitude neither is in keeping with our social nature nor does it show respect for the dignity of infertile couples as persons. A human being is spiritual as well as material. There is an integral unity between the physical, psychic, and

[47] Cf. B. ASHLEY – K. O'ROURKE, *Health Care Ethics, op. cit.*, p. 34.

[48] Ibid., pp. 35-36.

spiritual dimensions of the person, which any effort aimed at promoting human health cannot overlook. The fact that these three dimensions exert mutual influence in a way that affects an individual's overall well-being is well-recognized in the palliative care of terminally ill patients.[49] It is a well-known fact in the medical field that severe stress can reduce the body's immune system and compromise a person's health. As psychic and emoting organisms with ability to sense, imagine, and feel,[50] people who find themselves childless involuntarily are affected by the intolerance and negativity towards them, and this attitude is an indirect attack on their physical and mental health.

As Gbadegesin observes, Africans place a high premium on the practical demonstration of solidarity among the members of a community.[51] To show solidarity with childless couples, there should be an effort, perhaps a nationwide campaign, to correct the erroneous beliefs about infertility and to eliminate the social stigma and other negative attitudes that constitute an attack on their dignity. Such a campaign should seek to foster love, support, and respect for them instead of rejection and abuse. Most infertile couples in Nigeria and other African countries have strong religious affiliations; as a mark of solidarity, religious leaders should set aside a day in the year to speak about the problem and to offer prayers for them. Reflection should aim at offering them hope and providing them with the incentives to cope and patiently accept their condition. At the same time, it should educate the public on the need to exhibit more positive attitudes of understanding, love, and care towards childless people.

Above all, the religious community, family, and society should identify with them in their suffering and in their search for an ethically acceptable solution to their infertility. This expression of love and concern will reassure them that they are not alone, greatly alleviate their inner suffering, and make it easier for them to accept their situation. The need for such solidarity in African society is captured philosophically by Mbiti

[49] Cf. L. GORMOLLY, "Palliative Treatment and Ordinary Care," in J. CORREA – E. SGRECCIA (eds.), *The Dignity of the Dying Person, Proceedings of the Fifth Assembly of the Pontifical Academy for Life,* Vatican City, 24-27 February, 1999, Libreria Editrice Vaticana, Citta del Vaticano 2000.

[50] Cf. B. ASHLEY – K. O'ROURKE, *Health Care Ethics, op. cit.,* p. 39.

[51] Cf. S. GBADEGESIN, "Yoruba Philosophy: Individuality..., *op. cit.,* p. 132.

when he asserts that "the guiding principles of African people's ethical behaviour may be summed up in the consciousness that 'I' am because we are and since we are, therefore, 'I' am."[52] Supporting this communitarian maxim, Magesa states that "community should be re-established in a way that we will come to understand that what falls on one falls on all."[53]

[52] J. MBITI, *African Religions and Philosophy,* Heinemann Books, Oxford 1975, *op. cit.*, pp. 108-109.

[53] L. MAGESA, *African Religion…*, *op. cit.*, p. 65.

CREATING SUPPORT GROUPS

As a mark of solidarity with those traumatized by their childless condition, the state, religions, and charitable organizations should create support groups where such couples can be helped to cope with their situation as they continue to seek medical solutions. The nucleus of each support group should comprise professionals such as a psychologist and a medical doctor, a religious chaplain, and some social workers. The professional assistance, which should be voluntary, should be directed to the true good of the childless individuals in a way that respects their dignity and autonomy. Counselling should develop their coping skills and lead them to greater acceptance.

It is necessary, however, to remember that a true and genuine support is not necessarily that which is evasive of the problem or which offers false and empty hopes. Rather, an authentic support is that which gradually helps the childless couples to come to terms with the reality of their situation and to deal effectively with the numerous challenges posed by their childless state. Such a support should empower them to confront their fears and inner feelings of inadequacy and to acquire a more positive mental attitude towards themselves, their situation, their environment, and their life as a whole. It should lead them to harness all their energies and resources—physical, mental, and spiritual—towards an integral development of their personality and life. Expanding their horizon on life, it should prepare them for a more positive role in society and for greater service to humanity. To make such groups more goal-oriented, the coordinators should design practical and educative programmes that engage them in creative activities aimed at making them more productive in the various spheres of life. One possible problem is that some infertile couples may find it degrading and shameful to belong to such a group. Nigerian men may associate it with weakness, making it possible that the vast majority of childless individuals who attend such centres will be women.

SELF-TRANSCENDENCE: OPTING FOR ADOPTION

When confronted with the problem of involuntary childlessness, couples need to understand that to have a child is not a right and that a successful marriage depends more on their total fidelity to their marriage vocation. In the absence of a child that will be genetically related to them, they should avail themselves of the opportunity to adopt one. In doing so, they should recognize and give priority to the best interest and well-being of the child, which is also the expectation in natural conception.

The moral comparison often made between donor-conception and adoption is profoundly mistaken because the two cannot be equated. With regard to the underlying motive, the first aims at self-realization while the latter challenges the couple to transcend themselves and their desire to have a biological child. The primary aim of ART is to satisfy the couple's desire for a biological child, whereas the needy child is the primary concern in adoption. Adoption aims primarily at providing a home, a family, love, and care to an abandoned and needy child. When a couple resorts to it, they rescue a bad moral situation that they did not create, whereas in ART the couple consciously and freely creates the situation to satisfy their desire. Adoption involves self-transcendence and sacrifice when couples resort to it primarily for the sake of the child. But the same cannot be said about donor-conception and other techniques that jeopardize the personal identity and the future psycho-social well-being of the child. A couple's unrestrained determination to satisfy their desire for a biological child rather than adopt a child only reveals the couple's inability to transcend themselves in order to offer hope to one of the numerous children in need of parents. Taking such a step requires an expansion of the heart and a deeper vision of life based on love, which makes one ready to make sacrifices, and which is not really foreign to African culture and practices.

Adoption, as practiced in Western societies, may be strange to Africans because originally every child was born into a family, and the problem of abandoned or motherless babies did not arise. But in the face of the present reality, adoption can be a good way to deal with the vacuum created in a marriage by the problem of childlessness. In African culture, this practice can be covered by the recognition of every human life as a gift from God, solidarity with a helpless child in need of parents, and the emphasis on the unity of humanity as an extended family, which is integral to African ethics.[54] Besides, as Bujo asserts, the African universalistic concept of community cannot be founded exclusively on blood ties because an individual can be admitted as a member of a community through the marriage bond, friendship, or neighbourhood.[55]

To facilitate the cultural acceptance of adoption in Nigeria, civil leaders can embark on a nationwide campaign to enlighten and form the consciences of infertile couples and society, teaching them the need to transcend our narrow understanding of parenthood and adopt children in need of loving parents. Similarly, there is need to create a sociocultural climate in which adopted children are culturally recognized and accepted as full members of their new families and respective communities, with all the rights and privileges due to them. A mere constitutional recognition of adoption in Nigeria may not be enough, making the cultural acceptance of this reality a challenge in our society. Already, in some Nigerian communities, this sense of adoption is recognized and practiced with some minor restrictions. Among the Urhobo and some Igbo subcultures in Nigeria, an adopted child, once he is properly received as a member of a family, perhaps through the performance of certain traditional rites, has the right of inheritance and can become the head of the given family, although he cannot become the ruler of the entire community.

[54] Cf. B. BUJO, *Foundations of an African Ethic, op. cit.*, p. 85; See also P. IROEGBU, *Metaphysics…, op. cit.*, p. 349.

[55] Cf. B. BUJO, *Foundations of an African Ethic, op. cit.*, p.113; See also J. MUYA, "Benezet Bujo, "The Awakening of…, *op. cit.*, p. 125.

CREATING A HEALTHY ENVIRONMENT FOR CHILDREN

We are rational beings, and the act of bringing a child into existence should be neither a matter of instinct nor an exercise devoid of proper planning. Rather, it should flow out of a desire to love and care for the child. Most people will agree that the sexual relationship should be an act of love and mutual self-giving of couples. Children, who are fruits of such a union, are signs of that love and deserve adequate love and care from their parents. This implies that the desire to procreate should correspond to the responsibility to love and care for the child through the creation of a suitable environment that supports its personal development. This requires giving every child a basic formal education and adequate moral formation.[56,57]

The sufferings of childless couples should challenge today's society to rethink issues like abortion and the treatment of children as objects. If a child is so valuable that some childless couples desire to have one "at all cost," every structure in society that does not promote the integrity and dignity of the child should be eliminated. Reflecting on the trauma of involuntary childlessness, society needs to redress the issues of child labour, child hunger, childhood diseases, human trafficking, homicide, and other realities of our time that do not promote the dignity of children. Otherwise, it may be argued that there is no sense in seeking to have a child at all cost in the absence of a corresponding desire and plan to provide an environment that is conducive to its holistic development.

[56] Cf. *GS.* 35, 52.

[57] See T. BUERGENTHAL – D. SHELTON – D. STEWART, *International Human Rights in a Nutshell, Third Edition,* West Group Publishing Co., St. Paul, MN 2002, p. 38.

HUMANIZING SCIENCE AND TECHNOLOGY

When evaluating the morality of a human action, we consider not only the actor and his action but also the recipient of his act. For instance, most people will agree that cutting an insect in half does not carry the same moral significance as cutting a human being in half. The reason is that the two actions have different meanings in our minds. Every human endeavour must have a starting point, and this entails answering some fundamental questions: Who is man? Is he merely another animal? Does his life have a meaning? These questions are crucial because the answers they elicit will influence how we deal with him. Certainly, man is not the same as the animals and does not have an equal moral significance with them, as some authors wrongly suggest. If we accord the same moral status to them, on what ground do we expect man to observe laws, to take responsibility for his actions, or to behave in a certain ethically acceptable way when we do not require the same of animals? If there is no meaning in human life, it would be unreasonable to establish moral codes of conduct to determine how people should live, for instance, how and with whom they should express their sexuality. Most of us find incest and homosexuality to be morally reprehensible, but the nonhuman animals also practice these activities and are not judged to be moral or immoral. No one scrutinizes their behaviour or subjects them to a moral probe, and the same should apply to man if he is not different from them. If we agree that man is not merely another animal and that there is a meaning to his life, every technology, every medical intervention, and the concept of human progress as a whole must be evaluated on the basis of his fundamental identity. As such, the drive for scientific knowledge and technological progress, political motives, the disordered craze for economic power, and social domination cannot be the guiding principles of human progress.

Numerous examples of corruption and dishonesty in the medical-scientific field demonstrate that we cannot derive the concept of human progress solely from scientific, technological, and economic progress. We should acknowledge the value of science and technology, but we must note that what constitutes human progress should derive from a profound and objective reflection on "who man really is" and on the purpose of his life. This is the first and fundamental challenge that society needs to address, and every other thing should derive its significance from it. The values that correspond to man's identity and the purpose of his life should guide technological research and medicine, not vice versa. As the CDF rightly states in *Donum Vitae*, the fact that something is technologically possible does not make it ethically acceptable.[58] A human being is not merely body—he is a composite of body and soul. Any concept of human progress must take cognizance of this and aim at the integral and holistic development of the person in all his dimensions.

There is no doubt that science and technology can be part of our mastery and domination of nature, but a serious danger arises when man himself comes to be dominated by technology, which is the case when technology becomes the primary determinant of human progress or the sole guide of what is ethically acceptable. On account of this, there is need to draw an important dividing line between rationally using technology for our overall good and surrendering our control to it. The first involves humanizing technology to reflect our values, while the latter involves our becoming technologized by ceding control to technology and allowing our desires to determine our values. Science furnishes us with necessary information, but how this information guides human progress should be the fruit of philosophical and moral reflection on the meaning of the human person. To master technology, we must guide it by giving it a precise content in view of our identity rather than allow its benefits to enslave us. The latter will be the case if we accept that whatever is technically possible is ethically acceptable.

Man's rational domination of nature implies mastery over the means of such domination, which in this case is technology. We need to be weary of technology's subtle tendency to condition the way we think as individuals and as a society. Science and its technological application are not morally neutral.[59] To think that it is neutral and to accept everything that is technically possible solely because of noble intentions or good consequences will promote a public morality that justifies human actions

[58] *DV.* 2. This observation by *Donum Vitae* that we cannot derive criteria for guidance from mere technical efficiency should not be treated with levity or dismissed out right. Science can furnish us with necessary knowledge that can enlighten us in formulating certain values, but it cannot be the decisive guide of human values or progress.

[59] Cf. *DV.* 2.

without any consideration for the means that are used. To safeguard our common good in a way that also respects the reasonable wishes of the individual, we must reject the emerging temptation to approve every new invention in the name of scientific and technological progress. Rather, such approval must be subject to our reason and to a reflection on man's identity and purpose. Callahan arrives at the same conclusion:

> Technology itself has to be ethically assessed and rationally controlled. Faced with new reproductive technological imperative (what can be done should be done), fueled in this case by people's desires, decide the question whether a course of action is good or right.[60]

[60] Cf. S. CALLAHAN, "The Ethical Challenge of…, *op. cit.,* p. 510.

THE NEED TO PROMOTE MEDICINE OF NEEDS, NOT DESIRES

Amidst the rapid and dangerous advances in technology, we must insist on the traditional goal of medicine, which is to cure and care for the sick. This is opposed to the expanded version of this goal that includes the pursuit of desires without a medical basis. This approach is bound to end in chaos and a complete waste of resources that could support beneficial research. We should never forget that desires are unlimited and can never be completely satisfied. In fact, new successes in science and technology will only engender new desires. With regard to infertility, the real challenge to scientists and medical professionals is to uncover and treat the causes of infertility rather than treat mere desires, as we see in ART. As Mailaender remarks, when medical scientists use donated gametes to establish a pregnancy for an infertile couple rather than focus on the causes of their infertility, medicine is no longer treating a disease of either husband or wife. "Instead, what is being 'treated' is the couple's desire to have a child."[61] The use of medicine to satisfy desires in the realm of ART presents a serious danger. Every new technology leads to new desires. And since some desires are subjective,[62] it will be difficult to guarantee that the child will not be harmed in the couple's attempt to satisfy their desires. According to Meilaender, if it is the couple's desire that is being treated, we need to remember that they may not simply desire a child—they may also desire a healthy, beautiful, tall, intelligent child should human genetic enhancement design become scientifically feasible.[63]

---

[61] G. MEILAENDER, *Bioethics: Primer for Christians, op. cit.,* p. 15.

[62] Certain desires are based on what each person or society considers to be good at a given time, meaning that some desires can change as the taste of the individual or society changes.

[63] G. MEILAENDER. "A Child of One's own: At What Price…, *op. cit.,* p. 43.

THE LAST WORDS

Following an ethical appraisal of ART, our conclusions depend largely on the values we hold dear in ethical judgment and especially on our beliefs concerning the moral status of the human embryo. If we deny the personhood of the early embryo, or if we evaluate the moral rightness of an action solely from the standpoint of its utility, or if we judge actions on the basis of respect for procreative autonomy understood in an absolute sense, all the artificial reproductive technologies will be morally acceptable. But if we say that the early human embryo has a right to life and if we evaluate moral rightness from the perspective of the goodness of the end, the moral object, and the circumstances, we are bound to reject most of the ART procedures currently in use. The tendency to evaluate the various ART techniques according to compassion towards suffering childless couples, their practical utility for the agent, and respect for an exaggerated procreative autonomy has some serious limitations. It implies that everything that is technically possible is morally acceptable. This makes objective moral evaluation impossible by reducing morality to the subjective autonomy of the individual.

Renowned bioethicist Gonzalo Miranda speaks of the "vacuum of sense" that some individuals experience in certain situations in their life as the main reason underlying the demand for euthanasia.[64] But this vacuum of sense is not only restricted to requests for assisted suicide and euthanasia—it also applies to procreation. The root cause is the inability of most human beings to reflect on the meaning and the purpose of human life. Although the desire to have one's own child is powerful and has a biological basis, it can be rationally controlled when it is impossible to fulfil it in an ethically acceptable way. To measure the meaning of one's life, one's personal worth, or the success of one's marriage according to the ability to have a child reflects a vacuum of sense.

Some people claim that their life is meaningless in the absence of a child they can call their own. On the contrary, there is no situation that is beyond the capacity of our will to accept, provided we adopt a positive mental attitude towards life and all that it brings. Experience shows that

[64] G. MIRANDA, "The Meaning of Life and the Acceptance of Death," in J. CORREA – E. SGRECCIA (eds.), *The Dignity of the Dying Person, op. cit.*, p. 297.

there are infertile couples who have not only accepted their condition as a challenge, but indeed have succeeded in diverting their time and their physical, mental, and spiritual resources to other creative and socially productive activities. The fact that childless couples in this category do not wish to do "everything technically possible" in their quest for a child and still find meaning and fulfilment in life shows that there can be meaning in a childless marriage. The idea that underpins this position is that our life is not a chance or an accident, and it has meaning beyond our personal feelings and existential condition. As Miranda maintains, our value does not depend on our condition; rather, we have value because we are.[65] Our life has meaning even in the worst condition of suffering provided we can maintain a more positive mental attitude towards our unalterable condition. Viktor Frankl puts this more succinctly when he states that

> We must never forget that we may also find meaning in life even when confronted with a hopeless situation, when facing a fate that cannot be changed. For what then matters is to bear witness to the uniquely human potential at its best, which is to transform a personal tragedy into triumph, to turn one's predicament into a human achievement. When we are no longer able to change a situation—just think of an incurable disease such as inoperable cancer—we are challenged to change ourselves.[66]

Commenting further on this point, Miranda argues that finding meaning in one's life enables a person to transform into a service a situation which, humanly speaking, seems to be a dead end.[67] In support of this view, he cites Frankl who asserts that a person who sees meaning even in the worst situation can always transform it into a victory, into an authentic service.[68] In the face of childlessness, we must seek self-

[65] Ibid., p. 311.

[66] V. FRANKL, *Man's Search for Meaning,* Pocket Books, New York 1984, p. 135.

[67] G. MIRANDA, "The Meaning of Life..., *op. cit.,* p. 309.

[68] V. FRANKL, *La sofferenza di una vita senza senso,* Elle Di Ci, Leumann Torino 1978. Cited in G. MIRANDA, "The Meaning of Life..., *op. cit.,* p. 309; ID.,

transcendence rather than insist on self-realization. To insist on the latter when the object of our desire (a child) is beyond our reach will only lead to tension and interior suffering. On the other hand, an inner attitude of acceptance and resignation overcomes the trauma of infertility. Fulton Sheen makes this point exceedingly clear: "What we consider constrictions can be made opportunities for growth provided we become the masters of our circumstances rather than its victim."[69] Similarly, John Paul II maintains that physical sterility can be for spouses the occasion for other important services in the areas of adoption, care of handicapped children, assistance to poor families, and various forms of educational work.[70]

The above assertions have implications for childless couples and for all humans in their daily search for meaning and happiness in marriage, work, and other challenges of life. Everyone desires happiness, but this is only possible when a person finds meaning in his life, for it is impossible to be happy when one is overcome by a vacuum of sense. Although bearing children can bring parents some measure of satisfaction, it neither constitutes happiness nor determines the meaning of one's life. Meaning is not externally derived; it is intrinsically connected with our inherent dignity as persons. This is why meaning and happiness are possible in the absence of a genetic child and even amidst the most difficult situations in life. Moreover, if having a child is what gives meaning to life and constitutes happiness, then without exception the life of every childless couple or individual ought to be unhappy and meaningless—but of course this is not the case.

Even with ART and human cloning,[71] every couple cannot satisfy the desire for a biological child because not all cases of infertility can be resolved. It would be a personal tragedy to lose the sense of intrinsic worth, dignity, and meaning because of incurable childlessness. In like

---

Man's Search for Meaning, op. cit., p. 133. In the face of childlessness, it is possible to seek self-transcendence rather than insist on self-realization.

[69] F. SHEEN, *From the Angel's Blackboard,* Asian Trading Corporation, Bangalore 1998, p. 7.

[70] *CF.* 14.

[71] Even if human "reproductive" cloning is achieved, it may still not guarantee that every infertile couple will have a child.

manner, it would be tragic and shameful on the part of society to stigmatize and ostracize people in such a situation, thereby leading them to an "existential distress or vacuum of sense."[72] A child is a fundamental good of marriage, but couples need to realize that it is not an absolute good. The distinction between the two is crucial: When we make a child an absolute good, the only option for an infertile couple is to do "everything that is technically possible" to have one. But if we view it as a fundamental good, we are saying that infertile couples should limit themselves only to "necessary means," or to what is ethically acceptable. It is an ethically bad choice to sacrifice fundamental and absolute moral values in the quest for a child or any other human good. Because a child is a gift from God, infertile couples should confine themselves to technical assistance that is ethically acceptable and that promotes the notion of a child as a gift.[73]

In the final analysis, the incidence of infertility remains a problem. Society must strive to find a holistic and ethically acceptable solution in order to relieve the suffering of infertile couples. Although suffering itself is undoubtedly a part of our existential reality, this does not justify insensitivity and inaction. As a response to the problem of infertility and other unresolved conditions that cause intense suffering, we must rediscover the values of love and solidarity, which correspond to our human dignity and social nature. This solidarity must be practical and should translate into an active service that uses our gifts, energies, and positions to serve childless couples who suffer.[74] It requires us to confront and eliminate every man-made structure and antisocial attitude that treats the person—an infertile couple, a prospective child, a surrogate mother, or an egg

---

[72] Cf. V. FRANKL, *Man's Search for Meaning, op. cit.,* pp. 128-129. Such existential vacuum underlie the phenomenon of alcoholism, drugs, frustration, suicide, request for euthanasia and the like.

[73] This assertion applies more to those who believe that a child is a gift.

[74] Policy makers in the State should work on measures that will guarantee that childless people are not neglected to suffer in their old age. Even though the African culture attaches importance to the care of parents and elderly people at home, it may not be realizable in some cases. Hence, there should be provision for homes to take care of abandoned old people in their various communities where a particular family cannot cope financially. Such homes should be subsidized by government from a fund created for that purpose.

vendor—as a means in pursuit of economic profit, social and political ideologies, inordinate ambitions, or self-interest. Above all, we are called to rediscover the intrinsic value of every human life from conception until its last moment; we must defend the innocent child, family, and society from the new threat posed by techniques of ART that constitute an attack on human life and dignity. Because human life has intrinsic value and meaning in every existential condition, solidarity compels us to help childless couples rediscover the sense of meaning in their childless situation, for this is essential to authentic human existence, flourishing, and happiness.

BIBLIOGRAPHY

I. Encyclopedia and Dictionaries

AMMER, C., *A Concise Encyclopedia, The New A to Z of Women's Health, Fifth Edition,* Checkmark Books, New York 2005.

BONNICKSON, A., "Reproductive Technologies: In Vitro Fertilization," in W. REICH (ed.), *Encyclopedia of Bioethics,* Simon, Schuster Macmillan, New York 1995, 2216-2221.

DANTO, A., "Person," in P. EDWARDS (ed.), *The Encyclopedia of Philosophy, Vol. 5,* Macmillan Publishing Co. Inc. and the Free Press, New York 1965, 110-114.

FLETCHER, J., "Reproductive Technologies," in J. MACQUARRIE – J. CHILDRESS (eds.), *A New Dictionary of Christian Ethics,* SCM Press, London 1967, 535-539.

FREY, R., "Utilitarianism and Bioethics," in S. POST (ed.), *Encyclopedia of Bioethics, Vol. 5,* Macmillan Reference USA, New York 2004, 2531-2534.

JUENGST, E., "Human Enhancement Uses of Biotechnology, Ethics, The Ethics of Enhancement," in T. MURRAY - M. MEHLMAN (eds.), *Encyclopedia of Ethical, Legal and Policy Issues in Biotechnology, Vol. 2,* John Wiley and Sons Inc., New York 2000, 503-507.

LEROY, B., "Reproduction, Ethics, Sex Selection," in T. MURRAY – M. MEHLMAN (eds.), *Encyclopedia of Ethical, Legal and Policy Issues in Biotechnology, Vol. 2,* John Wiley and Sons Inc., New York 2000, 969-977.

MASTROIANNI JR. L., "Reproductive Technologies: Introduction," in W. REICH (ed.), *Encyclopedia of Bioethics,* Simon, Schuster Macmillan, New York 1995, 2207-2212.

MASTROIANNI JR. L., "Reproduction Technologies: Introduction, in S. POST (ed.), *Encyclopedia of Bioethics, Vol. 4,* Macmillan Reference USA, New York 2004, 2261-2267.

McCLURE, M., "Infertility," in SHENFIELD F. - SUREAU, C. (eds.), *Encyclopedia of Applied Ethics,* Vol. 2, Academic Press, San Diego 1998, 673-678.

MCMILLAN, J., "Reproductive Technologies: Sex selection," in S. POST (ed.), *Encyclopedia of Bioethics, 3rd Edition, Vol.* Macmillan Reference USA, New York 2004, 2267-2271.

ODERBERG, S., *Applied Ethics: A Non-Consequentialist Approach,* Blackwell Publishers Ltd., Oxford 2000.

RESNIK, D., "Genetic Engineering, Human," in S. POST (ed.), *Encyclopedia of Bioethics, Vol. 2,* Macmillan Reference USA, New York 2004, 959-966.

SEIDEL JR. G., "Cloning: Scientific Background," in S. POST (ed.), *Encyclopaedia of Bioethics, 3rd Edition, Vol. 1,* Macmillan Reference USA, New York 2004, 447-454.

SHARMA, R., *The Family Encyclopedia of Health: A Guide to Integrated Medicine,* Hammersmith, Thorsons, London 2000.

SMART, J., "Utilitarianism," in P. EDWARDS (ed.), *The Encyclopedia of Philosophy, Vol. 7,* Macmillan Publishing Co. Inc. & The Free Press New York 1967, 206-212.

TONG, R., "Reproductive Technologies: Surrogacy," in W. REICH (ed.), *Encyclopedia of Bioethics,* Simon, Schuster Macmillan, New York 1995, 2225-2229.

WACHBROIT, R., "Human, Enhancement Uses of Biotechnology," in T. MURRAY - M. MEHLMAN (eds.), *Encyclopedia of Ethical, Legal and Policy Issues in Biotechnology, Vol. 2,* John Wiley and Sons Inc., New York 2000, 549-552.

WADLINGTON, W., "Reproductive Technologies: Artificial Insemination," in REICH, W. (ed.), *Encyclopedia of Bioethics,* Simon, Schuster Macmillan, New York 1995, 2216-2221.

WEHMEIER, S. (ed.), *Oxford Advance Learner Dictionary of Current English, Sixth Edition,* Oxford University Press, Oxford 2000, See "Assistance" and "Substitute"

WERTZ, D., "Reproductive Technologies: Sex Selection," in REICH, W. (ed.), *Encyclopedia of Bioethics,* Simon, Schuster Macmillan, New York 1995, 2212-2216.

II. Church and Papal Documents and Discourses

PIUS XII, Address to Catholic Doctors, September 29, 1949: *AAS* 4, 1949, 559-560.

_____, Address to those taking part in the second Naples World Congress on Fertility and Human Sterility, 19 May 1956: *AAS* 48 1956, 467-474.

PAUL VI, *Humanae Vitae, Of Human Life,* 25 July 1968: *AAS* 60 1968, 481-503.

VATICAN COUNCIL II, *Gaudium et Spes, Pastoral Constitution on the Church in the Modern World,* 7 December 1965: *AAS* 58 1996, 1023-1120.

JOHN PAUL II, *Catechesi Tradendae, On Catechesis in our Time,* 16 October 1979: *AAS* 74 1979, 1277-1340.

______, *Familiaris Consortio, On the Role of the Christian Family in the Modern World,* 22 November, 1981: *AAS* 74 1982, 81-191.

______, Address to the participants at the 35th General Assembly of the World Medical Association, 29 October 1983: *AAS* 76 1984, 389-395.

______, *Mulieris Dignitatem, On the Dignity and Vocation of Women,* 15 August 1988: *AAS* 80 1988, 1653-1729.

______, *Veritatis Splendor, On the Splendour of Truth,* 6 August 1993: *AAS* 85 1993, 1133-1228.

______, *Ecclesia in Africa, The Church in Africa,* 14 September 1995: *AAS* 88 1996, 5-82.

______, *Evangelium Vitae, The Gospel of Life,* 25 March 1995: *AAS* 87 1995,

SACRED CONGREGATION FOR THE DOCTRINE OF THE FAITH, *Declaration on Procured Abortion,* 18 November 1974: AAS 66 1974, 730-747.

______, *Declaration on Certain Questions Concerning Sexual Ethics,* 29 December 1975: *AAS* 68 1976, 77-96.

______, *Iura et Bona, Declaration on Euthanasia,* 5 May 1980: *AAS* 72 1980, 542-552.

______, *Donum Vitae, Instruction on Respect for Human Life in its Origin and on the Dignity of Procreation: Replies to Certain Questions of the Day,* 22 February 1987: *AAS* 80 1988, 70-102.

______, *Dignitas Personae, Instruction on Certain Bioethical Questions,* The Incorporated Catholic Truth Society, London 2009.

CATECHISM OF THE CATHOLIC CHURCH, *Popular and Definitive Edition,* Burns & Oats, London 2000.

III. Books

ALPER, M. - TURKINGTON, C., *Understanding Fertility and Infertility,* Checkmark Books, New York 2003.

AMMER, C., *The New A to Z of Women's Health, Fifth Edition,* Checkmark Books, New York 2003.

AQUINAS, Thomas., *Summa Theologica I,* trans. English Dominican. Fathers, Beninger Brothers, New York 1948.

ASHLEY, B. - O'ROURKE, K., *Ethics of Health Care, Third Edition,* Georgetown University Press, Washington, D.C. 2002.

ATADO, J., *African Marriage Customs and Church Law: A Case Study of the Igbos,* Modern Printers Limited, Kano, Nigeria 1998.

AYASI, E., *An Introduction to the Study of African Culture,* East African Educational Publishers, Nairobi 1992.

BAYER, S. - ALPER, M. - PENZIAS, A., *The Boston IVF Handbook of Infertility,* The Pantheon Publishing Group, New York 2002.

BAYLIS, F., "Human Embryonic Stem Cell Research: A Comment on the NBAC Report," in S. HOLLAND - K. LEBACQZ - L. ZOLOTH (eds.), *The Human Embryonic Stem Cell Debate,* A Bradford Book: MIT Press, Cambridge 2001.

BEAUCHAMP, T. - CHILDRESS, J., *Principles of Biomedical Ethics, Fifth Edition,* Oxford University Press, New York 2001.

BELL, R., *Understanding African Philosophy,* Routledge, New York 2002.

BELLER, R., *Life, Person and Community in Africa: A Way Towards Inculturation with the Spirituality of the Focolare,* Paulines Publication Africa, Nairobi 2001.

BENNETT, R. - ERIN, C. et al., "Bioethics, Genethics and Medical Ethics," in N. BUNNIN - E. TSUI-JAMES (eds.), *The Blackwell Companion to Philosophy, Second Edition,* Blackwell Publishing Ltd., Malden, MA 2003, 499-516.

BEN-RAFAEL, Z. - ORVIETO, R., "Infertility due to Defective Ovulation," in O. RODRIGUEZ-ARMAS - B. HEDON - S. DAYA, *Infertility and Contraception,* The Pantheon Publishing Group, New York 1998, 22-36.

BENTLEY, G. - MASCIE-TAYLOR, C. (eds.), *Infertility in the Modern World: Present and Future Prospects,* Cambridge University Press 2000.

BEWAJI, J., "Ethics and Morality in Yoruba Culture," in K. WIREDU (ed.), *A Companion to African Philosophy,* Blackwell Publishing Ltd., Oxford 2004, 396-403.

BEYLEVELD, D. - BROWNSWORD, R., *Human Dignity in Bioethics and Biolaw,* Oxford University Press, New York 2001.

BILLINGS, E. - WESTMORE, A., *The Billings Method, Revised Edition,* Gracewing Publishing, Herefordshire, UK 2000.

BITTLES, A. - MATSON, L., "Genetic Influences on Human Infertility," in G. BENTLEY - C. MASCIE-TAYLOR (eds.), *Infertility in the Modern World: Present and Future Prospects,* Cambridge University Press 2000, 46-81.

BLANK, R. - MERRICK, J., *Human Reproduction, Emerging Technologies, and Conflicting Rights,* CQ Press, Washington D.C. 1995.

BOHR, D., *Revised Catholic Moral Tradition,* Our Sunday Visitor Publishing Division, Indiana 1999.

BOONIN, D., *A Defense of Abortion,* Cambridge University Press, New York 2003.

BOURDILLON, M., "Witchcraft and Society," in J. OLUPONA (ed.), *African Spirituality: Forms, Meanings and Expressions,* The Crossroad Publishing Company, New York 2000, 176-197.

BROWN, L., "Understanding and Ontology in Traditional African Thought," in L. BROWN (ed.), *African Philosophy: New and Traditional Perspectives,* Oxford University Press, Inc., New York 2004.

BUBEK, D., "Sex Selection: The Feminist Response," in J. BURLEY - J. HARRIS (eds.), *A Companion to Genethics,* Blackwell Publishing Ltd., Malden, MA 2004, 216-228.

BUERGENTHAL, T. - SHELTON, D. - STEWART, D., *International Human Rights, Third Edition,* West Group, St Paul, Minnesota 2002.

BUJO, B., *African Christian Morality at the Age of Inculturation,* Paulines Publications Africa, Nairobi Kenya 1990.

______, *African Theology in its Social Context,* Paulines Publications Africa, Nairobi Kenya 1992.

______, *Foundations of An African Ethic,* Paulines Publications Africa, Nairobi Kenya 2003.

BURLEY, J. - HARRIS, J. (eds.), *A Companion to Genethics,* Blackwell Publishing Ltd., Malden, MA 2004.

BURLEY, J., (ed.), *The Genetic Revolution and Human Rights,* Oxford University Press, New York 1999.

CALLAHAN, S., "The Ethical Challenge of the New Reproductive Technology," in S. LAMMERS - A. VERHEY (eds.), *On Moral Medicine, Second Edition,* Wm. B. Eerdmans Publishing Co., Cambridge 1998, 509-518.

CARLSON, B., *Patten's Foundation of Embryology, 5th* (ed.), McGraw-Hill New York, 1988.

CATALDO, J., "Beginning of Life Issues: Catholic Teaching on Reproductive Technologies," in P. CATALDO - A. MORACZEWSKI (eds.), *Catholic Health Care Ethics: A Manual for Ethics Committees,* The National Catholic Bioethics Center, Boston, Massachusetts 2001, 9/1- 9/7.

CHARLESWORTH, L., *The Couple's Guide to In Vitro Fertilization,* Da Capo Lifelong Books, Massachusetts 2004.

CLAYTON, M., "Individual Autonomy and Genetic Choice," in J. BURLEY - J. HARRIS (eds.), *A Companion to Genethics,* Blackwell Publishing Ltd., Malden, MA 2004, 191-205.

COLEMAN, G., *Human Sexuality,* Alba House, New York 1992.

COLOMBO, R., "The Identity of the Human Embryo," in G. MIRANDA, (ed.), *The Stem Cell Dilemma For the Good of all Human Beings?* Guile Foundation Press, Rome 2002, 75-79.

COLSON, C. - CAMERON, N. (eds.), Human *Dignity in Biotech Century: A Christian Vision for Public Policy,* InterVarsity Press, Illinois 2004.

COOK, R. - SCLATER, S. - KAGANAS, F. (eds.), *Surrogate Motherhood: International Perspectives,* Hart Publishing, Oregon 2003.

COOPER-HILBERT, B., *Infertility and Involuntary childlessness,* W.W. Norton & Company, Inc., New York 1998.

DAWKINS, M., "The Scientific Basis for Assessing Suffering in Animals," in P. SINGER (ed.), *In Defense of Animals, The Second Wave,* Blackwell Publishing Ltd., Oxford 2006, 26-39.

DEGRAZIA, D., "On the Question of Personhood Beyond Homo Sapiens," in P. SINGER (ed.), *In Defense of Animals, The Second Wave,* Blackwell Publishing Ltd., Oxford 2006, 40-53.

DEVERAUX, L. - HAMMERMAN, A., *Infertility and Identity,* Jossey-Bass Publishers, San Francisco 1998.

DRIVER, J., *Ethics: The Fundamentals,* Blackwell Publishing Ltd., Oxford 2006.

EHRLICH, A. - SCHROEDER, C., *Medical Terminology for Health Professions, Fifth Edition,* Thomson Delmar Learning, New York 2005.

ENGELHARDT, H., *The Foundations of Bioethics, 1st Edition,* Oxford University Press, New York 1986.

______, "The Sanctity of Life and the Concept of a Person" in L. POJMAN (ed.), *Life and Death: A Reader in Moral Problems,* Wadsworth Publishing Co., Belmont, CA 2002.

EVANS, D. (ed.), *Creating the Child: The Ethics, Law and practice of Assisted Procreation,* Martinus Nijhoff Publishers, The Hague, The Netherlands, 1996.

EVANS, R. "The Moral Status of Embryos," in KILNER, J. – CUNNINGHAM, P. - HAGER, D. (eds.), *The Reproduction Revolution,* Wm. B. Eerdmans Publishing Co., Cambridge, UK 2000, 60-76.

FLAMAN, P., *Genetic Engineering: Christian Values and Catholic Teaching,* Paulist Press, New York 2002.

FORD, N., *The Prenatal Person,* Blackwell Publishers Ltd., Oxford 2002.

______, *When Did I Begin?* Cambridge University Press, New York 1988.

FRANKL, V., *Man's Search for Meaning,* Pocket Books, New York 1984.

FURROW, D., *Ethics: Key Concepts in Philosophy,* Continuum, London 2005.

GBADEGESIN, S., "Yoruba Philosophy: individuality, community and the moral order" in E. EZE (ed.), *African Philosophy: An Anthology,* Blackwell Publishing Ltd., Oxford 1998, 130-141.

GBUJI, A., *The Pastoral Care of Marriage and Family Life in Nigeria,* Snaap Press Limited, Enugu 1998.

GETUI, M., "The Evolution of the Family in Africa," in TANGAZA OCCASIONAL PAPERS/VOL. 3, *Theology of the Church as Family,* Paulines Publications Africa, Nairobi 1997, 39-47.

GILBERT, S., *Development Biology, 6th Edition,* Sinecure Associates, Sunderland, MA 2000.

GIUGNON, C. (ed.), *The Existentialists,* Rowman and Littlefield Publishers, Inc., Maryland 2004.

GREEN, R., *The Human Embryo Research Debates: Bioethics in the Vortex of Controversy,* Oxford University Press, New York 2001.

GRUDZINSKAS, J. - YOVICH, J. (eds.), *Gametes – The Spermatozoon,* Cambridge University Press 1995.

HARRIS, J. - HOLM, S. (eds.), *The Future of Human Reproduction,* Clarendon Press, Oxford New York 1998.

HARRIS, J., "Rights and Reproductive Choice," in J. HARRIS - S. HOLM (eds.), *The Future of Human Reproduction: Ethics, choice and Regulation,* Oxford University Press, Oxford 1998, 5-37.

_____, "The Ethical Use of Human Embryonic Stem Cells in Research and Therapy," in J. BURLEY - J. HARRIS (eds.), *A Companion to Genethics,* Blackwell Publishing Ltd., Malden, MA 2004, 158-174.

HILGERS, T., *Medical Applications of Natural Family Planning,* Pope Paul VI, Institute Press, Omaha 1991.

HOLLAND, S., *Bioethics,* Polity Press, Cambridge 2003.

HOLLINGER, G., "Sexual Ethics and Reproductive Technologies," in J. KILNER - P. CUNNINGHAM - W. HAGER (eds.), *The Reproductive Revolution,* Wm. B. Eerdmans Publishing Co., Grand Rapids, Michigan 2000, 79-91.

HUI, E., *At the Beginning of Life: Dilemmas in Theological Bioethics,* Intervarsity Press, Illinois 2002.

IDOWU, B., *African Traditional Religion: A Definition,* SCM Press, London 1973.

IGLESIAS, T., "Using Donor Egg and Sperm," in J. KILNER - P. CUNNINGHAM - W. HAGER (eds.), *The Reproductive Revolution,* Wm. B. Eerdmans Publishing Co., Grand Rapids, Michigan 2000, 92-112.

IGWEGBE, I., *The Meaning of the Beginning,* Snaap Press, Enugu 2002.

INHORN, M., *Local Babies, Global Science: Gender, Religion and In Vitro Fertilization in Egypt,* Routledge, New York 2003.

INHORN, M. - BALEN, F. (eds.), *Infertility around the Globe,* University of California Press, Ltd., London 2002.

IROEGBU, P., *Metaphysics: The Kpim of Philosophy,* International University Press, Owerri 1995.

JONES, R., *Human Reproductive Biology, Second Edition,* Academic Press, San Diego, California 1997.

JONSEN, A. - V EATCH, R. - WALTER, L. (eds.), *Source Book in Bioethics: A Documentary History,* Georgetown University Press, Washington D.C. 1998.

KAGABO, L., "Alexis Kagame: The Trail of African Theology," in B. BUJO - J. MUYA (eds.), *African Theology in the 21st Century, Vol. 2,* Paulines Publications Africa, Nairobi 2006, 13-44.

KALBIAN, A., "Stem Cells and the Catholic Church," in M. RUSE – C. PYNES (eds.), *The Stem Cell Controversy,* Prometheus Books, Amherst, New York 2003.

KALU, O., "Ancestral Spirituality and Society in Africa," in J. OLUPONA (ed.), *African Spirituality: Forms, Meanings and Expressions,* The Crossroad Publishing Company, New York 2000, 54-84.

KANT, Immanuel. *Critique of Practical Reason,* Translated. L. BECK, Bobbs-Merrill, Indianapolis 1956.

______, *Foundations of the Metaphysics of Morals,* Translated. L. WHITE BECK, Bobbs-Merrill Company, Indianapolis 1959; *The Doctrine of Virtue, Part II of the Metaphysics of Morals,* Translated by M. GREGOR, University of Pennsylvania Press, Philadelphia 1964.

______, *Grounding for the Metaphysics of Morals,* Translated by J. ELLINGTON, Hackett, Indianapolis 1981.

KAPLAN, L. - C. KAPLAN., "Natural Reproduction and Reproduction-Aiding Technologies," in K. ALPERN , (ed.), *Ethics of Reproductive Technology*, Oxford University Press, New York 1992, 15-31.

KASS, L., Life, *Liberty and Defence of Dignity: The Challenges for Bioethics,* Encounter Books, San Francisco 2002.

______, *Toward a More Natural Science,* The Free Press, New York 1985.

KASS, L. - WILSON, J. *The Ethics of Human Cloning,* The AEI Press, Washington, D.C. 1998.

KAZCOR, C., *The Edge of Life: Human Dignity and Contemporary Bioethics,* Springer Publication, Dordrecht, The Netherlands 2005.

KEARON, K., *Medical Ethics: An Introduction,* The Columba Press, Dublin 1999.

KIMBRELL, A. *The Human Body Shop, Second Edition,* Regnery Publishing, Inc.,Washington, D.C. 1997.

KISEMBO, B. - MAGESA, A. - SHORTER, A., *African Christian Marriage,* Kenya: Pauline Publications Africa, Nairobi 1988.

LAMMERS, S. - VERHEY, A. "Technological Reproduction," in S. LAMMER - A.VERHEY, (eds.*), On Moral Medicine, Second Edition,* Wm. B. Eerdmans Publishing Co., Grand Rapids, Michigan 1998

LARSEN, J., *Human Embryology, Third Edition,* Churchill Livingstone, Philadelphia 2001.

LEBOVIC, I. - GORDON, J. - T AYLOR, R., *Reproductive Endocrinology and Infertility,* First Edition, Scrubhill Press, Inc., Arlington, VA 2005.

LEE, P., *Abortion and Unborn Human Life*, The Catholic University of America Press, Washington, D. C. 1996.

LIPSHULTZ, L. - HOWARDS, S. (eds.), *Infertility in the Male, Third Edition*, Mosby Publication, St. Louis 1997.

LOCKE, John., *An Essay Concerning Human Understanding,* Edited by A. WOOZLEY, World, Cleveland, Ohio, 1964.

LUCAS, R., *Bioetica per Tutti,* Edizione San Paolo s.r.l., Milano 2002.

MAGESA, L., *African Religion: The Moral Traditions of Abundant Life,* Orbis Books, Maryknoll New York 1997.

MAHLSTEDT, P., "Psychological Issues of Infertility and Assisted Reproductive Technology" in L. LIPSSHULTZ - S. HOWARDS, *Infertility in the Male, Third Edition,* Mosby Publication, St. Louis 1997, 462-475.

MANN, J. - GRUSKIN, S., et al. (eds.), *Health and Human Rights,* Routledge, New York and London 1999.

MARTIN-SCHRAMM, J. - STIVERS, R., *Christian Environmental Ethics, A Case Method Approach,* Orbis Books, Maryknoll, New York 2003.

MAY, W., *Catholic Bioethics and the Gift of Human Life,* Our Sunday Visitor Publishing Division, Huntington, Indiana 2000.

______, "The Gestated and Sold," in S. LAMMERS - A. VERHEY (eds.), *On Moral Medicine, Second Edition,* Wm. B. Eerdmans Publishing Co., Cambridge 1998, 519-524.

MAZOR, M. "Emotional Reaction to Infertility," in K. ALPERN (ed.), *The Ethics of Reproductive Technology,* Oxford University Press, New York and Oxford 1992.

______,"Emotional Reaction to Infertility," in MAZOR, M. - SIMONS, H. (eds.), *Infertility: Medical, Emotional and Social Considerations,* Human Sciences Press, New York 1984.

MBITI, J., *African Religions and Philosophy,* Heinemann Books, Oxford 1975.

______, *Introduction to African Religion,* Heinemann Books, Oxford 1991.

MCFARLAND, I., "Who is My neighbor? The Good Samaritan as a Source for Theological Anthropology," in N. MESSER (ed.), *Theological Issues in Bioethics,* Darton, Longman and Todd Ltd, London 2002, 76-84.

MCDOWELL, J., "Ethical Implications of In Vitro Fertilization," in S. LAMMERS - A. VERHEY (eds.), *On Moral Medicine, Second Edition,* Wm. B. Eerdmans Publishing Co., Cambridge 1998, 505-508.

MEILANDER, G., *Bioethics, Second Edition,* Wm. B. Eerdmans Publishing Co., Cambridge, UK. 2005.

______, "A Child of One's Own: At What Price?" in J. KILNER - P. CUNNINGHAM - W. HAGER (eds.), *The Reproductive Revolution,* Wm. B. Eerdmans Publishing Co., Grand Rapids, Michigan 2000, 36-45.

MENIKOFF, J., *Law and Bioethics: An Introduction,* Georgetown University Press, Washington, D.C. 2001.

MENKITI, I., "On the normative conception of a person," in K. WIREDU (ed.), *A Companion to African philosophy,* Blackwell Publishing Ltd., Oxford 2004, 324-331.

MESSER, N. (ed.), *Theological Issues In Bioethics,* Darton, Longman and Todd, Ltd., London 2002.

METUH, E., *African Religions in Western Conceptual Schemes: The Problem of Interpretation, Second Edition,* IMICO Press, Jos, 1991.

______, *God and Man in Africa Religion,* Geoffrey Chapman, London 1981.

MILL, John Stuart., (1859) *On Liberty and other Essays,* Edited by J. GRAY (ed.), Oxford University Press, Oxford 1991.

MILSTEN, R. - SLOWINSKI, J., *The Sexual Male: Problems and Solution,* W. W. Norton and Company, New York 1999.

MOORE, K. - PERSUAD, T., *The Developing Human: Clinically Oriented Embryology, 6th Edition*, W. B. Saunders, Philadelphia, 1988.

______, *The Developing Human : Clinically Oriented Embryology, Seventh Edition,* W. B. Saunders, Philadelphia 2003.

MORACZEWSKI, A., "The Ethics of Pain Management," in P. CATALDO - A. MORACZEWSKI (eds.), *Catholic Health Care Ethics: A Manual for Ethics Committees,* The National Catholic Bioethics Center, Boston, Massachusetts 2001, Part 14/2.

MOSLEY, A., "Witchcraft, Science and the Paranormal in Contemporary African Philosophy," in L. BROWN (ed.), *African Philosophy: New and Traditional Perspectives,* Oxford University Press, Inc., New York 2004.

MUYA, J., "Benezet Bujo: The Awakening of a Systematic Authentically African Thought," in B. BUJO - J. MUYA (eds.), *African Theology in the 21st Century, Vol. 1,* Paulines Publications Africa, Nairobi 2003, 107-149.

MUZOREWA, G., *The Origins and Development of African Theology,* Orbis Books, Maryknoll, New York, 1985.

NIEDERBERGER, C. - LAMB, D., "Spermatogenesis in the Adult" in L. LIPSHULTZ - S. HOWARD, *Infertility in the Male, Third Edition,* Mosby Publication, St. Louis 1997, 106-122.

NKEMNKIA, M., *African Vitalogy: A Step Forward in African Thinking,* Paulines Publications Africa, Nairobi 1999.

OBORJI, F., *Towards a Christian Theology of African Religion: Issues of Interpretation and Mission,* AMECEA Gaba Publications, Kenya 2005.

O'DONNELL, T., *Medicine and Christian Morality,* Alba House, New York 2002.

O'ROUKE, K. (ed.), *A Primer For Health Care Ethics, Essays For A Pluralistic Society, Second Edition,* Georgetown University Press, Washington D.C. 2000.

O'RAHILLY, R. - MULLER, F., *Human Embryology and Teratology, 3rd Edition,* Wiley-Liss, New York 2001.

PALMER, M., *Moral Problems in Medicine, A Practical Course Book,* Lutterworth Press, Cambridge, UK 1999.

PARIS, P., *The Spirituality of African Peoples: The Search for a Common Moral Discourse,* Fortress Press, Minneapolis, 1995.

PINON JR., R., *Biology of Human Reproduction,* University Science Books, Sausalito, California 2002.

POLLARD, I., *Life, Love and Children: A Practical Introduction to Bioscience Ethics and Bioethics,* Kluwer Academic Publishers, Massachusetts 2002.

PURDY, L., "Surrogacy Mothering," in KUSHE - P. SINGER (eds.), *Bioethics: An Anthology,* Blackwell Publisher Ltd., Oxford 1999, 103-112.

PUTNAM, H. "Cloning People," in J. BURLEY. (ed.), *The Genetic Revolution and Human Rights,* Oxford University Press, Inc., New York 1999, 1-13.

RAE, S., "Surrogate Motherhood," in J. KILNER - P. CUNNINGHAM - W. HAGER (eds.), *The Reproductive Revolution,* Wm. B. Eerdmans Publishing Co., Grand Rapids, Michigan 2000, 113-123.

RAHNER, K., *"The Problem of Genetic Manipulation,"* in S. LAMMERS - A. VERHEY (eds.), *On Moral Medicine, Second Edition,* Wm. B. Eerdmans Publishing Co., Cambridge 1998, 542-547.

REYNOLDS, J., *Understanding Existentialism,* Acumen Publishing Ltd., Chesham 2006.

RICHARDS, J., "Ethical Issues – The Major Faiths: A Personal View," in D. SINGER - M. HUNTER (eds.), *Assisted Human Reproduction,* Whurr Publishers Ltd., London 2003, 41-57.

ROBERTSON, J., *Children of Choice: Freedom and the New Reproductive Technologies,* New Jersey University Press, Princeton, New Jersey 1994.

RODRIGUES-ARMAS, O. - HEDON, B. - DAYA, S., *Infertility and Contraception,* The Panthenon Publishing Group, New York 1998.

SADLER, T., *Langman's Medical Embryology, Ninth Edition,* Lippincott Williams and Wilkins, Baltimore 2004.

SAMPLE, R. - MILLS, C. - STERBA, J. *Philosophy: The Big Questions,* Blackwell Publishing Ltd., Malden, MA 2004.

SARTRE, Jean-Paul, *Being and Nothingness: An Essay on Phenomenological Ontology,* H. BARNES (trans.), Routeledge, London 1994, p. 554.

______, "Existentialism is a Humanism," in R. SAMPLE - C. MILLS - J. STERBA, *Philosophy: The Big Questions,* Blackwell Publishing Ltd., Malden, MA 2004, pp. 313-321.

SASS, H., "The moral significance of brain life criteria," in F. BELLER - R. WEIR (eds.), *The Beginning of Human Life,* Kluwer Academic Publishers, Dordrecht 1994.

SAUNDERS, W., "The Human Embryo in Debate," in Human *Dignity in Biotech Century: A Christian Vision for Public Policy,* InterVarsity Press, Illinois 2004, 115-135.

SEIBEL, M. - CROCKIN, S. (eds.), *Family Building through Egg and Sperm Donation: Medical, Legal and Ethical Issues,* Jones and Bartlett Publishers, Massachusetts 1996.

SGRECCIA, E., *Manuale Bioetica,* Vol. 1, Terza Edizione, V e P Università, Milano 1999.

SHANNER, L., "Bioethics Through the Back Door: Phenomenology, Narratives and Insights into Infertility," in L. SUMMER - J. BOYLE (eds.), *Philosophical Perspectives on Bioethics,* University of Toronto Press, Toronto - Buffalo - London 1996, 115-143.

SHANNON, T., "Reproductive Technologies: Ethical and Religious Issues" in SHANNON, T. (ed.), *Reproductive Technologies,* Rowman & Littlefield Publishers, Inc., New York 2004, 37-55.

______, *An Introduction to Bioethics, Third Edition,* Paulist Press, New York/Mahwah, N.J. 1997.

______, "Ethical Issues in Genetics," in SHANNON, T. - J. WALTER, (eds.), *The New Genetic Medicine,* Rowman and Littlefield Publishers, Inc., Maryland 2003, 18-40.

SHANNON, T. - WOLTER, A., "Reflections on the Moral Status of the Preembryo," in SHANNON, T. - J. WALTER, (eds.), *The New Genetic Medicine,* Rowman and Littlefield Publishers, Inc., Maryland 2003, 41-63.

SHEFIELD, F., "Issues of gamete donation and sex selection: a clinician's view," in D. SINGER - M. HUNTER (eds.), *Assisted Human Reproduction,* Whurr Publishers Ltd., London 2003, 28-40.

SHENFIELD, F. - SUREAU, C., (eds.), *Ethical Dilemmas in Reproduction,* The Parthenon Publishing Group, New York 2002.

SHER, G. - DAVIS, V. - STOESS, J., *In Vitro Fertilization: The Art of Making Babies, Updated Edition,* Facts on File, Inc., New York 1998.

SHORTER, A., *African Culture, An Overview,*: Paulines Publication Africa, Nairobi Kenya 2001.

SINGER, D. - HUNTER, M. (eds.), *Assisted Human Reproduction,* Whurr Publishers Ltd., London 2003.

SINGER, P., "New Assisted reproductive Technology," in H. KUHSE - P. SINGER (eds.), *Bioethics: An Anthology,* Blackwell Publisher Ltd., Oxford 1999, 99-102.

______, *Rethinking life and Death,* Oxford University Press, Oxford 1994.

SONG, R., *Human Genetics,* Darton, Longman and Todd, Ltd., London 2002.

SPAGNOLO, A. - GAMBINO, G. (eds.), Woman's Health Issues, Società Editrice Universo, Rome 2003.

SPEROFF, L. - GLASS, R. - KASE, N., *Clinical Gynecologic Endocrinology and Infertility, Sixth Edition,* Williams and Wilkins Lippincott, Baltimore 1996.

SPEROFF, L. - FRITZ, M., *Clinical Gynecologic Endocrinology and Fertility, Seventh Edition,* Lippincott Williams and Wilkins, Philadelphia 2005.

STEINBOCK, B., "Preimplantation Genetic Diagnosis and Embryo Selection" in J. BURLEY - J. HARRIS (eds.), *A Companion to Genethics,* Blackwell Publishing Ltd., Malden, MA 2004, 175-190.

______, "Respect for Human Embryos," P. LAURITZEN, (ed.), *Cloning and the Future of Human Embryo Research,* Oxford University Press, Inc., New York 2001.

______, "Sex Selection: Not Obviously Wrong," in SHANNON, T. (ed.), *Reproductive Technologies,* Rowman & Littlefield Publishers, Inc., New York 2004, 57-66.

STRONG, C., *Ethics in Reproductive and Perinatal Medicine: A New Framework,* Yale University Press, New Haven and London 1997.

STUMPF, S. - FIESER, J., *Philosophy: History and Problems, Sixth Edition,* McGraw-Hill Higher Education, New York 2003.

TANGWA, G., "Some African Reflections On Biomedical And Environmental Ethics," in K. Wideru (ed.), *A Companion to African Philosophy,* Blackwell Publishing Ltd., Oxford 2004, 387-395.

TONG, R., *Feminist Approaches to Bioethics,* Westview Press, Colorado 1997.

TOOLEY, M., "Abortion and Infanticide," in H. KUHSE - P. SINGER (eds.), *Bioethics: An Anthology,* Blackwell Publisher Ltd., Oxford 1999, 21-35.

TURKINGTON, C. - ALPER, M., *Understanding Fertility and Infertility,* Checkmark Books, New York 2003.

VERLINSKY, Y. - KULIEV, A., *An Atlas of Preimplantation Genetic Diagnosis, Second Edition,* Taylor and Francis Group, London 2005.

WARNOCK, M., *A Question of Life, The Warnock Report on Human Fertilization and Embryology,* Basil Blackwell Ltd, London 1985.

______, *Nature and Morality,* Continuum, London - New York 2003.

WARREN, M., *Moral Status,* Oxford University press, Inc., New York 1997.

______, "The Moral Status of the Gene," in J. BURLEY- J. HARRIS (eds.), *A Companion to Genethics,* Blackwell Publishing Ltd., Malden, MA 2004, 175-190.

______, "The Personhood Argument in Favour of Abortion," in L. POJMAN (ed.), *Life and Death: A Reader in Moral Problems,* Wadsworth Publishing Co., Belmont, CA 2000.

WATERS, B. - COLE-TURNER, R., (eds.), *God and the Embryo: Religious Voices on Stem Cell and Cloning,* Georgetown University, Washington, D.C. 2003.

WATT, H., *Life and Death in Health Care Ethics: A Short Introduction,* Routledge, London 2000.

WESTERLUND, "Spiritual Beings as Agents of Illness," in J. OLUPONA (ed.), *African Spirituality: Forms, Meanings and Expressions,* The Crossroad Publishing Company, New York 2000, 152-175.

WILDERS, K. (ed.), *Infertility: A Crossroad of Faith, Medicine and Technology,* Kluwer Academic Publishers, Dordrecht 1997.

WIREDU, K., *African Religions and Philosophy,* East African Educational Publishers, Nairobi 2002.

WISOT, A. - MELDRUM, D., *Conceptions and Misconceptions, Second Edition,* Hartley and Marks Inc., WA 2004.

WILLIAMS, T., *Who is My Neighbor? Personalism and the Foundation of Human Rights,* The Catholic University of America Press, Washington, D.C. 2005.

IV. Reports of Commissions/ Proceedings/ Publications of Professional Bodies

AMERICAN COLEGE OF OBSTETRICIANS AND GYNECOLOGISTS, "Smoking and Women's Health," *Education Bulletin,* No. 240, 1997.

ASRM ETHICS COMMITTEE REPORT, AMERICAN SOCIETY OF REPRODUCTIVE MEDICINE, "Family members as gamete donors and surrogacy," *Fertility and Sterility 80,* No. 5, November 2003.

______, "Sex Selection: final word from the ASRM Ethics Committee on the use of PGD (American Society of Reproductive Medicine: pre-implantation genetic diagnosis)," *The Hastings Centre Report,* March 1, 2006.

EUROPEAN SOCIETY OF HUMAN REPRODUCTION AND EMBRYOLOGY "Preimplantation Genetic Diagnosis" Consortium Data collection III, May 2002, *Hum Reprod,* 17, 2002, 233-246.

GORMALLY, L., "Palliative Treatment and Ordinary Care," in J. CORREA - E. SGRECCIA (eds.), *The Dignity of the Dying Person,* Proceedings of the Fifth Assembly of the Pontifical Academy for Life, Vatican City, 24-27 February, 1999, Libreria Editrice Vaticana, Citta del Vaticano 2000, 252-266.

GRISEZ, G., "When Do People Begin?" *Proceedings of the American Catholic Philosophical Association 63,* 1990, 27-47.

HERRANZ, J., "The Dignity of the Human Person and Law," in J. CORREA - E. SGRECCIA (eds.), *The Nature and Dignity of the Human Person as the Foundation of the Right to Life,* Proceedings of the Eighth Assembly of the Pontifical Academy for Life, Vatican City February 25-27, 1997, 21-37.

KABORE, E., "Identity and Status of the Human Embryo in African Traditional Societies," in J. CORREA - E. SGRECCIA (eds.), *Identity and Statute of the Human Embryo,* Proceedings of the Third Assembly of the Pontifical Academy for Life, Vatican City, February 14-16, 1997.

MIRANDA, G., "The Meaning of Life and the Acceptance of Death," in J. CORREA - E. SGRECCIA (eds.), *The Dignity of the Dying Person,* Proceedings of the Fifth Assembly of the Pontifical Academy for Life, Vatican City, 24-27 February, 1999, Libreria Editrice Vaticana, Citta del Vaticano 2000, 297-312.

NATIONAL ACADEMY OF SCIENCES, *Scientific and Medical Aspects of Human Reproductive Cloning,* National Academy Press, Washington, D.C. 2002.

NATIONAL ACADEMY OF SCIENCES - NATIONAL ACADEMY OF ENGINEERING - INSTITUTE OF MEDICINE - NATIONAL RESEARCH COUNCIL, *Scientific and Medical Aspects of Human Reproductive Cloning,* National Academy Press, Washington, D.C. 2002.

NATIONAL RIGHT TO LIFE COMMITTEE, "Bone Fragments Left from Aborted Babies Can Cause Infertility," *National Right to Life News (Magazine/Journal), Vol. 30, Issue: 50*, May 1, 2003.

NIGERIAN FERTILITY SOCIETY, "Communiqué from the First International Workshop on Assisted Conception," Held on 7th to 9th of November, 2005, at The Eko Hotel, Lagos, Nigeria.

PALAZZANI, L., "The Meanings of the Philosophical Concept of Person and their Implications in the Current Debate on the Status of the Human Embryo," in J. CORREA - E. SGRECCIA (eds.), *Identity and Statute of the Human Embryo,* Proceedings of the Third Assembly of the Pontifical Academy for Life, Vatican City February 14-16, 1997, 74-95.

SERRA, A. - COLOMBO, R., "Identity and Status of the Human Embryo: The Contribution of Biology," in J. CORREA - E. SGRECCIA (eds.), *Identity and Statute of the Human Embryo,* Proceedings of the Third Assembly of the Pontifical Academy for Life, Vatican City February 14-16, 1997, 128-177.

THE REPORT OF A WORKING PARTY OF THE CATHOLIC BISHOPS' JOINT COMMITTEE ON BIOETHICAL ISSUES, *Genetic Intervention on Human Subjects,* The Catholic Bishops Joint Committee on Bioethical Issues, London 1996.

THE REPORT OF THE PRESIDENT'S COUNCIL ON BIOETHICS, *Human Cloning and Human Dignity,* Public Affairs, New York 2002.

UNITED NATIONS ORGANIZATION, Universal Declaration of Human Rights, adopted and proclaimed by the General Assembly of the United Nations Organization Meeting in Paris on December 10, 1948.

WATT, H., "Parenthood and New Reproductive Technologies: Anthropological Considerations," in J. CORREA - E. SGRECCIA (eds.), *The Dignity of Human Procreation and Reproductive Technologies: Anthropological and Ethical Aspects,* Proceedings of the Tenth Assembly of the Pontifical Academy for Life, Vatican City February 20-22, 2004, 33-42.

WORLD HEALTH ORGANIZATION, "Infertility," WHO *Progress in Reproductive Health Newsletter* – Issue No. 63.

______, *Laboratory Manual for Examination of Human Semen and Sperm-cervical Mucus Interaction, 2nd Edition,* University Press, Cambridge 1992.

V. Journals/ Magazines/ Lectures

AKINTOYE, S. - ANENE, F., "Five Hospitals Acquire Capability for Test-tube Babies," *The Guardian on Sunday Newspaper,* Nigeria, November 15, 1998.

ANNAS, G., "Death without Dignity for Commercial Surrogacy: The Case of Baby M," *The Hastings Centre Report 18,* 1998, 22.

"Noninvasive prenatal diagnostic technology: medical, market, or regulatory model?" *Annals of the New York Academy of Sciences 731,* 1994, 262-268.

AUGOOD, C. et al., "Smoking and Female Infertility: A Systematic Review and Meta-analysis," in *Human Reproduction*, 3(6), 1998, 1532-1539.

AUSTRALIAN BUREAU OF STATISTICS, "Lifetime Childlessness," in *The Australian Demographic Statistics,* Sept. Quarter, 1999, ABS Catalogue no. 3101.0.

AWOYOKUN, D., "Perils of IVF and Surrogacy Motherhood," *Vanguard Newspaper,* Nigeria, Monday, September 29, 2003.

BARTON, J. - BERGAUER, N. et al., "Does advanced maternal age affect pregnancy outcome in women with mild hypertension remote from term?" *American Journal of Obstetrics and Gynecology,* Vol. 176, Issue 6, June 1997, 1234-1240.

BAUM, F., *Choosing not to have Children,* Vol. 2, No. 3, 1994, 22- 25.

______, "Orientation Towards Voluntary Childlessness," *J. Biosoc Sci. 15*(2), April, 1983, 153-164.

BECKWITH, F., "Defending Abortion Philosophically: A Review of David Boonin's A Defense of Abortion," *Journal of Medicine and Philosophy 31,* 2006, 177-203.

CAMPELL, A., "Reproductive Medicine – The ethical issues in the twenty-first century," *Human Fertility 5,* (suppl): S33-S36.

CHUKWUDEBELU, W. - ESEGE, N. - MEGAFU, U., "Aetiological factors in infertility in Enugu, Nigeria," *Pub Med: Infertility,* 1979; 2 (2):193-200.

DAMSCHEN, G. - A. GOMEZ-LOBO - D. SCHONECKER., "Sixteen Days? A reply to B. Smith and B. Brogaard on the Beginnings of Human Individuals," *Journal of Medicine and Philosophy, 31,* 2006, 165-175.

DOERFLER, J., "Technology and Human Reproduction," *Ethnics & Medics 24,* 8, August 1999, 3-4.

DONCEEL, J., "Immediate Animation and Delayed Hominization," *Theological Studies 31,* 1970, 76-105.

DYBAN, A. - FREDINE, M. - SEVEROVA, E. et al., "Detection of aneuploidy in human oocytes and corresponding first polar bodies by FISH," *J Assist Reprod Genet,* 13, 1996, 72-77.

DYER, S. et al., "Men leave me as I cannot have children: women's experiences with involuntary childlessness," in *Human Reproduction 17,* 6: 2002, 1663-1668.

EHUSANI, G., "Childlessness should not Invalidate a Marriage," in *The Guardian on Sunday, Newspaper,* Nigeria, November 26, 2000.

ESANGBEDO, J., "'Caution on IVF,' – A Rejoinder," in *The Guardian Newspaper,* Nigeria, April 18, 1999.

______, "Facts, 'Fears' about Test-tube Babies," in *Sunday Times Newspaper,* Nigeria, September 9, 1990.

EUROPEAN SOCIETY OF HUMAN REPRODUCTION AND EMBRYOLOGY "Preimplantation Genetic Diagnosis," Consortium Data collection III, May 2002, *Hum Reprod,* 2002, 17: 233-46.

FELDMAN, D., "The Jewish response to surrogate motherhood," *Women's League Outlook* 57, 4: 1987, 9-10.

FISHER, A., "When Did I Begin? Revisted," *Linacre Quarterly 58,* 1991, 59-68.

GIWA-OSAGIE, O., "ART in Developing countries with particular references to sub- Saharan Africa," in *WHO Progress in Reproductive Health Newsletter* 63, 2003, 22-27.

______, "Assisted Reproductive Technology or Medically Assisted Conception," A paper delivered in the Department of Obstetrics and Gynecology, College of Medicine, University of Lagos Teaching Hospital, Lagos, March 2004.

GIWA-OSAGIE, O. et al., "Aetiologic Classification and Sociomedical Characteristics of Infertility in 250 Couples," *International Journal of Fertility* 29, 1984,104-108.

______, "Clinical Profile, Assessment for IVF and the outcome of IVF in Lagos," 12th World Congress of Fertility and sterility, 1986, Abstracts p.737.

______, "Human Oocyte Recovery for In Vitro Fertilization: The Use of Cervical Mucus and Plasma Oestrodiol as Indices of Follicular Development," *West African Journal of Medicine,* 1988, 7: 136-139.

GIWA-OSAGIE, O. - KAYODE, B., "A Rational Approach to Increasing Access to ART Procedures in Low Resource Countries: Meeting the Challenges of a Public Health and Human Rights Issues," A Lecture delivered at the Department of Obstetrics and Gynaecology, University of Lagos, Nigeria, April 2003.

GOLDENRING, J., "The Brain-Life Theory: Towards a Consistent Definition of Humanness," *Journal of medical ethics 11,* 1985, 198-204.

GRISEZ, G., "When Do People Begin?" Proceedings of the American Catholic Philosophical Association 63, 1990, 27-47.

GRODSTEIN, F. et al., "Infertility in Women and Moderate Alcohol Use," *American Journal of Public Health,* 84(9), 1994, 1429-1432.

HAKIM, R.et al., "Alcohol and Caffeine Consumption and Decreased Fertility," *Fertility and Sterility,* 70(4), 1998, 632-637.

HARRIS, J., "In Vitro Fertilisation: The Ethical Issues," *Philosophical Quarterly 33,* 1983: 224.

HARRIS, R., "Delivering Public Policy: The Status of the Embryo and Tissue Typing" in *Studies in Christian Ethics, Public Theology and Bioethics,* Vol. 18, No. 1, Sage Publications, London 2005.

HASSOLD, T. et al., "Recombination and Maternal Age-Dependent Non-disjunction: molecular Studies of Trisomy 16," *American Journal of Human Genetics* 57: 867-874.

IKECHUKWU, J. - ADINMA, B. et al., "High Prevalence of Male Fertilty in South-Eastern Nigeria," *Journal of Obstretics and Gynaecology,* 23(6), 2003, 657-659.

INHORN, M., "Making Muslim Babies: Sunni versus Shi'a Approaches to IVF and Gamete Donation," Being an address to the Department of Human Behavior and Human Education School of Public Health, II, University of Michigan; Also presented at Session 108 on "Infertility and New Reproductive Technologies" IUSSP Annual Conference Tours, France, July 2005.

JOBANPUTRA, V. - SOBRINO, A. et al., "Multiplex interphase FISH as a screen for common aneuploidies in spontaneous miscarriages," *Hum Reprod,* 17: 1166, 2002.

KIDD, S. - ESKENAZI, B., - WYROBEK, A., "Effects of male age on semen Quality and Fertility: A Review of the literature," *Fertile Steril,* 75:237, 2001.

KOCK-HERSHENON, K. "Totipotency, Twining and Ensoulment at Fertilization," *The Journal of Medicine and Philosophy, Vol. 31,* no. 2. April 2006, 139-164.

KUKU, S. - D. OSEGBE., "Oligo/azoospermia in Nigeria", *Archives of Andorology,* 1989, 22: 233-238.

KULIEV, A. - VERLINSKY, Y., "Thirteen Years Experience of Preimplantation Genetic Diagnosis" *Reprod Biomed Online,* 2002; 4:183. I.

KUNZLE, R. et al., "Semen Quality of Male Smokers and Nonsmokers in Infertility Couples," *Fertiity anld Sterility,* 79(2), 2003, 287-291.

LAURENT, S. - THOMPSON, S. et al., "An Epidemiologic Study of Smoking and Primary Infertility in Women," *Fertility and Sterility,* 57, 1992.

LEWIS, C. - PINEL, T. et al., "Controlling misdiagnosis errors in preimplantation genetic diagnosis: a comprehensive model encompassing extrinsic and intrinsic sources of error," *Hum Reprod,* 16:43, 2001.

"Lifetime Childlessness," *Australian Demographic Statistics, 2002, Population,* Sept. Quarter (1999).

McALLISTER, F. - CLARKE, L., "Choosing Childlessness," in *Findings by the Family Policy Studies Centre,* Ref. 738, July 1998.

MORALES, P. et al., The Relationship between the motility and morphology of spermatozoa in human semen," *Fertile Sterile* 54: 513, 1990.

MORENO, J., "The Name of the Embryo," in *The Hastings Centre Report, Vol. 36. No. 5,* September – October 2006, 3.

MUNNE, S., "Preimplantation Genetic Diagnosis of Numerical and Structural Chromosome Abnormalities," *Reprod Biomed Online,* 4: 2002, 183-196.

MUNNE, S. - SANDALINAS, M. et al., "Improved Implantation after Preimplantation Genetic Diagnosis of Aneploidy," *Reprod Biomed Online,* 2003, 7:91-97.

NWOFOR, A. - UGEZU, A. (eds.), "The Difficulties Encountered in the Management of Male infertility in Nnewi, Nigeria," *Nigerian Medical Journal 45,* 1: 2003, 1.

OBORJI, F., "African Traditional Religion Between Pluralism and Ultimate Reality," *Studies in Interreligious Dialogue, PEETERS,* February 14, 2004, 129-159.

OGEDENGBE, O. - GIWA-OSAGIE, O. - OGUNYEMI, D., "The Implications of Pattern of Tubal Disease for Microsurgery and In Vitro Fertilization in Lagos, *Journal of National Medical Association,* 79: 1987, 510-512.

OKAFOR, U., "Caution on IVF," in *The Guardian Newspaper,* Nigeria, April 4, 1999.

ONUEKWUESI, N., "Special Issues on Infertility," A Paper Presented at the Training of Trainers Workshop on Natural Family Planning for Catholic Health Services Workers and Family Life Promoters, Lagos, Nigeria, October 25, 2002.

O'ROURKE, K., "The Embryo as Person," in *The National Catholic Bioethics Quarterly 6,* (2): 2006, 241-251

PALAZZANI, L., "The Concept of Person between Bioethics and Biolaw". Being a Lecture-Handout at the Faculty of Bioethics, Pontifica Universita Regina Apostolorum, Oct., 2004 – Feb., 2005.

PARAZZINI, F. et al., "Alcohol Consumption is not related to fertility in Italian Women," *British Medical Journal* (1999) 318-397.

PARENS, E. "Is better always good?" *Hastings Cent Rep,* 1998; 28: (1): S-1-S-17.

PENNINNGS, G., "Ethics of sex selection for family balancing: family balancing as a morally acceptable application of sex selection," *Human Reproduction,* 11, 1996.

PETRELLI, G. - MANTOVANI, A., "Environmental Risk factors and Male Fertility and Reproduction," *Contraception,* 65 (2002) 297-300.

ROBERTSON, J., "Preconception Gender selection" *American Journal of Bioethics,* 1, 2001, 1:2-9.

ROMANO, L., "Infertilità," Lecture-slides at Università Pontificia Regina Apostolorum, November 2004.

SMITH, B. - BROGAARD, B., "16 days,' *Journal of Medicine and Philosophy, 28,* 2003, 45-78.

STILLMAN, R. - ROSENBERG, M. - SACHS, B., "Smoking and Reproduction," in *Fertility and Sterility,* 46, 1986.

SUAREZ, A., "Hydatidiform Moles and Teratomas Confirm the Human Identity of the Prermplantation Embryo," *Journal of Medicine and Philosophy 15,* 1990, 627-635.

SUTTON, A., "The New Genetics: Facts, Fictions and Fear," *Linacere Quarterly,* August 1995, 76-87.

THONNEAU, P. et al., "Occupational Heat Exposure and Male Fertility: A Review," *Human Reproduction,* 13(8), 1998, 2122-2125.

TRANSPLANT COMMUNICATION INC., "Ethical of preimplantation genetic diagnosis debated. (Brief Article)," *Transplant News (Newsletter), Vol. 12 Issue1.* January 12, 2002.

TUREK, W. et al., "Perioperative Complication Arising After Transvaginal Oocyte Retrieval," *Obstetrics and Gynaecology,* 81(4), 1993.

VERLINSKY, Y. - RECHITSKY, S. et al., "Preimplantation Diagnosis for Fanconi anemia combined with HLA matching" *J Am Med Assoc,* 2001, 285; 3130-3133.

WARREN, M., "On the Moral and legal status of abortion," *The Monist 57,* 1973, 43-61.

WHITEFORD, L. - GONZALEZ, L., "Stigma: The Hidden Burden of Infertility" *Social Science and Medicine* 40,1995, 27-32.

VI. Internet Sites

AJAYI, R., "Nigeria," *Fertility World.org : Country – Reports,* in http://www.fertilityworld.org/content/doc_8/o/en/version_i/doc.asp (Downloaded 23/12/2005).

BELKIN, L., "Getting the Girl," in *New York Times Magazine,* July 25 1999. Published in http://www.nytimes.com/library/magazine/home/19990725mag-sci-gender-choice.html (Downloaded 4/7/2006).

FEINMAN, M., "Preimplantation Genetic Diagnosis (PGD)," in *The Fertility Network,* http://www.fertilitynetwork.com/articles/articles-pgd.htm (Downloaded 26/3/2006).

"Health: Fertility Milestones," *BBC News World Edition,* 22 July, 2003, in http://www.newint.org/issue303/infertility (Downloaded 21/3/2005).

JICK, B., "Gender selection: The latest Techniques for choosing the sex of your child," (1999), in http://www.parenthoodwb.com/parentcfmfiles/pros.cfm/839 (13/4/2006).

MATETAKUFA, S., "Infertility is not just a problem in the West," in http://www.newint.org/issue303/infertility.html (17/3/2005).

MULLIS, K. - JOHNSON, P. - THOMAS JR., C., "Dissenting on AIDS: The Case Against The HIV–Causes–AIDS Hypothesis," The San Diego Union-Tribune 15 May 1994. Published in http://www.virusmyth.net/aids/data/kmsdtrib.htm (Downloaded 26/3/2005).

NEWSWEEK INTERACTIVE, "The science of sex selection," in *New Babies – Newsweek Health* – MSNBC, in http://www.msnbc.com/id/3990134 (Downloaded 5/5/2005).

NZEAGWU, "Making Pregnancy a Natural Experience," An article published in This Day Online of 16/11/2004, in http://www.thisdayonline.com/archive/2004/10/200410plu01html (Downloaded 17/4/2006).

OBI, C., "Marriage Among the Igbo of Nigeria," in *ATR Special Topics,* in http://www.africaworld.net/afrel/igbo-marriage.htm (Downloaded 16/7/2006).

OKONOFUA, F., in "Health, IVF: An African Dream," *BBC News World Edition,* July 2003, in http://www.newint.org/issue303/ infertility (Downloaded 24/4/2005).

PENNEY, L., "Unexplained Infertility," The Fertility Network, in http://www.fertilitynetwork.com/articles/articles-unexplained.htm (Downloaded 12/3/2006).

"Reproduction Issues," in http://www.themodernreligion.com/misc/sex/srepro.htm (Downloaded 16/8/2005).

ABOUT THE AUTHOR

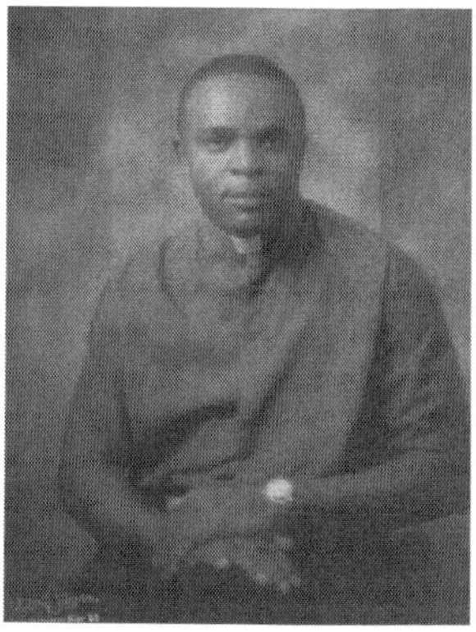

Paschal John Chibuzo Nwaezeapu is a priest of the Catholic Archdiocese of Lagos, Nigeria. After obtaining degrees in Philosophy and Theology, he specialized in Bioethics at the *Universita Pontifica Regina Apostolorum* in Rome. He has practical experience in seven parishes since his ordination, including years of general pastoral counselling of couples. He also has specific experience counselling infertile couples. This experience, coupled with his studies, has greatly enriched him to speak authoritatively on the problems of "Childlessness and Artificial Reproduction."

About Leonine Publishers

Leonine Publishers LLC makes fine Catholic literature available to Catholics throughout the English-speaking world. Leonine Publishers offers an innovative "hybrid" approach to book publication that helps authors as well as readers. Please visit our web site at www.leoninepublishers.com to learn more about us. Browse our online bookstore to find more solid Catholic titles to uplift, challenge, and inspire.

Our patron and namesake is Pope Leo XIII, a prudent, yet uncompromising pope during the stormy years at the close of the 19th century. Please join us as we ask his intercession for our family of readers and authors.

Do you have a book inside you? Visit our web site today. Leonine Publishers accepts manuscripts from Catholic authors like you. If your book is selected for publication, you will have an active part in the production process. This informative book is an example of our growing selection of literature for the busy Catholic reader of the 21st century.

www.leoninepublishers.com